Resistance
of
Pseudomonas
aeruginosa

Resistance
of
Pseudomonas aeruginosa

Edited by

M. R. W. Brown

Department of Pharmacy,
The University of Aston in Birmingham

A Wiley–Interscience Publication

JOHN WILEY & SONS

London · New York · Sydney · Toronto

Copyright © 1975, by John Wiley & Sons Ltd.

Library of Congress Cataloging in Publication Data:

Brown, Michael Robert Withington, 1931–
Resistance of *Pseudomonas aeruginosa*.

'A Wiley-Interscience publication.'
1. *Pseudomonas aeruginosa*. 2. Drug resistance in micro-
organisms. I. Title.
DNLM: 1. Drug resistance, Microbial. 2. *Pseudomonas
aeruginosa*—Drug effects. QW148 B879r
QR82.P78B76   616.01'4   74–30224

ISBN 0 471 11210 0

Printed in Great Britain by J. W. Arrowsmith Ltd.,
Winterstoke Road, Bristol.

Contributors

BERGAN, T.

Microbiology Department,
University of Oslo, Blindern,
Oslo 3, Norway

BROWN, M. R. W.

Department of Pharmacy,
University of Aston in Birmingham,
Birmingham, England

EAGON, R. G.

Department of Microbiology,
University of Georgia, Athens,
Georgia 30602, U.S.A.

GILLELAND JR H. E.

Department of Microbiology,
University of Georgia, Athens,
Georgia 30602, U.S.A.

JONES, R. J.

M.R.C. Industrial Injuries and Burns Unit,
Birmingham Accident Hospital,
Birmingham, England

LOWBURY, E. J. L.

M.R.C. Industrial Injuries and Burns Unit,
Birmingham Accident Hospital,
Birmingham, England

MELLING, J.

Microbiology Research Establishment,
Porton Down,
Salisbury, England

RICHARDS, R. M. E.

Department of Pharmacy,
(P.O. Box M.P.167),
The University of Rhodesia, Mount Pleasant,
Salisbury, Rhodesia

RICHMOND, M. H.

Department of Bacteriology,
University of Bristol, Medical School,
University Walk, Bristol, England

v

STINNETT, J. D.   *Department of Microbiology,*
                                  University of Georgia,
                                  Athens, Georgia 30602, U.S.A.

WILKINSON, S. G.   *Department of Chemistry,*
                                  University of Hull,
                                  Kingston-upon-Hull, England

Preface

Pseudomonas aeruginosa causes a wide variety of problems *in vivo* as well as *in vitro*. Recently there have been considerable advances in knowledge about the genetics as well as the envelope structure of Gram-negative bacteria in general. In particular, new light has been cast on resistance mechanisms. The position of *P. aeruginosa* among Gram-negative bacteria as an opportunist, drug-resistant pathogen and spoilage organism is notorious and pre-eminent. The purpose of this book is to give some idea of the dimensions of the problem, and especially to consider the fundamental mechanisms by which *P. aeruginosa* has achieved this position. Thus, in addition to chapters directly on the resistance mechanisms of this bacterium there are contributions on epidemiological typing as well as on the eradication of the organism *in vivo* and *in vitro*. A related book, *Genetics and Biochemistry of Pseudomonas*, edited by Professor Patricia H. Clarke and Professor Mark H. Richmond, has been published by John Wiley and Sons Ltd.

MICHAEL BROWN

Contents

CHAPTER 1

Antibiotic Inactivation and its Genetic Basis

M. H. RICHMOND

ANTIBIOTIC INACTIVATION AS A
METHOD OF ACHIEVING RESISTANCE

Bacteria generally protect themselves against antibiotic action, where they are able to do so, by one of three basic molecular processes: either they modify some target site within themselves to render it insensitive to antibiotic attack, or they synthesize some macromolecular layer that hinders access to the target, or they elaborate an enzyme specifically to destroy the antibacterial agent. All three methods may be effective at a physiological level but destruction of the antibiotic is likely to be the safest since no inhibitor remains to cause trouble if circumstances change for any reason; indeed this method is used by many bacteria, both Gram-positive and Gram-negative, to protect themselves. In this chapter we will concentrate on antibiotic destruction as it occurs as a means of resistance in *Pseudomonas aeruginosa* and related species. Modification of the organisms to achieve resistance—often by alteration of their surface properties—will only be touched on here. It is, however, dealt with extensively later in the book.

1

Although all antibiotic-destroying enzymes have the common property of converting the inhibitor to an inactive product, they are not acting in isolation. In all cases the organisms that produce them have to be considered and this fact may have a profound influence on the action of the enzymes and the conditions under which they exert their optimal effect. In practice, all bacterial enzymes are of two main types: intracellular (or cell bound) and extracellular, and antibiotic-destroying enzymes are no exception.

Extracellular Enzymes

As their name implies, these enzymes are released into the growth medium either as the culture grows or as it enters the stationary phase (Pollock, 1963). Since the enzymes are liberated into the medium surrounding the organisms they are greatly diluted in the process and therefore relatively large amounts are needed if protection is to be effective over a wide zone; particularly since motility (or even Brownian movement) will ensure that the bacteria to be protected do not remain continually in the same position, and diffusion will dilute the enzyme even if the organisms do not move. Furthermore, to be effective it is imperative that the concentration of the antibiotic in the surrounding medium be reduced to a low level so that the growth inhibitory concentration for the bacteria is not exceeded. In practice, both these requirements are met by the production characteristics of many extracellular antibiotic destroying enzymes. The β-lactamase of *Staphylococcus aureus*, for example, sometimes amounts to 0·5% by weight of the total dry weight of the bacterial population that synthesizes it (Richmond *et al.*, 1964) and its affinity for naturally occurring penicillins like benzyl penicillin is about 10^{-7} M (Richmond, 1963). This ensures that the β-lactamase will continue to work at full rate at concentrations of benzyl penicillin as low as 0·3 μg/ml, an essential property if the MIC of *Staph. aureus* is not to be reached.

Another consequence of the extracellular production of enzymes is that the protective effect on bacterial cultures is populational. Since the enzyme is free in the growth medium all cells produce the enzyme and all cells share in its effect. A consequence is therefore that resistance is much more effective at high cell densities than at low: a phenomenon encountered by many who test the effectiveness of antibiotics as an 'inoculum effect'.

The need for the production of large quantities of extracellular antibiotic-destroying enzymes also has its consequences in the physiological characteristics of synthesis (Citri & Pollock, 1966). Many extracellular enzymes of this class are inducible and, in teleological terms at least, the reason is not far to seek. It would seem advantageous to the bacteria to produce large amounts of enzyme only when the need exists.

Cell-bound enzymes

Examination of practical examples shows that cell-bound antibiotic-inactivating enzymes need not be present in the bacteria at such high concentrations as their extracellular counterparts. Moreover, the reason is not far to seek. Being located in restricted positions in the bacteria (Neu, 1968; Heppel, 1971), the cell-bound enzymes can exert their effects without the dilution and diffusion problems that confront enzymes liberated from the cell surface. As an example of this lower level of synthesis one need only look at the level of expression of the β-lactamases of Gram-negative species and compare them with those already described in the previous section (Table 1). While extracellular enzymes are frequently expressed at levels of about 0·5% of the dry weight of the culture (see above) the cell-bound enzymes rarely reach 1/50th of this value, and are often much more dilute.

Table 1. Typical levels of expression of β-lactamase genes in Gram-positive and Gram-negative species

Species	Enzyme production	Enzyme expression	
		units/mg dry wt	% by wt
Bacillus cereus	EC	1500*	0·5
Bacillus licheniformis	EC	1200*	0·4
Staphylococcus aureus	EC	1000*	0·3
Escherichia coli R⁺	CB	7·5	0·003
Klebsiella aerogenes	CB	1·5	0·0005
Pseudomonas aeruginosa	CB	4·0*	[0·015]

Abbreviations: EC, Extracellular; CB, cell-bound; *, fully induced; bracketed value is tentative.

In practice no bacterial strains seem to carry their antibiotic-destroying enzymes directly on the cell surface. In all cases the enzymes are either in the periplasmic space (Figure 1) or bound more or less tightly in or on the cytoplasmic membrane (Heppel, 1971). Whichever the case, however, the enzymes commonly lie between the 'outside' of the bacterial cell and the antibiotic-sensitive targets, the majority of which are either firmly embedded within the inner membrane or inside that structure (Gale *et al.*, 1973). This location ensures that the enzymes are well placed to intercept any antibiotic on its way into the cell, and this strategic location is almost certainly one of the reasons why relatively few of these cell-bound enzymes are needed to protect Gram-negative bacteria.

Whether the antibiotic-destroying enzyme is in the periplasmic space or on the surface of the inner membrane, a glance at Figure 1 will show that a macromolecular layer, the outer membrane, lies between the enzyme and the surrounding medium. Nor is this layer inert as far as access of antibiotics to the target and to any destructive enzyme in the periplasmic space is concerned. Often the layer considerably restricts access; this has frequently been demonstrated by the phenomenon of 'crypticity' (Richmond & Sykes, 1973; Richmond & Curtis, 1974). This parameter of enzyme behaviour in bacterial cells is

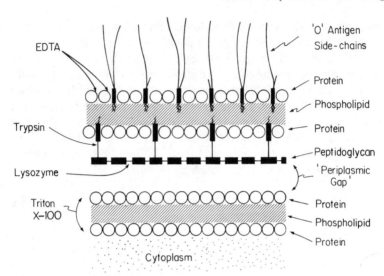

Figure 1. The organization of the surface layers of a typical Gram-negative bacteria. Reproduced with permission from C. A. Schnaitman, *J. Bacteriol.*, **108**, 553–563 (1971)

defined as the quotient obtained when the activity of a broken cell preparation is divided by the activity of an equal number of intact cells; values of 100 or more are not uncommon for some antibiotics and some antibiotic-destroying enzymes. On the other hand, some antibiotics do not seem to be impeded by these layers and crypticity values of 1·0 may also occur (see later).

Since the outside membrane impedes the access of many antibacterial substances it itself achieves some degree of resistance to many antibiotics. This subject will be dealt with in great detail in subsequent chapters since the properties of the outside membrane certainly contribute significantly to the 'intrinsic', i.e. non-enzymic, resistance of Gram-negative bacteria (see New York Academy Symposium, 1974). However, the manner in which the outer membrane interacts functionally with the enzymes that lie within it, to give a much higher level of resistance than either is capable of alone, is dealt with later in this chapter.

In an earlier passage, dealing with extracellular enzymes produced in large quantities, it was pointed out that such enzymes are frequently inducible—presumably to spare the protein synthesizing systems of the bacterial cell when challenging antibiotic is absent. As would be expected from the lower level of expression, the cell-bound enzymes are much more commonly constitutive, although there are exceptions. Among penicillinases, for example, only the Types Id (Sabath, Jago & Abraham, 1965) and Ia (Hennessey, 1967) in the classification given by Richmond & Sykes (1973) are ever synthesized inducibly and even in the latter case this pattern of synthesis is by no means universal.

Although many antibiotic-destroying enzymes may be classified with some accuracy as being either extracellular or cell-bound (Heppel, 1971), it is important to realize that this distinction may be over-simple and even perhaps misleading. Indeed, one example to be found in *P. aeruginosa* is a case in point. The Type Id enzyme found universally among clinical isolates of this strain (Sykes & Richmond, 1971) is cell-bound during the exponential growth phase but substantial liberation may take place as the culture enters the stationary phase (Nordström & Sykes, 1974). It is quite uncertain at present whether this liberation has a physiological role to play in the life of the population, since it is difficult to discover whether the release occurs under natural conditions, or whether it is merely fortuitous. Whatever the case, however, it is tempting to think that this organism may have evolved a system to give the best of both types of antibiotic-destroying enzyme: the cell-bound and the extracellular.

THE ENZYMES

Before starting on a detailed description of the various antibiotic-destroying enzymes to be found among isolates of *P. aeruginosa* it is important to define the limits of our concern here. This is particularly important since it is now clear that R-factors are relatively common among clinical isolates of this species and that some limited flow of genetic information between *P. aeruginosa* and members of the Enterobacteriaceae is possible (Sykes & Richmond, 1970; Bryan, van den Elzen & Tseng, 1972; Olsen & Shipley, 1973). This means that all the antibiotic-destroying enzymes found among members of the Enterobacteriaceae might be expected to occur in *P. aeruginosa*. However, even without the help of enzyme destruction, *P. aeruginosa* is very resistant to the action of many antibacterial substances (see other chapters of this book) and the addition of an enzyme makes little difference to the overall resistance of the culture. Discussion in this chapter will therefore be limited primarily to enzymic activity against antibiotics effective against *P. aeruginosa*, and the reader will be referred elsewhere for the details of enzymes that may, almost by accident, be found in this species because they happen to be specified by an R-factor that has crossed the taxonomic boundary between the Enterobacteriaceae and the Pseudomonadales.

β-Lactamases

General Properties

The *β*-lactamases are a group of enzymes that open the *β*-lactam bond of both the penicillin and cephalosporin nucleus (Figure 2), although not all enzymes are active against every antibiotic of this general class. When the *β*-lactam of a penicillin opens the corresponding penicilloic acid is produced: a compound that is devoid of antibiotic activity. With penicillins the reaction is complete at this point and the penicilloic acid may provide a convenient means

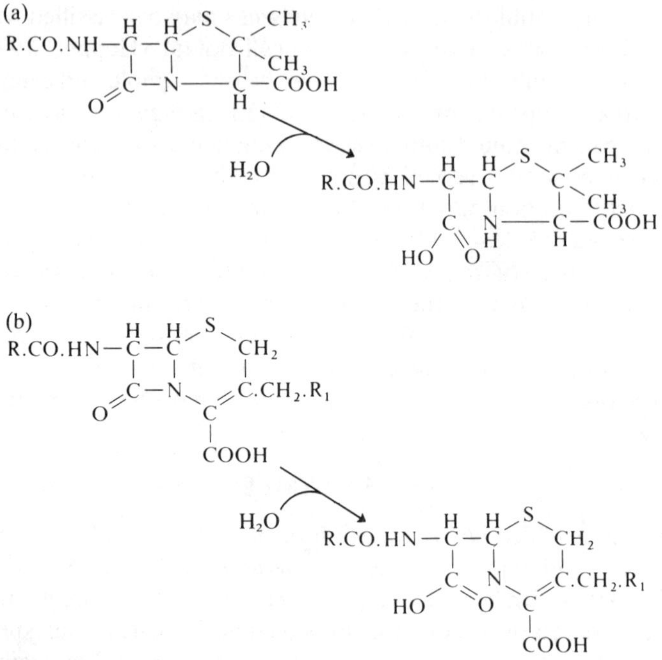

Figure 2. β-Lactamase action on typical penicillins and cephalosporins

of assaying the action of β-lactamase with penicillins as substrates. With cephalosporins, however, the situation is more complex. Not only is the 'cephalosporanoic acid' that might form an intermediate in the breakdown path very unstable if formed at all, the nuclear substituents in those cephalosporins that have leaving groups in the 3-position may be liberated following the rupture of the β-lactam bond (Hamilton-Miller, Newton & Abraham, 1970; Hamilton-Miller, Richards & Abraham, 1970). This gives a much more complex pattern of degradative products and consequently the activity of β-lactamase against cephalosporins is best measured by following the disappearance of substrate rather than the appearance of products. However, none of this alters the essential fact that β-lactamases inactivate many cephalosporins regardless of their nuclear substituents.

Examination of the β-lactamases synthesized by Gram-negative bacteria has shown that at least 14 different types are known if they are characterized in terms of their substrate profiles, electrophoretic mobilities and sensitivities to β-lactamase inhibitors (Jack & Richmond, 1970a; Richmond & Sykes, 1973). Of these enzymes only three have been found among isolates of *P. aeruginosa*. These are the Type Id enzyme, sometimes called the Sabath and Abraham enzyme: an enzyme with a primarily cephalosporinase profile (Sabath, Jago & Abraham, 1965); the Type Vd enzyme, a β-lactamase notable for a high relative rate of hydrolysis of carbenicillin: a penicillin specifically developed for the treatment of infections involving *P. aeruginosa* (Newsom, Sykes &

Richmond, 1970); and the Type IIIa enzyme, a general purpose β-lactamase active against a wide range of penicillins and cephalosporins (Sykes & Richmond, 1970; Fullbrook, Elson & Slocombe, 1970). The substrate profiles of these three enzymes are summarized in Table 2 and some of their other properties in Table 3.

Table 2. Substrate profiles of the three β-lactamases encountered so far in strains of *P. aeruginosa*

Enzyme class	Enzyme type	Substrate profile					
		Pen G	Amp	Carb	Clox	CER	CEX
I	d	100	10	0	0	600	80
III	a	100	180	10	0	140	<10
V	d	100	180	80	0	40	<10

Abbreviations: Pen G, benzyl penicillin; Amp, ampicillin; Carb, carbenicillin; Clox, cloxacillin; CER, cephaloridine; CEX, cephalexin. Data from Richmond & Sykes (1973).

Table 3. Further characteristics of the three β-lactamases found so far among strains of *P. aeruginosa*

Enzyme class	Enzyme type	Inhibited by				Electrophoretic mobility	M.W.
		*p*CMB	Clox	Meth	Carb		
I	d	R	S	S	S	+0·3	29,000
III	a	R	S	S	R	−1·6	25,000
V	d	R	R	R	R	−0·8	25,000

Electrophoretic mobility determined at pH 8·5.
Abbreviations: Meth, methicillin; *p*CMB, *p*-chloromercuribenzoate. Others as in Table 2. Data from Richmond & Sykes (1973).

Type Id Enzyme

The substrate profile of Type Id enzyme shows that it is predominantly active against cephaloridine but that it has detectable activity against most penicillins and cephalosporins as well. The exceptions encountered so far are methicillin, cloxacillin and carbenicillin. The first two of these antibiotics are powerful non-competitive inhibitors of the enzyme (Sabath, Jago & Abraham, 1965). Inhibition by these compounds may be reversed, but only by prolonged dialysis against antibiotic free solutes, and even under these conditions reactivation is not always complete. Carbenicillin, on the other hand, is a powerful competitive inhibitor. Indeed it is possible that this property, or at least its rigid resistance to hydrolysis by Type Id enzyme, is a very important component of its therapeutic action against strains of *P. aeruginosa* (Sykes & Richmond, 1971; Garber & Friedman, 1970; Nordström & Sykes, 1974).

Recently Zyk, Kalkstein & Citri (1972) have reported a purification procedure for Type Id enzyme involving chromatography on CM-Sephadex. Unfortunately the criteria for purity are not given in great detail and it is difficult to judge, at a specific activity of 5·5 units/μg protein, whether the protein is pure. Certainly this specific activity is considerably less than values reported elsewhere for other β-lactamases of bacterial origin (Table 4).

Table 4. Specific enzymic activities of some β-lactamases

Enzyme class and type	Specific activity units/μg protein	Reference
S. aureus β-lactamase A	310	Richmond (1963)
B. cereus β-lactamase I	355	Citri & Pollock (1966)
B. licheniformis	325	Citri & Pollock (1966)
Type Ia	75	Hennessey & Richmond (1967)
Type Id	5·5 (28)	Zyk *et al.* (1972); McPhail & Furth (1973)
Type IIIa	85	Datta & Richmond (1966)

Bracketed value is due to McPhail & Furth (1973).

Abraham and his colleagues (Sabath, Jago & Abraham, 1965) originally published some kinetic parameters on Type Id enzyme and Citri's group have now published further information about their purified preparations (Zyk *et al.*, 1972). These values are set out in Table 5. Perhaps the most interesting point in these data is that although Type Id enzyme has a relatively high V_{max} against cephaloridine and cephalothin, the K_m values for these substrates are also high, indicating that the enzyme has a relatively low physiological efficiency, at least in the isolated state, against cephalosporins.

Table 5. Kinetic constants for Type Id enzyme as determined by Zyk, Kalkstein & Citri (1972). The relative values of hydrolysis are expressed in relation to a value of 100 for cephalothin

	Relative rate of hydrolysis	Affinity constants (μM)	
		K_m	K_i
6APA	0	—	4000
Benzyl penicillin	17	500	—
Ampicillin	3·5	5·5	4·0
Carbenicillin	0	—	1·0
Methicillin	3·5	—	3·0
Cloxacillin	2·3	—	0·55
7ACA	0	—	460
Cephaloridine	63	1800	—
Cephalothin	100	750	—

McPhail & Furth (1973) have also studied purified Type Id enzyme although these workers have used a two-step separation procedure involving chromatography on CM-50 Sephadex and on DEAE-cellulose. The specific activity of the purified preparation is 28 units/μg protein, a value about 5·5 times higher than that reported by Zyk and her colleagues (Zyk *et al.*, 1973). However, the measurements of specific activity obtained by the Oxford and Israel groups were not identical and the large difference in specific activity obtained may not necessarily mean that the enzyme obtained by Zyk, Kalstein & Citri was not pure. Furth & McPhail do not quote Michaelis constants for their purified enzyme although they do give the amino acid analysis of the protein. This data (Table 6) shows that the enzyme seems quite distinct from those whose amino acid analysis has been published earlier (Jack & Richmond, 1970b).

Table 6. Amino acid composition of Type Id β-lactamase from *P. aeruginosa* NCTC 8203. The amino acid composition was determined after hydrolysis for 24, 48 and 72 hr at 105 °C, and the values given are based on an assumed molecular weight of 42,000

Amino acid	Residues/mole
Asp	34
Thr	16
Ser	16
Glu	39
Pro	27
Gly	35
Ala	44
Val	20
Met	4
Ile	14
Leu	50
Tyr	19
Phe	12
Lys	20
His	8
Arg	26
Trp*	8
Cys	1

*Determined spectrophotometrically.

In the most complete survey published so far, Sykes & Richmond (1971) found Type Id enzyme in all 56 clinical isolates of *Pseudomonas aerogenes* isolated from clinical sources although the enzyme was absent from isolates of *Pseudomonas thomasii* and *Pseudomonas cepacia* (M. H. Richmond, unpublished observations). Wherever strains of *P. aeruginosa* were found to make two types of β-lactamase (6/56 examples examined by Sykes & Richmond, 1971), the Type Id enzyme was present although the pattern of its synthesis was sometimes modified by the presence of the second enzyme in the same bacterial cell.

Type Id enzyme production seems to be confined to strains of *Ps. aeruginosa* and when the enzyme occurs its synthesis is always inducible. In the early work on this enzyme it seemed that induction occurred in a cell that was completely without β-lactamase until induction commenced. However, it is now certain that most if not all strains of *Ps. aeruginosa* synthesize a basal level of about 0·2 enzyme units/mg dry wt in the absence of inducer, a quantity of enzyme difficult to detect with certainty by conventional means (Richmond & Curtis, 1974).

Recently Nordström and his colleagues (Nordström & Sykes, 1972, 1974) have studied the induction of this enzyme and taken their cue for many of their experiments from the pioneer work on this enzyme of Sabath, Jago & Abraham (1965). The induction kinetics of Type Id enzyme are somewhat unusual when viewed against the classic pattern of β-galactosidase in *Escherichia coli*. Not only are the kinetics of induction non-linear from the time of first appearance of the enzyme, there is also a lag period following addition of inducer which may last for as much as an hour before enzyme is detectable. In fact, these kinetics are not so different from those obtained with other inducible β-lactamases (e.g. Bacilli: Citri & Pollock, 1966; Staphylococci: Richmond, 1968) and it seems that this broadly autocatalytic response to the addition of inducer is a typical response of β-lactamases in bacteria and not a quirk of this particular enzyme in *P. aeruginosa*.

When benzyl penicillin is used as inducer of Type Id enzyme synthesis in *P. aeruginosa* the maximum induction ratio obtained is 100-fold or more but very large concentrations of inducer (500 μg/ml or more) are needed to obtain this response and at this concentration of antibiotic there is a considerable effect on growth with some lysis (Nordström & Sykes, 1972). Perhaps the best inducer for this species is 6-aminopenicillanic acid. Here a maximal response may be obtained with 400 μg/ml but there is very little growth inhibition (Rosselet & Zimmerman, 1973). It should perhaps be mentioned in passing that cloxacillin and methicillin give very poor induction of Type Id enzyme not because they are poor inducers but because they are powerful non-competitive inhibitors of the Type Id enzyme (see Table 3). Enzyme activities measured in the presence of these antibiotics is therefore always substantially less than might have been expected.

Csányi and his colleagues have suggested that the autocatalytic induction kinetics obtained with many β-lactamases implies the presence of an intermediate step between the addition of the inducer and the appearance of active enzyme (Figure 3) (Csányi, Jacobi & Straub, 1967). Some hypotheses require that a modification of the inducer to an active molecule is the intervening process (Figure 3a) while others suggest it may be the refashioning of some proto-enzyme (Figure 3b). Whether any intermediate process of this type occurs in *P. aeruginosa* is unknown at present. Attempts to obtain mutants that synthesize Type Id enzyme constitutively have all failed (M. H. Richmond, unpublished results; K. G. H. Dyke, unpublished results; K. Nordström,

(a)

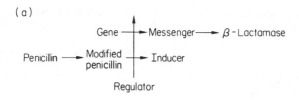

(b)

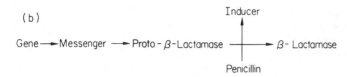

Figure 3. Two models to explain the autocatalytic induction kinetics of β-lactamases in *Bacillus cereus*. (a) The modification of the inducer to an active intermediate. (b) Modification of a 'proto-enzyme'

unpublished results) and this must be taken to suggest that the induction mechanism in this system differs from that for β-galactosidase in *E. coli* where constitutive mutants may readily be isolated (Cohen-Bazire & Jolit, 1953). Indeed, the only type of mutants that effect synthesis of Type Id enzyme that have been isolated so far are mutants in which the enzyme is uninducible (Rosselet & Zimmerman, 1973).

Before leaving the subject of the Type Id enzyme, it is important to try to assess its importance in the resistance of *P. aeruginosa* to β-lactam antibiotics. Sabath & Abraham (1964) concluded that the enzyme did play some part in resistance of this organism to cephalosporin C (the only cephalosporin readily available at that time) since mixtures of this cephalosporin with cloxacillin were synergistic when tested as a growth inhibitor. Since cloxacillin is a potent inhibitor of Type Id enzyme the synergy was interpreted as being an inhibition of the enzyme leading to a sparing of the cephalosporin C for antibacterial action. Latterly, the importance of the Type Id enzyme in the resistance of *P. aeruginosa* to β-lactam antibiotics seems to have been confirmed. Synergism between cloxacillin and cephaloridine is clear-cut (Nordström & Sykes, 1974) and similar results, though less striking, are found with cloxacillin and other β-lactam antibiotics.

The importance of Type Id enzyme to resistance of *P. aeruginosa* can be assessed directly by comparing the MIC values obtained with an uninducible mutant (see above) with those found with the unmutated parent in which the synthesis of Type Id enzyme is fully inducible. The ability to induce the enzyme causes a sharp increase in MIC value for all penicillins and cephalosporins save carbenicillin (Table 7) (Rosselet & Zimmerman, 1973). The failure of enzyme induction to affect the MIC values obtained with carbenicillin is quite understandable since this penicillin is completely insensitive to hydrolysis by

Table 7. β-lactamase production and sensitivity to β-lactam antibiotic of mutants of *P. aeruginosa* defective in the induction mechanisms in comparison with the parental strain

β-lactamase activity (units/mg dry wt bacteria)		Induction ratio	MIC (μg/ml)				
Strain	Uninduced Induced		6APA	Pen G	Amp	Carb	CER
2126 wt	0·48	18·0	37·5	550	1000	250	40	>1000
2126 mutant	0·48	0·81	1·7	250	70	30	50	30

Abbreviations: 6APA, 6-aminopenicillanic acid; Pen G, benzyl penicillin; Amp, ampicillin; Carb, carbenicillin; CER, cephaloridine. Data from Rosselet & Zimmerman (1973).

Type Id enzyme (Table 2). Indeed it is a powerful competitive inhibitor of the enzyme (Garber & Friedman, 1970). To some extent, therefore, this reinforces one's view of the importance of this enzyme in the resistance of *P. aeruginosa* to β-lactam antibiotics.

Type Vd Enzyme

Type Vd β-lactamase is relatively rare among isolates of *P. aeruginosa*. Nor has the enzyme yet been detected in any other bacterial species. The enzyme was first encountered in a clinical specimen obtained from a patient with an oesophageal tumour (Newsom *et al.*, 1970) although it has subsequently been reported from two other hospitals (see a footnote in Sykes & Richmond, 1971; Jephcott, Lowbury & Richmond, 1973). It is an all-purpose β-lactamase with a strong relative rate of hydrolysis of carbenicillin (Table 2). In none of the reported cases of isolation does the enzyme seem to have caused serious problems as far as the treatment of the underlying pathology went and there must be some doubt as to how important this enzyme is (at the moment at least) from the clinical point of view.

An interesting observation about the strains that produce this type of enzyme is that they also produce Type Id enzyme 'underneath' the Type Vd. However, the latter enzyme is produced constitutively and its presence substantially modifies the characteristics of Type Id enzyme synthesis since the presence of the Type Vd component destroys any β-lactam compound added with the objective of inducing Type Id enzyme. This phenomenon of the constitutive production of one enzyme phenotypically repressing the induction of another will be encountered again in reference to the Type IIIa enzyme (see p. 13).

Type IIIa enzyme

This enzyme is a constitutive β-lactamase with a wide range of activities against many penicillins and cephalosporins (Table 2). Type IIIa β-lactamase has been purified and its amino acid composition and molecular weight well established by a number of groups of workers. The only penicillins that seem resistant to hydrolysis are cloxacillin and methicillin, both of which are powerful competitive inhibitors of the hydrolysis of most other β-lactam substrates (Table 3). Carbenicillin is hydrolysed by this enzyme but only at about 10% of the rate of that found with benzyl penicillin. In fact the point is important since this enzyme is the cause of most of the clinically significant carbenicillin resistance that has been encountered so far (Lowbury *et al.*, 1969; Ingram, Richmond & Sykes, 1973).

Perhaps the most important aspect of the Type IIIa enzyme is that it is almost invariably R-factor mediated and therefore also commonly to be found among members of the Enterobacteriaceae (Jack & Richmond, 1970a). In fact it was the realization that an enzyme responsible for carbenicillin resistance in clinical strains of *P. aeruginosa* was indistinguishable in substrate profile, physicochemical properties and immunological cross-reaction from a common β-lactamase of *E. coli* that first suggested that the R-factors that specified the synthesis of this enzyme (Lowbury *et al.*, 1969) might be able to cross the intergeneric boundary between the Pseudomonadales and the Enterobacteriaceae (Sykes & Richmond, 1970; Fullbrook, Elson & Slocombe, 1970). In fact this particular class of R-factor (the so-called P-compatibility class: Datta *et al.*, 1972) can be transferred extremely widely among Gram-negative species; but this point has already been discussed at length here and also by Stanisich & Richmond (1974).

When P-compatibility class R-factors like RP1 and RP4 are carried by strains of *P. aeruginosa* the carbenicillin resistance they confer is extremely high. Table 8 compares the MIC values for carbenicillin obtained with

Table 8. Resistance of *P. aeruginosa* Ps18 carrying RP1 to β-lactam antibiotics compared with the same strain lacking the R-factor

Strain	Single cell resistance (MIC) (μg/ml)			
	Pen G	Amp	Carb	CER
P. aeruginosa 18R⁻	400	200	40	400
P. aeruginosa 18(RP1)	~10,000	2500	5000	5000

Abbreviations: As in Table 7. Data from Richmond & Sykes (1973).

P. aeruginosa Ps18R⁻ (RP1) (Sykes & Richmond, 1970). The presence of the R-factor raises the MIC values with carbenicillin from about 30 μg/ml to about 5 mg/ml. In view of the poor relative rate of hydrolysis of carbenicillin by Type IIIa enzyme (see Table 2), it is a little surprising that possession of this enzyme can make so much difference to the MIC values obtained with carbenicillin. This mystery has to some extent been solved by the discovery of genes on certain of the P-class R-factors which influence the intrinsic resistance of the bacteria that carry them, even when no β-lactamase is being expressed by the cells (Curtis, Richmond & Stanisich, 1973). This gene was discovered by examining the properties of mutant R-factors from which the β-lactamase gene had been deleted. The β-lactamase-less mutant of the R-factor RP1 (designated RP1amp1) still specifies a resistance of about 600 μg carbenicillin/ml to strains of *P. aeruginosa* that carry it while the unmutated RP1 gives an MIC of about 30 mg/ml and the R-factor-less strain an MIC of about 30 μg carbenicillin/ml. Thus the greatly enhanced resistance to carbenicillin shown by cells expressing Type IIIa enzyme is due to an interplay between a β-lactamase and increased intrinsic resistance (almost certainly an increased impermeability to carbenicillin). Such an interplay is particularly effective at achieving resistance to β-lactam antibiotics; but this phenomenon was discussed in detail at the beginning of this chapter.

Aminoglycoside Inactivating Enzymes

The details of the various types and activities of these enzymes in Gram-negative bacteria are extremely complex, partly because of the various types of inactivation reactions catalysed and partly because of the large number of different enzymes that have been detected, this last point being itself much complicated by the fact that few commercially available preparations of these antibiotics consist of a single molecular species. Therapeutic preparations of streptomycin are usually homogeneous, but two of the amino glycosides particularly relevant to *P. aeruginosa*, namely kanamycin and gentamicin, are normally sold as mixtures of two or more components. Since the various inactivating enzymes have different actions on the various components the overall pattern of resistance, or partial resistance, of bacterial strains may be difficult to define accurately. Indeed, there is currently much discussion as to whether there is complete cross-resistance between gentamicin and tobramycin (Crowe & Sanders, 1972) and the conclusion is likely to depend on which resistance enzyme is involved (Benveniste & Davies, 1973). The structures of the various aminoglycosides discussed here are shown in Figure 4. The topic has recently been reviewed by Benveniste & Davies (1973).

Although there are a relatively large number of different enzymes that achieve complete or partial resistance to aminoglycoside antibiotics, the chemical basis of the inactivation falls into one of three classes: acetylation, phosphorylation or adenylylation. For the first the source of the substituent group is acetyl-CoA and for the last two ATP. The overall reactions are summarized in Figure 5. In all cases the enzymes inactivate by substitution of a key residue in the antibiotic (an —OH or a —NH$_2$) and never by opening of any of the rings which are present in all aminoglycosides.

As far as *P. aeruginosa* is concerned, the therapeutically important aminoglycosides are gentamicin, tobramycin, kanamycin, lividomycin and BBK-8, a semi-synthetic kanamycin derivative that has recently been described (Kawaguchi *et al.*, 1972). However, since many of the aminoglycoside-

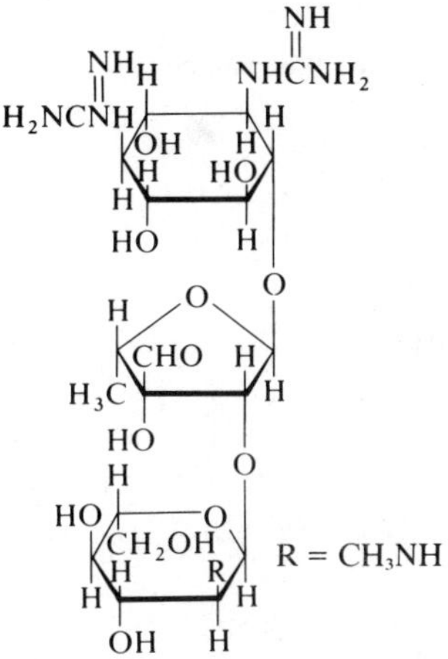

Streptomycin

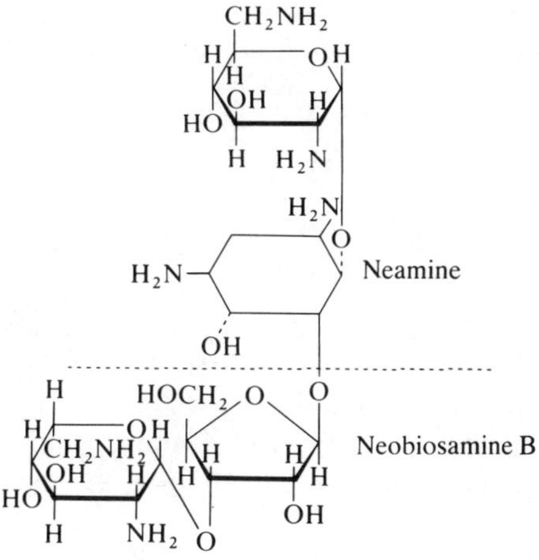

R = CH₃NH

Neomycin B

Neamine

Neobiosamine B

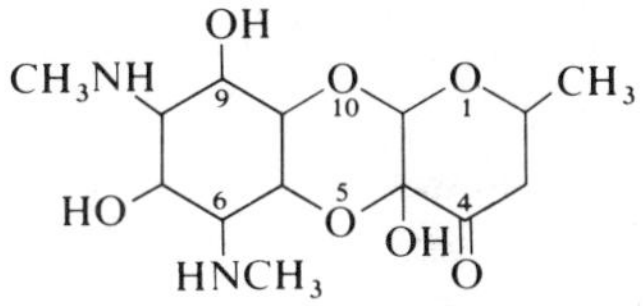

Kanamycin

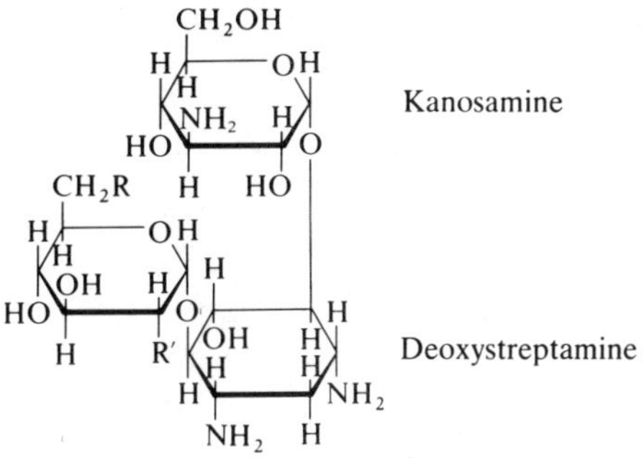

Kanosamine

Deoxystreptamine

Spectinomycin

Gentamicin

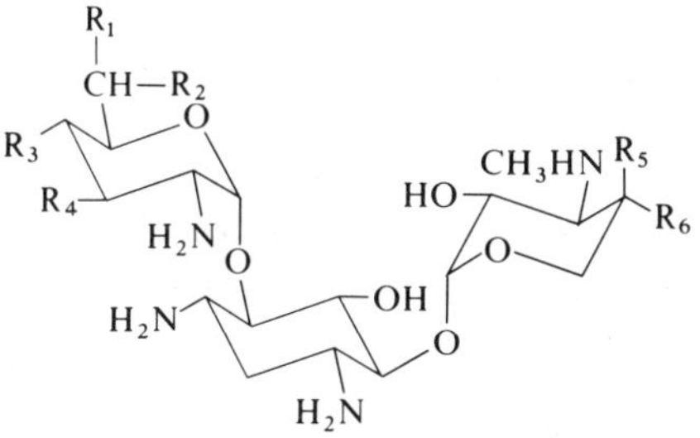

		R₁	R₂	R₃	R₄	R₅	R₆
Gentamicins	A	H	OH	OH	OH	H	OH
	C₁ₐ	H	NH₂	H	H	OH	CH₃
	C₂	CH₃	NH₂	H	H	OH	CH₃
	C₁	CH₃	NHCH₃	H	H	OH	CH₃

fig. 4 continued on next page.

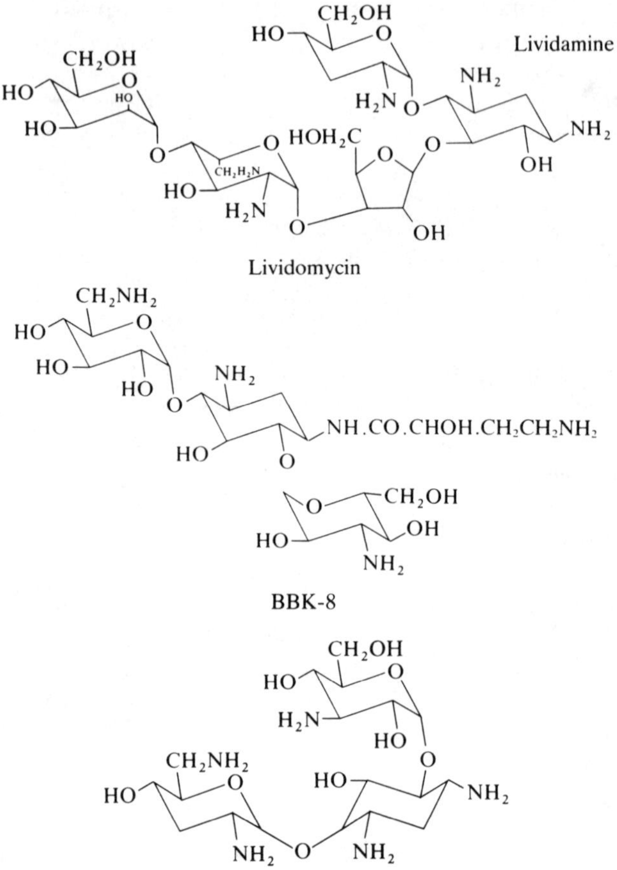

Figure 4. The structures of various aminoglycosides discussed in this article

Acetylation

$$- NH_2 + CH_3CO.SCoA \longrightarrow NH- CO.CH_3 + CoASH$$
$$- OH + CH_3CO.SCoA \longrightarrow O - CO.CH_3 + CoASH$$

Phosphorylation

$$- OH + ATP \longrightarrow - O - Phosphate + ADP$$

Adenylylation

$$- OH + ATP \longrightarrow - O - adenylyl + PP$$

The three basic inactivation reactions catalysed by enzymes with aminoglycosides as substrates.

Figure 5. The three types of reaction that can lead to the inactivation of the aminoglycoside antibiotics

inactivating enzymes are R-factor mediated, the situation already mentioned in connexion with β-lactamases may occur: enzymes prevalent among members of the Enterobacteriaceae may be found in strains of *P. aeruginosa* not because they cause clinically significant levels of resistance but because their genes are linked on an R-factor to other genes which do specify a therapeutically important resistance. For example, the P-class R-factor RP1 specifies Type IIIa β-lactamase (carbenicillin resistance) as well as carrying the gene for a neomycin/kanamycin phosphotransferase (Grinsted *et al.*, 1972). Table 9

Table 9. Aminoglycoside modifying enzymes

Enzyme	Modification
Kanamycin acetyltransferase (KacT)	6-Amine group of an amino hexose acetylated
Gentamicin acetyltransferase I (GacTI)	3-Amino group of 2-deoxy streptamine acetylated
Gentamicin acetyl transferase II (GacTII)	2-Amino group of an amino hexose is acetylated
Streptomycin–spectinomycin adenylyl transferase (SadT)	Hydroxyl group of a D-*threo* methylamino alcohol acetylated
Gentamicin adenylyl transferase (GadT)	2-Hydroxy of an amino-hexose adenylylated
Streptomycin phosphotransferase (SpT)	3-Hydroxy group of N-methyl-L-glucosamine phosphorylated
Neomycin–kanamycin phosphotransferase (NpT)	3-Hydroxyl of an amino hexose phosphorylated
Lividomycin phosphotransferase (LvpT)	5-Hydroxyl group of D-ribose phosphorylated

Data from Beneviste & Davies, 1973.

summarizes the properties of the aminoglycoside-inactivating enzymes already described as R-factor mediated in members of the Enterobacteriaceae. So far there are certainly eight, perhaps nine: Streptomycin/spectinomycin adenylate synthetase; Streptomycin phosphotransferases; two distinct Neomycin/kanamycin phosphotransferases; Neomycin/kanamycin acetyl transferase; Kanamycin/gentamicin adenylate synthetase; and two Gentamicin acetyl transferases; and possibly Lividomycin phosphotransferase (Benveniste & Davies, 1973). Of these, three are particularly important for the inactivation of gentamicin and/or tobramycin (antibiotics of particular relevance to *P. aeruginosa*: Table 10) and two others for the inactivation of kanamycin (Table 10). So far only one enzyme, neomycin/kanamycin acetyl transferase, has any activity against BBK-8. Lividomycin phosphotransferase is claimed by Mitsuhashi and his colleagues (Kobayashi, Yamaguchi & Mitsuhashi, 1972) to be a distinct enzyme from those acting on other aminoglycosides, but this conclusion has been questioned by Dr. J. Davies (unpublished experiments).

Table 10. Enzymic inactivation of some aminoglycoside antibiotics

	Enzyme				
	GacTI	GacTII	GadT	NpTI	KacT
Kanamycin A	−	−	+	+	+
B	−	−	+	+	(+)
C	−	−	+	+	−
Neomycin B or C	−	−	−	+	(+)
Paromomycin	−	−	−	+	−
Lividomycin B	?	?	?	+	−
Gentamicin C1$_a$	+	+	+	−	(+)
C$_2$	+	+	+	−	(+)
C$_1$	+	+	+	−	−
A	−	+	+	+	−
Tobramycin	−	+	+	−	(+)
Streptomycin	−	−	−	−	−
Spectinomycin	−	−	−	−	−
BBK-8	−	−	−	−	+

+, Active; −, inactive; (+) not active enough to give significant resistance.
Enzyme abbreviations: GacTI, GacTII, gentamicin acetyl transferase; GadT, gentamicin adenyl transferase; NPT, neomyin phosphotransferase; KacT, kanamycin acetyl transferase. Data from Benveniste & Davies, 1973.

Since the R-factors that specify these enzymes are often compatible (see p. 5), bacterial strains that express more than one of these enzymes are not uncommon. For example Benveniste & Davies (1971) have reported the existence of a strain of *Klebsiella aerogenes* that specifies three distinct aminoglycoside-inactivating enzymes which give resistance to all the clinically available aminoglycosides (Benveniste & Davies, 1973), and similar examples of multiple resistance patterns in *P. aeruginosa* are quoted elsewhere (Davies, Brzezinska & Benveniste, 1971).

Little work has been reported so far on the physiological expression of the aminoglycoside-inactivating enzymes. All appear to give MIC values against the antibiotics they inactive of about 1000 μg/ml, although the level of expression of the various enzymes is not identical (Dr. J. Arrand, unpublished experiments). However, all the enzymes do appear to be constitutive.

Experiments to locate the aminoglycoside-inactivating enzymes in Gram-negative bacteria are not so far advanced as those with β-lactamases (Heppel, 1971; Richmond & Curtis, 1974). However, Davies and his colleagues have shown that the streptomycin phosphorylating enzyme is periplasmic in strains of *E. coli* carrying the appropriate R-factors (Ozanne *et al.*, 1969) and similar results have been reported for the streptomycin/spectinomycin adenylylating enzyme (Benveniste, Yamada & Davies, 1970).

Other Inactivating Enzymes

The only other antibiotic-inactivating enzyme that has been studied in any detail is chloramphenicol acetyl transferase (see review by Shaw, 1972). This enzyme inactivates chloramphenicol by acetylation of the two available hydroxyl groups in the molecule (Figure 6). However, strains of *P. aeruginosa* are very resistant to chloramphenicol even without the benefit of the acetyl transferase enzyme and the relevance of this enzyme to the resistance of these strains is dubious.

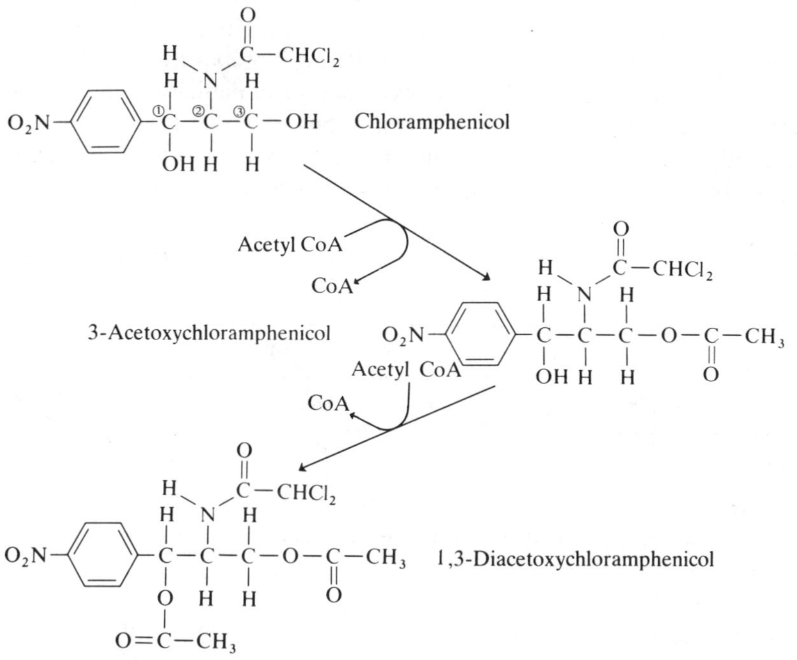

Figure 6. The action of chloramphenicol acetyl transferase on chloramphenicol

Apart from these examples all other resistance mechanisms are due either to impermeability of bacterial cells to the antibiotic or to modification of the target protein to achieve resistance. As such they are outside the scope of this chapter and anyway are of dubious importance as far as *P. aeruginosa* is concerned. The mechanisms have been reviewed recently by Benveniste & Davies (1973) and by Gale and his colleagues (Gale *et al.*, 1972).

INTERACTION OF ENZYMES AND INTRINSIC FACTORS

Much of what is described in other parts of this book is primarily concerned with the nature of the superficial layers of *P. aeruginosa* and the way they play a part in the resistance to antibacterial substances. As far as is known at the moment the spatial arrangement shown in Figure 1 represents the structure of the surface of *P. aeruginosa* as well as other Gram-negative species (Meadow, 1974). Nevertheless, there is some evidence that the detailed properties of the surface layers of this species are somewhat different from other Gram-negative species; and this probably contributes to their exceptional 'intrinsic' resistance to antibacterial agents (see Chapters 3, 4 and 5).

Some idea of the way in which the surface properties may differ is given by crypticity studies; that is by measurements to determine the ease with which molecules penetrate to the periplasmic space of the bacteria (Sykes & Richmond, 1973; Richmond & Curtis, 1974). As mentioned previously (see p. 3) this parameter of bacterial function may be measured by comparing the rate of destruction of an antibiotic by broken cell preparations and by intact bacteria. Determinations of this kind with a range of penicillins and cephalosporins with *P. aeruginosa* and *E. coli* show that the two species differ significantly (Table 11). Although the difference in crypticity towards penicillins is not too different for the two species, there is a sharp contrast between the

Table 11. Crypticity values obtained with Type IIIa β-lactamase in *P. aeruginosa* and *E. coli*

Host strain	Substrate			
	PenG	Amp	Carb	CER
P. aeruginosa	80	60	60	50
E. coli	30	65	125	1

Abbreviations: PenG, benzyl penicillin; Amp, ampicillin; Carb, carbenicillin; CER, cephaloridine. Data from Richmond & Sykes (1973).

values obtained for cephaloridine. Crypticity values for this antibiotic of about 1·0 were common with *E. coli* strains, but much higher crypticities are found with *P. aeruginosa*. The later species therefore either has a difference or an additional layer in its outer membrane, the structure controlling access to the periplasmic space from without.

The importance of the 'intrinsic' resistance afforded by the superficial layers of *P. aeruginosa* is reinforced by the finding that the resistance due to the possession of an antibiotic-destroying enzyme is greatly enhanced by its being situated within a barrier that restricts the flow of antibiotics. The β-lactamases of most Gram-negative species, *P. aeruginosa* included, lie within the outer membrane (Heppel, 1971) and either in the periplasmic space or in the surface of the inner membrane. In this position, therefore, they are ideally placed to intercept any antibacterial agent on its way to a target in the bacterial cell.

The experiments that go to show this cooperation all involve a comparison of the resistance of R-factor carrying and R⁻ bacteria before and after mutation of their surface properties (Richmond & Sykes, 1973). Most of the experiments have been carried out with *P. aeruginosa* Ps18 and the R-factor RP1: a plasmid that confers resistance to penicillins and cephalosporins, to neomycin and kanamycin and to tetracycline (Grinsted *et al.*, 1972). Furthermore, the evidence for cooperativity between enzymes and the surface layers primarily concerns β-lactamase and intrinsic resistance to β-lactam antibiotics, although there would be no difficulty in principle about getting similar information about the neomycin/kanamycin phosphotransferase and intrinsic resistance to these two aminoglycoside antibiotics.

The experimental approach that has been used is to take a strain of *P. aeruginosa* which lacks RP1 and which therefore relies for its resistance to 'intrinsic' factors and to obtain mutants which are inordinately sensitive to penicillins—usually carbenicillin but often ampicillin. These mutants are then tested for their MIC values towards various β-lactam antibiotics. Insertion of RP1 then allows crypticity measurements to be made on the mutant bacteria and these values are then compared to the unmutated parent. The examination is completed by studying the effect of the addition of the β-lactamase on the MIC values. The results in Tables 12 and 13 show that β-lactamases are considerably less effective at protecting *P. aeruginosa* against β-lactam antibiotics when the intrinsic components of the system have been impaired than when they are intact.

Table 12. Crypticity values for unmutated *P. aeruginosa* and for mutants inordinately sensitive to β-lactam antibiotics when lacking the R-factor RP1

Strain	Crypticity factor			
	PenG	Amp	Carb	CER
P. aeruginosa Ps18 wild type	75	60	55	50
P. aeruginosa Ps18 mutant 1	30	27	40	13
P. aeruginosa Ps18 mutant 3	30	28	48	20

For definition of crypticity factor, see text and Richmond & Sykes, 1973.
Abbreviations: PenG, benzyl penicillin; Amp, ampicillin; Carb, carbenicillin; CER, cephaloridine.

Table 13. MIC values obtained for unmutated *P. aeruginosa* and for mutants inordinately sensitive to β-lactam antibiotics when lacking the R-factor RP1.

Strain	Single cell resistance (μg/ml)			
	PenG	Amp	Carb	CER
P. aeruginosa Ps18 wt (R$^-$)	500	500	80	500
P. aeruginosa Ps18 mutant (R$^-$)	25	6·2	5	12·5
P. aeruginosa Ps18 wt (RP1)	1250	1250	1250	2500
P. aeruginosa Ps18 mutant (RP1)	312	312	625	312

Data from Richmond & Sykes (1973).

There have been a number of hypotheses to interpret this synergistic effect between the two resistance mechanisms in these bacteria. The first argued that the β-lactamase was placed strategically at a precisely defined place in the bacterial cell and that this was precisely on the path that the antibiotic would have to take on its way to its target in the cell (see Figure 6 in the review by Richmond & Sykes, 1973). In practice such a precise location of the components would seem to be unlikely. First calculation of the amount of β-lactamase synthesized by the bacteria, taken in conjunction with the probable size of the enzyme and the bacterial cells which expresses it, leads to the conclusion that there is too much enzyme in most R-factor carrying bacteria for the limited distribution required by the above model (Rosselet, unpublished experiments). Secondly, it is possible to show theoretically that apparent crypticity may follow whenever an enzyme is made to function within a diffusion barrier, and moreover that the numerical value of crypticity should vary as the amount of enzyme within the barrier varies, as undoubtedly it does in practice (Rosselet & Zimmermann, unpublished data). The more recent proposal, therefore, is to suggest that the enzyme is confined to the periplasmic space in the bacteria and that the very rigid spatial model proposed earlier is too precise. The synergy between the enzyme and the outer layers can still be said to be due to the action of an enzyme behind a structure giving a slow feed of substrate without the very precise spatial requirements of the earlier model. Yet, nevertheless, it is still important that the enzyme should be between the outside of the cell and the target within or inside the membrane.

The whole question of the interplay of enzymes and intrinsic factors has been made more complex by the discovery that certain R-factors, and RP1 is one of them, specify some intrinsic resistance to penicillins (but not to cephalosporins) as well as mediating Type IIIa β-lactamase synthesis (Curtis, Richmond & Stanisich, 1973). This conclusion is reached by experiments in which the β-lactamase gene of RP1 is deleted by mutagenesis and the resulting R-factor tested for its effect on *P. aeruginosa*. One of these mutant RP1 factors (RP1*amp*1) continues to confer resistance to $600\,\mu g$ ampicillin/ml to Pseudomonas strains that carry it, whereas the unmutated RP1 gives value of more than $5000\,\mu g$/ml. The same *P. aeruginosa* strain lacking the R-factor has an MIC against ampicillin of about $160\,\mu g$/ml (see Table 13). Work on these interesting R-factors is continuing. At present it seems clear that they also specify some increase in crypticity to penicillins but not to cephalosporins, some resistance to rifampicin and actinomycin D to mutants of *E. coli* that are sensitive to these antibiotics, and some chemical modifications to the surface layers of the cells that carry them.

The intrinsic resistance of *P. aeruginosa* to β-lactam antibiotics may be altered by the cultural conditions under which the bacteria are grown (see also Brown & Melling, 1969a,b). In particular, limitation in the supply of Mg^{2+} ions increases the penicillin sensitivity to bacteria that do not express β-lactamase. Insertion of R-factors specifying β-lactamase synthesis in strains grown in limiting Mg^{2+} ion concentrations results in strains which are hardly more resistant than the β-lactamase-less variants when grown in 0·08 mg MgCl$_2$/ml (F. Flett and M. Richmond, unpublished results).

In summary, therefore, strains of *P. aeruginosa* already have a relatively high resistance to many antibiotics because of as yet poorly understood properties of their surface layers. Expression of β-lactamase in the periplasmic space of the bacteria leads to very high levels of penicillin resistance provided (a) that the enzyme is capable of destroying the antibiotic concerned and (b) that the intrinsic barrier acts to give a slow feed of the antibiotic to the enzyme.

GENETIC BASIS OF ANTIBIOTIC RESISTANCE

Although the antibiotic-inactivating enzymes described in previous sections are all, of course, specified by genes, it is important to distinguish those where the genes are chromosomal from those which are present on a bacterial extrachromosomal element or plasmid. This is because the evolutionary potential of a gene is often significantly altered by its genetic location in the cell, particularly when the plasmid concerned is transmissible. This point is touched on briefly here (see p. 5) but dealt with more extensively elsewhere (Richmond, 1969, 1970; Stanisich & Richmond, 1974; Richmond & Wiedeman, 1974; Holloway, 1974; Richmond & Clarke, 1974).

Bacterial plasmids that specify resistance to antibiotics (the so-called R-factors) are commonly encountered among members of the Enterobacteriaceae (see Meynell, 1972) and they seem to be particularly prevalent in clinical isolates (Datta, 1969; Moorhouse, 1969; Linton *et al.*, 1972). Such plasmids have been known for about 15 years but their incidence seems to have been increasing latterly—probably in response to the use of antibacterial agents for therapy (Anderson, 1968). A number of distinct β-lactamases (Richmond, Jack & Sykes, 1972), several aminoglycoside-inactivating enzymes (Benveniste & Davies, 1973) and chloramphenicol acetyltransferase (Shaw, 1972) may all be plasmid mediated, although this is not invariable, and latterly a number of resistance traits (for example resistance to trimethoprim, admittedly not due to enzymic destruction) have appeared to be R-factor mediated (Datta & Hedges, 1972).

R-factors have been reported in strains of *P. aeruginosa* for a number of years (Lebek, 1963; Smith & Armour, 1966) but it is only relatively recently that they have been widely investigated. The impetus for this work came from the claim by Lowbury and his colleagues (Lowbury *et al.*, 1969) that an R-factor which specified β-lactamase synthesis was responsible for an outbreak of carbenicillin resistant *P. aeruginosa* that had occurred in the Burns Unit of the Birmingham Accident Hospital (see Chapter 8 and also p. 26). Lowbury's conclusion was confirmed by a number of workers and the ability of the plasmids to transfer to a wide range of different Gram-negative species—both members of the Enterobacteriaceae (Sykes & Richmond, 1970) and Pseudomonadales (Bryan *et al.*, 1972)—rapidly established. It is not intended here to go into great detail of the properties of these plasmids and those that have been isolated elsewhere since this has already been done in a related volume (Holloway, 1974; Stanisich & Richmond, 1974). What is intended now is merely to summarize the characteristics of the plasmids as they affect the clinical potential of *P. aeruginosa*. The properties of the R-factors that have been reported recently are summarized in Table 14.

Table 14. Characteristics of the R-factors isolated in *P. aeruginosa* and studied at a molecular level

R-factor	M.W. ($\times 10^{-6}$)	Marker pattern	G + C	Reference
RP1	40	P.N/K.T.	59	Grinsted *et al.* (1972)
RP4	40	P.N/K.T.	59	Grinsted unpublished; Bryan *et al.* (1973)
RP8	61	P.N/K.T.	59	Saunders & Grinsted (1972)
RP1-1	NP	P	NP	Ingram *et al.* (1972)
R55				
R931	25	ST	59	Bryan *et al.* (1973)
R1822	40	P.N/K.T.	59	Olsen & Shipley (1973)
R2/72	NP	Sm.P.K	NP	
R38/72	NP	T.Sm	NP	

NP: Estimations not possible because covalently closed circular DNA cannot be detected in these transferring strains.

Abbreviations: P, β-lactamase synthesis; N/K, neomycin/kanamycin phosphotransferase; T, tetracycline resistance; S, sulphonamide resistance; Sm, streptomycin resistance; K, kanamycin acetyl transferase.

The plasmids encountered in the series of strains studied by Lowbury (Lowbury *et al.*, 1969; Roe, Jones & Lowbury, 1971) all shared the property of being able to transfer readily between strains of *P. aeruginosa* and also were able to cross into a wide range of other enteric species. Even ecologically relatively distinct species like *Neisseria* and *Rhizobium* could be infected by these plasmids (Olsen & Shipley, 1973; Pühler, Burkhardt & Neumann, 1972); and there was some circumstantial evidence that they may have reached *P. aeruginosa* in the burned patients from other enteric species such as *Klebsiella* or *Proteus* (Ingram, Richmond & Sykes, 1973). All the plasmids of this outbreak specified the same marker pattern—namely Type IIIa β-lactamase, the neomycin/kanamycin phosphotransferase and tetracycline resistance (Grinsted *et al.*, 1972)—and were classified in compatibility group P (Datta *et al.*, 1972). A very similar plasmid was detected in a strain isolated at about the same time in Glasgow (Black & Girdwood, 1969). However, it has a rather larger molecular weight (60×10^6 as against 40×10^6 for the Birmingham isolates) despite its similar marker pattern (Saunders & Grinsted, 1972).

Following these reports, a relatively large number of other surveys showed R-factors to be present in *P. aeruginosa* although transfer to enteric bacteria is by no means universal even if transfer to other strains of *P. aeruginosa* occurred at reasonably high frequency. Indeed, only the plasmid R mentioned by Chabbert and his colleagues (Witchitz & Chabbert, 1971a,b; Chabbert *et al.*, 1972) makes this intergeneric transfer apart from those of the Lowbury series.

At the moment there is some preliminary evidence to suggest that various transfer systems in *P. aeruginosa* may differ significantly from the R-factors of *E. coli* and similar organisms. First, it has proved impossible to identify covalently closed circular DNA in some strains of *P. aeruginosa* that carry undoubted antibiotic resistance transfer properties (Ingram *et al.*, 1972). One example is the transfer system known as RP1-1 and the transfer system numbered 38/72 by Matsumoto and his associates (Kawakumi *et al.*, 1972) has the same properties. The other property that sets the antibiotic resistance transfer systems of *P. aeruginosa* somewhat apart from others that have been studied is their ability to mobilize chromosomal markers. Certain 'classical' R-factors (notably R1: Pearce & Meynell, 1968) and also the fertility factor F (Curtiss & Renshaw, 1969), can show this property in *E. coli* but in none is it so well developed as in RP1 and RP1-1 (Stanisich & Holloway, 1971). These systems are discussed in detail by Holloway (1974) and by Stanisich & Richmond (1974).

Perhaps the most interesting R-factors from the point of view of their clinical implication for *P. aeruginosa* are those that specify resistance to gentamicin, since this antibiotic is perhaps the best for the treatment of serious *P. aeruginosa* infections (Jackson, 1969). So far two classes of these elements have been detected by Chabbert and his colleagues (Witchitz & Chabbert, 1971a,b, 1972; Chabbert *et al.*, 1972). One specifies gentamicin acetyltransferase (Benveniste & Davies, 1973) and the other gentamicin and kanamycin adenylylation (Benveniste & Davies, 1971) (see p. 17). Rather little molecular work has been done on these two classes of element. However, Chabbert has put one of them into his compatibility group 6 and the other into group 4 on the basis of their co-existence properties with other bacterial plasmids.

The very rapid rise in the number and type of R-factor and related transfer system detected in strains of *P. aeruginosa* suggests that there will be much interest in the elements in the future and that their incidence may be increasing. Furthermore, many of their properties make them ideal instruments for investigating the molecular biology of this group of organisms (Holloway, 1974; Stanisich & Richmond, 1974). As far as the clinical picture is concerned, it is worth stressing that all the types of enzyme capable of destroying antibiotics that have been encountered in strains of *P. aeruginosa* so far can be plasmid mediated, although it is still not certain whether this is always the case.

SOME CLINICAL EXAMPLES

The presence of transmissible plasmids specifying resistance to antibiotics in strains of *P. aeruginosa* suggests that some outbreaks of antibiotic resistance in this species may be epidemiologically related, and this is indeed the case. Two examples have been well investigated in this species although other examples are to be found among other species of enteric bacteria (Anderson, 1968; 1971). The two situations concerning *P. aeruginosa* have been alluded to already: they are the outbreak of carbenicillin resistance in the Burns Unit of the Accident Hospital in Birmingham, England, and the two unrelated outbreaks of resistance to gentamicin that have been followed in France by Chabbert and his colleagues.

R-Factor Mediated Resistance to Carbenicillin

This sequence of events has been analysed in increasing depth in a number of reports (Lowbury *et al.*, 1969; Sykes & Richmond, 1970; Roe, Jones & Lowbury, 1971; Ingram, Richmond & Sykes, 1973).

Up to March 1969 few carbenicillin-resistant strains of *P. aeruginosa* had been detected in the Burns Unit in Birmingham, and certainly none of them owed their resistance to β-lactamase production. About the middle of that month, however, carbenicillin resistant strains of *P. aeruginosa* which owed their resistance to an R-factor mediated β-lactamase appeared simultaneously in a number of sero- and phage-types of *P. aeruginosa* (Table 15) (Lowbury *et*

Table 15. Dates of isolation, serotypes and phage types of *P. aeruginosa* strains carrying R-factors isolated in the Burns Unit of the Accident Hospital, Birmingham

Serotype	Phage type	Date of isolation
NT	44/F8/109/119X/1214	March 3, 1969
8	7/21/68/119X	March 4, 1969

Up to the 3rd March, 1969, no R-factor carrying *P. aeruginosa* strains had been detected in the Burns' Unit.

al., 1969; Sykes & Richmond, 1970). So resistant were these organisms that the value of carbenicillin for therapy was severely undermined and alternative treatment had to be instituted. Carbenicillin was withdrawn in the Unit and the resistant pseudomonads disappeared: only sensitive strains could be isolated from the burns. After about six months without resistant strains being isolated and without carbenicillin being used, the antibiotic was administered once more and the resistant strains, many of them with different phage- and sero-types from those found before, appeared once more. The resistance was once again R-factor mediated. Withdrawal of carbenicillin resulted in a further disappearance of resistance, and it seems quite clear that the rise and fall of the incidence of R-factors in the pseudomonads in this Unit reflected the fluctuating selection pressure from an alternating policy for carbenicillin use.

Molecular studies on the nature of the R-factors in the two phases of carbenicillin resistance showed that the plasmids involved were extremely similar (Table 16). They all had a molecular weight of about 40×10^6, a G + C

Table 16. Characteristics of the plasmids isolated from the two phases of carbenicillin resistance in *P. aeruginosa* and from the intervening period in ampicillin resistant *K. aerogenes*

Plasmid	Species of isolation	Molecular weight	G + C of plasmid DNA (%)	Marker pattern				Phase of isolation
RP1	*P. aeruginosa*	40×10^6	60	Ap	Km	Ne	Tc	I
RP2	*P. aeruginosa*	40×10^6	60	Ap	Km	Ne	Tc	I
RK1	*K. aerogenes*	40×10^6	60	Ap	Km	Ne	Tc	Intermediate
RP9	*P. aeruginosa*	40×10^6	60	Ap	Km	Ne	Tc	II

Abbreviations: Ap, resistance to ampicillin and carbenicillin; Km, kanamycin resistance; Ne, neomycin resistance; Tc, tetracycline resistance.

content of the plasmid DNA of about 60%, a contour length under the electron microscope of about $19\mu m$ and a marker pattern Ap Ne Km Tc. Furthermore, the plasmids all had a similar base sequence to their DNA in that they almost entirely hybridized with one another (Ingram, Richmond & Sykes, 1973). Such a close similarity in properties was not detected in other groups of R-factors isolated in other circumstances, and it seemed probable that the same R-factor had infected strains of *P. aeruginosa* to produce an evolutionary change during two periods separated by about six months.

Since no carbenicillin-resistant pseudomonads were found in the Unit while this antibiotic was withheld, the question arose as to where the reservoir of this particular R-factor might be. After a prolonged search strains of *K. aerogenes* were found with an indistinguishable R-factor, and there was good evidence, in one patient at least, that *K. aerogenes* carrying the relevant R-factor appeared in his burns before the plasmid was detected in *P. aeruginosa*. Under these circumstances the circumstantial evidence for the transfer of this particular R-factor (RP1) from *K. aerogenes* to *Aerobacter aerogenes* in the burn was strong. Moreover, the pattern of events suggests that the plasmid in question was maintained in *Klebsiella* strains in the Unit, possibly in the gut of patients, by selection pressure afforded by ampicillin use (Ingram, Richmond & Sykes, 1973). The β-lactamase gene gives resistance to ampicillin in enteric species but this point is irrelevant for *P. aeruginosa* as this antibiotic is inactive against these strains. Ampicillin therefore selects R-factors in enteric bacteria while carbenicillin applies pressure to both enterics and *P. aeruginosa* (Lowbury, Babb & Roe, 1972).

R-Factor Mediated Resistance to Gentamicin

The first epidemic of R-factor mediated gentamicin resistance was described by Chabbert and his colleagues (Witchitz & Chabbert, 1972). The outbreak commenced in November 1969 and all but one of the strains were isolated in the Clinique de Réanimation of the Claude-Bernard Hospital in Paris. The R-factor concerned specified resistance to chloramphenicol, to sulphonamides, to penicillins and cephalosporins and to kanamycin and gentamicin. The aminoglycoside resistance was due to the gentamicin adenylylating enzyme (see p. 17). The plasmid was a member of Chabbert's compatibility group 6 (Chabbert *et al.*, 1972). In the period under discussion the R-factor appeared in seven different species: *E. coli, Enterobacter aerogenes, Klebsiella pneumoniae, Citrobacter, Proteus mirabilis, Providencia* and *P. aeruginosa*. The presence of a single plasmid with the full resistance pattern could be demonstrated by transduction of a single linkage group with all the markers by the phage P1kc. Although no detailed molecular studies have yet been reported with this plasmid it seems highly likely that all the isolates were members of the same plasmid clone which had become distributed through a wide range of Gram-negative species in this particular clinic, and since transferable gentamicin resistance had been sought but not found before November 1969 (Chabbert & Baudens, 1965; Datta & Waterworth, 1967) it suggests that this particular plasmid is likely to have evolved around this time. Eleven months after the first isolation in the Claude-Bernard Hospital gentamicin-resistant organisms with the same pattern appeared in the St-Joseph Hospital on the South Bank of the Seine, and thereafter similar strains have been isolated in Nantes, Lyons and Caen, the strains not being detected in Nantes and Lyons until 1972. One therefore has a good example of the spread of a single R-factor clone in a single country. The incidents are somewhat reminiscent of the occurrence in the Birmingham Burns Unit but in this case extended outside a single hospital. Of course, it is important to stress that Gram-negative species other than *P. aeruginosa* were isolated among this series of strain. However, the R-factor was isolated on at least one occasion from Pseudomonads.

The other type of R-factor mediated gentamicin resistance involves gentamicin acetyl transferase (see p. 17 and Witchitz & Gerbaud, 1972). *P. aeruginosa* strains expressing this type of gentamicin resistance do not form such a close ecological group as the ones described above and examples have been encountered outside France (Benveniste & Davies, 1973). This R-factor clone therefore seems to be more widely distributed than those of *com*6, and indeed there is some evidence to suggest that the enzyme concerned may have been encountered in clinical isolates over a longer period (Benveniste & Davies, 1973) even if there is evidence that the earlier strains did not carry R-factors. This second type of gentamicin resistant Gram-negative organism has also been extensively isolated in France. In her article in May 1973, Allain-Regnault mentioned occurrences of this strain in Lyons, Nantes, Angers, Caen and Lille as well as in Paris (Allain-Regnault, 1973). Of course these isolates may reflect, to a great extent, Chabbert's efforts to alert France's provincial microbiologists about gentamicin-resistant Gram-negative bacteria. Nevertheless, there is good evidence that two clones of Gram-negative bacteria specifying resistance to gentamicin, including Pseudomonads,·have become widespread in France.

In general, therefore, we find ourselves at a point where the incidence of antibiotic-destroying enzymes in strains of *P. aeruginosa* seems to be increasing. The fact that this rise appears to be some way behind that found with members of the Enterobacteriaceae is probably due to two causes: first, it is only relatively recently that antibiotics that are really effective against strains of *P. aeruginosa* have been developed; secondly, it is only recently that clinical procedures such as immune suppression have become at all widespread. In many ways we are moving from the period of clear infection with a single causative organism to one of multiple infections with organisms generally regarded as 'opportunistic' (Finland, Marget & Bartmann, 1971). *P. aeruginosa* is an 'opportunist' *par excellence*, and we must expect its importance and incidence in clinical infection to increase in the future. The expression of certain enzymes able to destroy agents effective against this species will therefore become more and more important, and we can expect a considerable increase in the incidence of the R-factors that specify them.

ACKNOWLEDGEMENTS

Much of the work mentioned here that originated in this Department has been supported by grants from the Medical Research Council, The Royal Society and The Smith, Kline and French Foundation. I am indebted to Glaxo Research Ltd., to Beecham Research Ltd., to Sterling-Winthrop Labs., and to CIBA-Geigy, Basel, for gifts of various antibiotics.

REFERENCES

Allain-Regnault, M. (1973). Les bactéries résistantes aux antibiotiques. *Le Monde*, 9th May, 1973.
Anderson, E. S. (1968). The ecology of transferable drug resistance among the Enterobacteria. *Annual Review of Microbiology*, **22**, 131–180.
Anderson, E. S. (1971). In *Recent Advances in Microbiology*, Proceedings of the Xth International Congress of Microbiology, Mexico City, p. 381. Asociacion Mexicana de Microbiologia, Mexico City.
Benveniste, R., Yamada, T. & Davies, J. (1970). Enzymatic adenylylation of streptomycin and spectinomycin by R-factor resistant *Escherichia coli*. *Infection and Immunity*, **1**, 109–119.
Benveniste, R. & Davies, J. (1971). R-factor mediated gentamicin resistance: a new enzyme which modifies aminoglycoside antibiotics. *FEBS Letters*, **14**, 293–296.
Benveniste, R. & Davies, J. (1973). Resistance to aminoglycoside antibiotics. *Annual Review of Biochemistry*, **42**, 471.
Black, W. A. & Girdwood, R. W. A. (1969). Carbenicillin resistance in *Pseudomonas aeruginosa*. *British Medical Journal*, **iv**, 234.

Brown, M. R. W. & Melling, J. (1969a). Loss of sensitivity to EDTA by *Pseudomonas aeruginosa* grown under conditions of Mg-limitation. *Journal of General Microbiology*, **54**, 439–448.

Brown, M. R. W. & Melling, J. (1969b). Role of divalent cations in the action of polymixin B and EDTA on *Pseudomonas aeruginosa*. *Journal of General Microbiology*, **59**, 263–274.

Bryan, L. E., Van Den Elzen, H. M. & Tseng, J. T. (1972). Transferable drug resistance in *Pseudomonas aeruginosa*. *Antimicrobial Agents and Chemotherapy*, **1**, 22–29.

Bryan, L. E., Semaka, S. D., Van Den Elzen, H. M., Kinnear, J. E. & Whitehouse, R. L. W. (1973). Characteristics of R931 and other *Pseudomonas aeruginosa* R-factors. *Antimicrobial Agents and Chemotherapy*, **3**, 625.

Chabbert, Y. A. & Baudens, J. G. (1965). Transmissible resistance to six groups of antibiotics in Salmonella infections. *Antimicrocial Agents and Chemotherapy* 1965, p. 380–383.

Chabbert, Y. A., Scavizzi, M. R., Witchitz, J. L., Gerbaud, G. R. & Bouanchaud, D. A. (1972). Incompatibility groups and the classification of fi⁻ resistance factors. *Journal of Bacteriology*, **112**, 66–675.

Citri, N. & Pollock, M. R. (1966). The biochemistry and functions of β-lactamase (penicillinase). *Advances in Enzymology and Related Subjects*, **28**, 237–323.

Cohen-Bazire, G. & Jolit, M. (1953). Isolation par sélection de mutants d'*Escherichia coli* synthétisant spontanément l'amylomaltase et la β-galactosidase. *Annales de l'Institut Pasteur, Paris*, **84**, 937–945.

Crowe, C. C. & Sanders, E. (1972). Is there complete cross-resistance of Gram-negative bacilli to Gentamicin and Tobramycin? *Antimicrobial Agents and Chemotherapy*, **2**, 415–416.

Csanyi, V., Jacobi, G. & Straub, B. F. (1967). The regulation of penicillinase synthesis. *Biochimica biophysica Acta*, **145**, 470–477.

Curtis, N. A. C., Richmond, M. H. & Stanisich, V. (1973). R-factor mediated resistance to penicillins which does not involve a β-lactamase. *Journal of General Microbiology*, **79**, 163–166.

Curtiss, R. & Renshaw, J. (1969). F⁺ strains of *E. coli* K12 defective in Hfr formation. *Genetics, Princeton*, **63**, 7–26.

Datta, N. (1969). Drug resistance and R-factors in the bowel bacteria of London patients before and after admission to hospital. *British Medical Journal*, **ii**, 407–411.

Datta, N. & Richmond, M. H. (1966). The purification and properties of a penicillinase whose synthesis is mediated by an R-factor in *Escherichia coli*. *Biochemical Journal*, **98**, 204–209.

Datta, N. & Waterworth, P. M. (1967). Resistance to aminoglycoside antibiotics. *Lancet*, **i**, 572–573.

Datta, N. & Hedges, R. W. (1972). Trimethoprim resistance conferred by W plasmids in Enterobacteriaceae. *Journal of General Microbiology*, **72**, 349–355.

Datta, N., Hedges, R. W., Shaw, E. J., Sykes, R. B. & Richmond, M. H. (1972). Properties of an R-factor from *Pseudomonas aeruginosa*. *Journal of Bacteriology*, **108**, 1244–1249.

Davies, J., Brzezinska, M. & Benveniste, R. (1971). Biochemical mechanisms of resistance to aminoglycosides. *Annals of the New York Academy of Sciences*, **182**, 226–233.

Finland, M., Marget, W. & Bartmann, K. (1971). *Bacterial Infections: Changes in their causative agents—Trends and possible basis*, Springer-Verlag, Berlin.

Fullbrook, P. D., Elson, S. W. & Slocombe, B. (1970). R-factor mediated β-lactamase in *Pseudomonas aeruginosa*. *Nature, London*, **226**, 1054–1056.

Gale, E. F., Cundliffe, E., Reynolds, P. E., Richmond, M. H. & Waring, M. (1973). In *The Molecular Basis of Antibiotic Action*, John Wiley, London.

Garber, N. & Friedman, J. (1970). β-lactamase and the resistance of *Pseudomonas aeruginosa* to various penicillins and cephalosporins. *Journal of General Microbiology*, **64**, 343–352.

Grinsted, J., Saunders, J. R., Ingram, L. C., Sykes, R. B. & Richmond, M. H. (1972). Properties of an R-factor which originated in a *Pseudomonas aeruginosa* 1822. *Journal of Bacteriology*, **110**, 529–537.

Hamilton-Miller, J. M. T., Newton, G. G. F. & Abraham, E. P. (1970). Products of aminolysis and enzymic hydrolysis of the Cephalosporins. *Biochemical Journal*, **116**, 371–384.

Hamilton-Miller, J. M. T., Richards, E. & Abraham, E. P. (1970). Changes in proton-magnetic resonance spectra during aminolysis and hydrolysis of cephalosporins. *Biochemical Journal*, **116**, 385–396.

Hennessey, T. D. (1967). Inducible β-lactamase of Enterobacter. *Journal of General Microbiology*, **49**, 277–285.

Hennessey, T. D. & Richmond, M. H. (1968). The purification and some properties of a β-lactamase (cephalosporinase) synthesised by *Enterobacter cloacae*. *Biochemical Journal* **109**, 469–473.

Heppel, L. (1971). In *The Structure and Function of Biological Membranes*, (Ed. L. Rothfield), Academic Press, London & New York, p. 223.

Holloway, B. W. (1974). In *The Biochemistry and Genetics of Pseudomonas*, Chapter 5 (Ed. P. H. Clarke & M. H. Richmond), John Wiley, London.

Ingram, L. C., Sykes, R. B., Grinsted, J., Saunders, S. & Richmond, M. H. (1972). A transmissible resistance element from a strain of *Pseudomonas aeruginosa* containing no detectable extrachromosomal DNA. *Journal of General Microbiology*, **72**, 269–279.

Ingram, L. C., Richmond, M. H. & Sykes, R. B. (1973). Molecular characterisation of the R-factors implicated in the carbenicillin resistance of a sequence of *Pseudomonas aeruginosa* strains isolated from burns. *Antimicrobial Agents & Chemotherapy*, **3**, 279–288.

Jack, G. W. & Richmond, M. H. (1970a). A comparative study of eight distinct β-lactamases synthesised by Gram-negative bacteria. *Journal of General Microbiology*, **61**, 43–61.

Jack, G. W. & Richmond, M. H. (1970b). Comparative amino acid contents of purified β-lactamases from enteric bacteria. *FEBS Letters*, **12**, 30–32.

Jackson, G. G. (1969). Introduction. *Journal of Infectious Diseases*, **119**, 341–342.

Jephcott, A. E., Lowbury, E. J. L. & Richmond, M. H. (1973). Non-transferable carbenicillin resistance of *Pseudomonas aeruginosa* from a burn. *Lancet*, **i**, 272.

Kawaguchi, H., Naito, T., Nakagawa, S. & Fujisawa, K. (1972). BBK-8, a new semi-synthetic aminoglycoside antibiotic. *Journal of Antiobiotics, Tokyo*, **25**, 695–708.

Kawakumi, Y., Mikoshiba, F., Nagasaki, S., Matsumoto, H. & Tazaki, T. (1972). Prevalence of *Pseudomonas aeruginosa* strain possessing R-factor in a hospital. *Journal of Antibiotics, Tokyo*, **25**, 607–609.

Kobayashi, F., Yamaguchi, M. & Mitsuhashi, S. (1972). Activity of lividomycin against *Pseudomonas aeruginosa*: its inactivation by phosphorylation induced by resistant strains. *Antimicrobial Agents and Chemotherapy*, **1**, 17–21.

Lebek, G. (1963). Ubertragung der Mehrfachsresistanz gegen Antibiotika und Chemotherapeutika von *E. coli* auf andere species gram-negativer Bakterien. *Zentralblatt für Bakteriologie, Parasitenkunde, Infektionskrankheiten und Hygiene*, **189**, 213–221.

Linton, K. B., Lee, P. A., Richmond, M. H., Gillespie, W. A., Rowlands, A. J. & Baker, V. N. (1972). Antibiotic resistance and R-factors in coliform bacilli isolated from hospitals and domestic sewage. *Journal of Hygiene, Cambridge*, **70**, 91–104.

Lowbury, E. J. L., Kidson, A., Lilly, H. A., Ayliffe, G. A. J. & Jones, R. J. (1969). Sensitivity of *Pseudomonas aeruginosa* to antibiotics: emergence of strains highly resistant to penicillins. *Lancet*, **ii**, 448–452.

Lowbury, E. J. L., Babb, J. R. & Roe, E. (1972). Clearance from a hospital of Gram-negative bacilli that transfer carbenicillin resistance to *Pseudomonas aeruginosa*. *Lancet*, **ii**, 941–945.

McPhail, M. & Furth, A. J. (1973). Purification and properties of an inducible β-lactamase from *Pseudomonas aeruginosa* NCTC 8203. *Biochemical Society Transactions*, **1**, 1260–1261.

Meadow, P. (1975). In *The Biochemistry and Genetics of Pseudomonas*, Chapter 3, (Ed. P. H. Clarke & M. H. Richmond), John Wiley, London.

Meynell, G. G., (1972). In *Bacterial Plasmids*, Macmillan, London.

Moorhouse, E. C. (1969). Transferable resistance in enterobacteria isolated from urban infants. *British Medical Journal*, **ii**, 405–407.

Neu, H. C. (1968). The surface Localization of Penicillinases in *Escherichia coli* and *Salmonella typhimurium*. *Biochemical and Biophysical Research Communications*, **32**, 258–263.

Newsom, S. W. B., Sykes, R. B. & Richmond, M. H. (1970). Detection of a β-lactamase markedly active against carbenicillin in a strain of *Pseudomonas aeruginosa*. *Journal of Bacteriology*, **101**, 1079–1080.

New York Academy Symposium, (1974). *Annals of the New York Academy of Sciences*, **235**.

Nordström, K. & Sykes, R. B. (1972). Induction of β-lactamase activity in *Pseudomonas aeruginosa*. *Journal of General Microbiology*, **73**, x–xi.

Nordström, K. & Sykes, R. B. (1974). *Antimicrobial Agents and Chemotherapy* **6**, 734–740; **6**, 741–746.

Olsen, R. H. & Shipley, P. (1973). Host range and properties of the *Pseudomonas aeruginosa* R-factor R1822. *Journal of Bacteriology*, **113**, 772–780.

Ozanne, B., Benveniste, R., Tipper, D. & Davies, J. (1969). Amino glycoside antibiotics: inactivation by phosphorylation in *Escherichia coli* carrying R-factors. *Journal of Bacteriology*, **100**, 1144–1146.

Pearce, L. E. & Meynell, E. M. (1968). Specific chromosomal affinity of a resistance factor. *Journal of General Microbiology*, **50**, 159–172.

Pollock, M. R. (1963). In *The Bacteria*, vol. 4, (Ed. I. C. Gunsalus & R. Y. Stanier), Academic Press, New York.

Pühler, A., Burkhardt, H. J. & Neumann, W. (1972). Genetic experiments with *Pseudomonas aeruginosa* R-factor RP4 in *Rhizobium lupini*. *Journal of General Microbiology*, **73**, xxvi.

Richmond, M. H. (1963). Purification and properties of the exopenicillinase from *Staphylococcus aureus*. *Biochemical Journal*, **88**, 452–459.

Richmond, M. H. (1968). The plasmids of *Staphylococcus aureus* and their relation to other extrachromosomal elements in bacteria. *Advances in Microbial Physiology*, **2**, 43–88.

Richmond, M. H. (1969). Extrachromosomal elements and the spread of antibiotic resistance in bacteria. *Biochemical Journal*, **113**, 225–234.

Richmond, M. H. (1970). Plasmids and chromosomes on prokaryotic cells. *Symposium of the Society for General Microbiology*, **20**, 249–277.

Richmond, M. H., Parker, M. T., Jevons, M. P. & John, M. (1964). High penicillinase production correlated with multiple antibiotic resistance in *Staphylococcus aureus*. *Lancet*, **i**, 293–296.

Richmond, M. H., Jack, G. W. & Sykes, R. B. (1972). The β-lactamases of Gram-negative bacteria including pseudomonads. *Annals of the New York Academy of Sciences*, **182**, 243–257.

Richmond, M. H. & Sykes, R. B. (1973). The β-lactamases of Gram-negative bacteria and their possible physiological role. *Advances in Microbial Physiology*, **9**, 31–88.

Richmond, M. H. & Clarke, P. H. (1975). In *The Biochemistry and Genetics of Pseudomonas*, Chapter 9, (Ed. P. H. Clarke & M. H. Richmond), John Wiley, London.

Richmond, M. H. & Curtis, N. A. C. (1974). The interplay of β-lactamases and intrinsic factors in the resistance of Gram-negative bacteria to penicillins and cephalosporins. *Annals of the New York Academy of Sciences*, **235**, 553–572.

Richmond, M. H. & Wiedeman, B. (1974). Plasmids and bacterial evolution. *Symposium of the Society for General Microbiology*, **24**, 59–85.

Roe, E., Jones, R. J. & Lowbury, E. J. L. (1971). Transfer of antibiotic resistance between *Pseudomonas aeruginosa*, *Escherichia coli* and other Gram-negative bacteria in burns. *Lancet*, **i**, 149–152.

Rosselet, A. & Zimmermann, W. (1973). Mutants of *Pseudomonas aeruginosa* with impaired β-lactamase inducibility and increased sensitivity to β-lactam antibiotics. *Journal of General Microbiology*, **76**, 455–457.

Sabath, L. & Abraham, E. P. (1964). Synergistic action of penicillins and cephalosporins against *Pseudomonas pyocyanea*. *Nature, London*, **204**, 1066–1069.

Sabath, L., Jago, M. & Abraham, E. P. (1965). Cephalosporinase and penicillinase activities of a β-lactamase from *Pseudomonas pyocyanea*. *Biochemical Journal*, **96**, 739–752.

Saunders, J. & Grinsted, J. (1972). Properties of RP4, an R-factor which originated in *Pseudomonas aeruginosa* S8. *Journal of Bacteriology*, **112**, 690–696.

Schnaitman, C. A. (1971). Effect of ethylenediaminetetraacetic acid, triton X-100, and lysozyme on the morphology and chemical composition of isolated cell walls of *Escherichia coli*. *Journal of Bacteriology*, **108**, 553–563.

Shaw, W. V. (1972). Enzymology of chloramphenicol resistance. *Annals of the New York Academy of Sciences*, **182**, 234–242.

Smith, D. H. & Armour, S. E. (1966). Transferable drug resistance in enteric bacteria causing infection of the genito-urinary tract. *Lancet*, **ii**, 15–18.

Stanisich, V. & Holloway, B. W. (1971). Chromosome transfer in *Pseudomonas aeruginosa* mediated by R-factors. *Genetical Research, Cambridge*, **17**, 169–172.

Stanisich, V. & Richmond, M. H. (1974). In *Biochemistry and Genetics of Pseudomonas*, Chapter 6, (Ed. P. H. Clarke & M. H. Richmond), John Wiley, London.

Sykes, R. B. & Richmond, M. H. (1970). Intergeneric transfer of a β-lactamase gene between *Pseudomonas aeruginosa* and *Escherichia coli*. *Nature, London*, **226**, 952–954.

Sykes, R. B. & Richmond, M. H. (1971). R-factors, beta-lactamase and carbenicillin resistant *Pseudomonas aeruginosa*. *Lancet*, **ii**, 342–344.

Witchitz, J. L. & Chabbert, Y. A. (1971a). High level transferable resistance to gentamicin. *Journal of Antibiotics, Tokyo*, **24**, 137–139.

Witchitz, J. L. & Chabbert, Y. A. (1971b). Résistance transférable à la gentamicine. I. Expression du charactère de résistance. *Annales de l'Institut Pasteur*, **121**, 733–742.

Witchitz, J. L. & Chabbert, Y. A. (1972). Résistance transférable á la gentamicine. II. Transmissions et liasons du charactère de résistance. *Annales de l'Institut Pasteur*, **122**, 367–378.

Witchitz, J. L. & Gerbaud, G. R. (1972). Classification de plasmides conferant la résistance à la gentamicine. *Annales de l'Institut Pasteur*, **123**, 333–339.

Zyk, N., Kalkstein, A. & Citri, N. (1972). Purification and properties of β-lactamase from *Pseudomonas aeruginosa*. *Israel Journal of Medical Science*, **8**, 1906–1911.

CHAPTER 2

The Effect of the
Bacterial Environment
on Resistance

J. MELLING and M. R. W. BROWN

INTRODUCTION

The Resistance of *Pseudomonas aeruginosa*

Pseudomonas infections in man, whether systemic or localized, have been found to be extremely refractory to chemotherapy (Feingold & Osk, 1965; Smith & Finland, 1968). Although polymyxins B and E as well as gentamicin, have been successful, their use is limited by the narrow range between toxic and effective doses (Darrell & Waterworth, 1967; Olesen & Madsen, 1967; Nishiura, Kawada, Tahara, Mizutani & Miyamura, 1967; Lowbury & Jackson, 1968). The semi-synthetic penicillin, carbenicillin, has proved quite effective *in vitro* (Acred, Brown, Knudsen, Rolinson & Sutherland, 1967; Bodey & Terrell, 1968) and *in vivo* for patients with infections of burns, respiratory and urinary tracts as well as generalized infections (Brumfitt, Percival & Leigh,

35

1967; Jones & Lowbury, 1967; Van Rooyen, Ross, Bethune & MacDonald, 1967).

In spite of the fact that resistance to the polymyxins has rarely been reported as arising during therapy (Brown, 1971), the emergence of strains resistant to the penicillins and aminoglycosides has proved troublesome (Weinstein, Drube, Moss & Waitz, 1971; Ayliffe, Lowbury & Roe, 1972). Information concerning the mechanisms of resistance, which is afforded by an examination of the effects of the bacterial environment, is therefore highly relevant in respect of these chemotherapeutic agents. As well as agents used *in vivo*, a similar study of the environment as it affects resistance to compounds employed for *in vitro* studies (EDTA, lysozyme and polysorbate) is also pertinent. Information on *in vivo* environmental circumstances affecting resistance is greatly lacking.

The Nature of Resistance to Chemotherapy

There are three ways in which micro-organisms resist the actions of antibacterial agents. Briefly, these are exclusion, degradation and target alteration. More fully, an organism becomes insensitive by excluding the agent as a result of some change in the permeability barrier, by modification of the agent so that it is no longer active or by some alteration in the target site of the agent. Concerning an alteration in the target site, except for the cell envelope, which we shall consider in relation to exclusion, there is no evidence that this resistance mechanism is affected by the phenotypic changes which result from modifications to the bacterial environment and it will not be considered separately. Alterations which do occur, such as the ribosomal change resulting in streptomycin resistance (Spotts & Stanier, 1961; Tanaka, 1970), are caused by mutations of the genome. It is tempting to speculate that variations in the relative amounts of DNA, RNA and the various proteins, lipids and carbohydrates, occurring as a consequence of environmental change, may so alter the stoichiometry between an agent and the site of action as to affect the survival of the cell, but evidence is lacking.

In the case of the remaining two major resistance mechanisms, it is clear that alterations in either the amount or the activity of some antibiotic-degrading enzyme and in the composition of the cell envelope can readily occur by the regulatory mechanisms available for phenotypic variation (see below). It is clear that the various observations could be classified according to the particular environmental parameter involved, but as this would involve discussing more than one resistance mechanism at once, the resistance mechanisms have been designated as the highest class and the environmental parameters are considered in relation to each of them.

The Bacterial Environment

Two distinct effects of the bacterial environment need to be considered in relation to the resistance of *P. aeruginosa*. Firstly, the influence of those factors in the growth environment which cause phenotypic changes in the bacterial cell. Secondly, those factors which may modify the response of bacteria to various agents through some interaction with the cell or agent, but which cannot be said to have induced a phenotypic change.

Although finally limited by the genotype, the extent of phenotypic variation exhibited by bacteria is wide. Indeed, unlike many eukaryotic cells whose environment is maintained in relative stability within the whole organism, bacterial cells must be able to adapt to a variety of conditions.

It has been estimated that a bacterium such as *Escherichia coli* contains some 2500 different enzymes whose relative concentrations and activities are subject to sensitive regulatory mechanisms. Such regulatory mechanisms may act at the cytoplasmic level by controlling enzyme activity through a system of end-product inhibition. Here the end-product of a series of reactions may affect the activity of an enzyme involved at an earlier point in the pathway as a result of the allosteric nature of some enzyme molecules (Monod, Changeux & Jacob, 1963). This type of control, although rapid, has the disadvantage for the organism that an unnecessarily large amount of enzyme may be produced, only to have its activity reduced later. Consequently, it is useful for bacteria to have the capacity to regulate enzyme synthesis at the genetic level in order to control the enzyme production according to the conditions pertaining. The mechanisms for regulating enzyme production include induction and repression such as has been described for the production of β-galactosidase (Jacob & Monod, 1961) and also catabolite repression (Magasanik, 1961).

In the struggle for survival bacteria are therefore well equipped in possessing the ability to vary their composition according to the prevailing environment, and consequently they achieve an enviable efficiency of operation. The levels of various enzymes may vary two, three or even several hundred-fold according to growth conditions, with a concomitant change in the products of metabolism. It has been known for some time that the composition of bacteria is not constant and alters markedly depending upon growth conditions (Herbert, 1961). Therefore, any definition of an organism's characteristics may only be valid if the growth conditions are stated. Consequently, it is hardly surprising that the resistance of bacteria to various agents should depend on the growth environment. Many workers in general have used chemically defined, simple salts media. Nevertheless, the nature of the nutrient finally limiting growth has rarely been specified (Brown & Hodges, 1974). This is especially important with regard to the structure and composition of the cell envelope, which is profoundly affected by the nature of the limiting nutrient (Brown & Melling, 1969a,b; Robinson & Tempest, 1973). Also, little attention has been given to the degree of excess of non-limiting nutrients. As well as defining bacterial resistance, particularly for pathogens, in relation to the environment, an investigation of these phenomena leads to an increased understanding of the mode of action of antibacterial substances.

The second class of environmental effects on resistance has been accorded less scientific attention than those involving phenotypic variation. However, further treatments of bacterial cultures may have a profound effect in any attempt to define the resistance of an organism or to investigate the effects of growth conditions on resistance (Farwell & Brown, 1971). Such treatments, or handling procedures, involved in a test system may themselves exhibit neither adverse nor favourable effects on the bacteria, but, as will be discussed, they do present problems arising from interactions either with the organism or with the agent which modifies the response. Therefore, just as the growth conditions have to be defined when discussing resistance, so do the conditions involved subsequent to the culture stage.

ENVIRONMENTAL CONDITIONS AFFECTING EXCLUSION OF ANTIBACTERIAL AGENTS

Cations

It is clear that there is still confusion about the role of cations, particularly calcium and magnesium, in the modification of the resistance of *P. aeruginosa* to various lethal agents. Two distinct but probably related effects are apparent, depending upon whether the effect of cations is examined in relation to the growth of this organism or to some test situation. Where, however, the growth and test situation are the same as, for example, in determining the minimum inhibitory concentration (MIC) of an agent, the two effects become inextricable. The influence of the magnesium concentration in the growth medium on the resistance of *P. aeruginosa* to EDTA and Polymyxin B was studied by Brown & Melling (1969a,b). *P. aeruginosa* was grown in batch culture in a glucose–salts medium without any added divalent cations except just sufficient magnesium to allow growth to proceed to the point where the carbon source was exhausted. Addition of either EDTA or polymyxin to the stationary phase

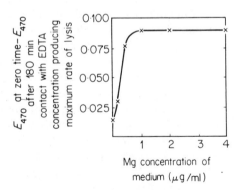

Figure 1. Maximum rate of lysis by EDTA of *P. aeruginosa* grown in media with different Mg concentrations. Reproduced with permission from M. R. W. Brown & J. Melling *J. gen. Microbiol.*, **54**, 439–444 (1969)

cultures indicated that *P. aeruginosa* grown under these conditions was highly resistant to both agents. Cultures grown with magnesium concentrations above the minimum showed increasing sensitivities to EDTA and to polymyxin as the magnesium content of the growth medium was raised (Figures 1, 2 and 3).

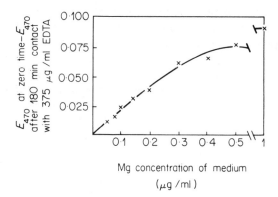

Figure 2. Relationship between maximum rate of lysis of *P. aeruginosa* by EDTA and Mg concentration in the medium: 375 µg EDTA/ml produced maximum rate of lysis over this Mg range. Reproduced with permission from M. R. W. Brown & J. Melling, *J. gen. Microbiol.*, **54**, 439–444 (1969)

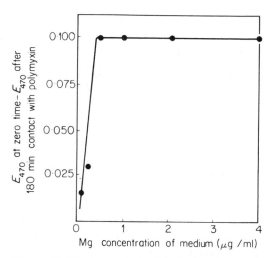

Figure 3. Maximum lysis (E_{470}) by polymyxin (units/ml) of *P. aeruginosa* grown in media containing graded Mg concentrations. Reproduced with permission from M. R. W. Brown & J. Melling, *J. gen. Microbiol.*, **59**, 263–274 (1969)

Other divalent cations, calcium in particular, appeared able to replace magnesium in its role concerning the sensitivity of *P. aeruginosa* to EDTA and polymyxin, although the minimum amount of magnesium required for growth always had to be included in the growth medium. The effect of raising the magnesium content of the medium was clearly shown to be a growth effect since addition of magnesium after growth had ceased (due to depletion of glucose) did not result in any increase in sensitivity to EDTA or to polymyxin. Magnesium-depleted and glucose-depleted cultures have also been examined for sensitivity to silver ions (Brown & Anderson, 1968). In contrast to the decrease in sensitivity to EDTA and polymyxin of magnesium-depleted cultures these were more sensitive to silver ions than glucose-depleted cultures (Figure 4).

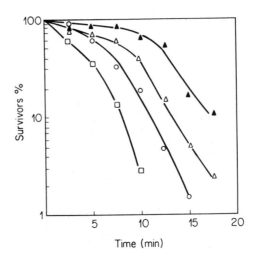

Figure 4. Rate of kill of *P. aeruginosa* in 1×10^{-5} M silver nitrate at 25°. ▲ Glucose-limited cells at pH 5·85. △ Glucose-limited cells at pH 6·25. ○ Glucose-magnesium-limited cells at pH 6·25. □ Magnesium-limited cells at pH 6·25. Reproduced with permission from M. R. W. Brown & R. A. Anderson, *J. Pharm. Pharmac.*, **20** Suppl., 15–35 (1968)

The results of Brown & Melling (1969a,b) were confirmed by Boggis (1971) who extended the studies on the effect of calcium and other cations in relation to the sensitivity of *P. aeruginosa* to EDTA, EGTA (a highly specific chelator of calcium ions) and polymyxin. The order of effectiveness of the cations in inducing sensitivity to EDTA was $Mg^{2+} > Mn^{2+} > Ca^{2+} > Ba^{2+} > Sr^{2+}$ with Zn^{2+} having no effect and Fe^{2+} having a protective effect. In addition, the kinetics of EDTA-induced lysis of culture grown in high magnesium concentrations suggested two sites of action for EDTA; one near the surface of the cell envelope and one less accessible, possibly the cytoplasmic membrane. This agrees with the finding of Cheng, Costerton, Singh & Ingram (1973) who found that spheroplasts of *P. aeruginosa* were insensitive to actinomycin D unless treated with EDTA. Thus, although EDTA affects the cell wall of *P. aeruginosa* and causes release of lipopolysaccharide (Gray & Wilkinson, 1965; Leive, Shovlin & Mergenhagen, 1968; Rogers, Gilleland and Eagon, 1969), a second site of action involving magnesium (and possibly other cations) and also susceptible to phenotypic variation would seem to exist.

Boggis (1971) also showed that the Mg^{2+} and Ca^{2+} contents of *P. aeruginosa* cell walls were related to the availability of these cations in the growth medium. Cell walls having low concentrations of Mg^{2+} and Ca^{2+} were derived from parent cultures insensitive to EDTA and polymyxin whilst walls containing high concentrations of Mg^{2+} or Ca^{2+}, or both, came from cultures showing high sensitivities to these agents. It was also shown that lysis by EGTA of *P. aeruginosa* grown in a calcium-plentiful, magnesium-deficient medium was depressed by the addition of magnesium to the growth medium. Although the Mg^{2+} content of the cell walls increased ($0\cdot16\%$ to $0\cdot25\%$) with such a change, the calcium content remained more constant at a higher level ($0\cdot28\%$ and $0\cdot34\%$ respectively). It was therefore suggested that high concentrations of Mg^{2+} in the medium might result in surface anionic groups being almost entirely associated with Mg^{2+}, while Ca^{2+} was associated with more deeply situated components within the cell envelope. With polymyxin the order of effectiveness of divalent cations in inducing sensitivity was Ca > Mg > Ba > Mn > Sr, but differences in the effectiveness of the various cations was less marked than for EDTA treatment. It was suggested that this indicated a relatively nonspecific association of cell walls with these cations. The greater differences seen for EDTA may therefore reflect the relative affinities of this compound for the different cations.

More recently, Melling, Robinson & Ellwood (1974) have found that the sensitivity to polymyxin of *P. aeruginosa*, grown in continuous culture, was reduced in magnesium-limited compared with carbon-limited or phosphate-limited culture. This agrees with the above findings and during the same work it was also found that magnesium limitation reduced the organism's sensitivity to EDTA, gentamicin, streptomycin and tetracycline. Other work, although involving less well-defined growth conditions, has also indicated that the resistance of *P. aeruginosa* depends on the growth environment. Carson, Favero, Bond & Peterson (1972) found that *P. aeruginosa* isolated from 'distilled' water showed greater resistance to acetic acid ($0\cdot25\%$), chlorine dioxide (67 p.p.m.) and a quaternary ammonium compound when grown in 'ripened' distilled water compared with the same strain grown in freshly distilled water. The ripened distilled water was distilled water which had been allowed to stand for several days and was then filter sterilized. Weisner, Asscher & Wimpenny (1968) reported that the resistance of *E. coli*, *P. aeruginosa* and *Proteus mirabilis* to penicillin, ampicillin, tetracycline and chloramphenicol was reversed by EDTA. The experiments involved determinations of the MIC of the particular antibiotic by growing cultures for 18 hr at 37 °C in nutrient broth + EDTA + antibiotic. In view of the work of Brown & Melling (1969a,b), the results may relate to growth in cation-depleted conditions owing to chelation of some of the available cations in the medium and EDTA can clearly not have been present in excess since otherwise no magnesium would have been available for growth. It is significant that addition of $0 \cdot 1$ M Mg^{2+} or Ca^{2+} prevented this effect of EDTA. The authors suggested that the effect of EDTA was to increase the permeability of the cell wall to the antibiotics but since free EDTA was probably not present this seems unlikely. Quite distinct from the effect of divalent cations in the growth medium is their presence in the test medium. Newton (1954) observed that addition of divalent cation (in order of effectiveness; $Mg^{2+} > Sr^{2+} > Ca^{2+} > Ba^{2+}$) protected washed *P. aeruginosa* against polymyxin B. Trivalent cations were even more effective and uranyl ions gave maximum protection. It was proposed that the protective action of these cations resulted from competition between them and polymyxin for phosphate groups near the cell surface. In this series of experiments it was clear that no phenotypic variation occurred. Similar results using polymyxin E have been reported by Davis, Ianetta & Wedgwood (1971a,b). Serum obtained from volunteers after injection of therapeutic doses of colistin was highly bactericidal for *E. coli*, but showed no activity against *P. aeruginosa* unless the calcium concentration was decreased either by dilution with nutrient broth or the addition of chelating agents. The six strains of *P. aeruginosa* used were insensitive to EDTA alone even when grown in nutrient broth. In a later study, Davis & Ianetta (1972a) showed that calcium was less antagonistic to the action of gentamicin than to colistin. It is interesting that extrapolation of these *in vitro* results to the *in vivo* situation is supported by the report of Hepding (1967), who found that gentamicin was more effective than colistin or polymyxin B in the treatment of experimental *Pseudomonas* infections in mice. The effectiveness of gentamicin for treatment of *Pseudomonas* keratinitis in rabbits was increased by EDTA (Wilson, 1970), but the author suggested that EDTA reduced tissue damage caused by calcium-dependent proteases rather than carrying out a synergistic antibacterial action. The proteolytic activity of cell-free extracts was reduced by the addition of EDTA—Na salt. The interpretation of *in vivo* experiments is difficult and it should be appreciated that, for example, polymyxin resistance may be influenced by divalent cations acting in both the growth and test situations.

A considerable amount of the work on the assessment of the effect of antibiotics has been done by determining the MIC of the antibiotic; therefore an assessment of the role of divalent cations is complicated. However, in view of the relatively high concentrations of divalent cations usually found in growth media ($>10^{-3}$ M) compared with the concentrations of $<10^{-5}$ M necessary to cause phenotypic variation, it is highly probable that in these cases the effect of the cations is related to exclusion of antibiotics from otherwise sensitive bacteria, which are growing in a physiological excess of cations.

Tseng, Bryan & Van Den Elzen (1972) reported that the magnesium content of the growth medium affected the sensitivity of *P. aeruginosa* to streptomycin. The inclusion of $0 \cdot 1$ M $MgCl_2$ into a low phosphate (concentration unspecified) medium gave a 3-fold increase in the MIC and reduced the uptake of streptomycin 8-fold. Unfortunately, no information was given about the effect of the addition of magnesium to 'high phosphate' cultures which exhibited higher MICs than 'low phosphate' cultures. Similarly, Davis & Ianetta (1972b) observed an antagonistic effect of Ca^{2+} (10^{-3} M) and of 20% human serum on the activity of tobramycin against *P. aeruginosa*. No such effect occurred with *E. coli*, not in the case of carbenicillin treatment of *P. aeruginosa*. These authors reported that the Ca^{2+} and serum antagonism of tobramycin was reversed by Mg—EDTA; this is contrary to the findings of Brown & Richards (1965) who found, in comparable experiments, that Mg—EDTA had no synergistic effect in combination with polymyxin, unlike Na—EDTA. In fact, saturation of cation-chelating agents by excess cation in the medium is another factor for consideration in designing test systems. A similar increase in the MIC of tobramycin against *P. aeruginosa* on addition of Ca^{2+} to the medium was reported by Dienstag & Neu (1972). They found Ca^{2+} more effective than Mg^{2+} in this respect.

There is considerable evidence of the antagonistic effects of calcium and magnesium on the activity of gentamicin against *P. aeruginosa*. Waitz & Weinstein (1969) observed that disc-sensitivity testing of *P. aeruginosa* produced variable zone diameters depending upon the medium used. Garrod & Waterworth (1969) found a 32-fold variation in the sensitivity of *P. aeruginosa* to gentamicin, depending upon the medium constituents and the type of agar used for producing solid media. In general, increasing the Mg^{2+} content of the medium resulted in an increased MIC of the antibiotic. Such variations in sensitivity were small in parallel tests using *E. coli*. Washington, Ritts & Martin (1970) described considerable (4-fold) increases in the MIC of gentamicin against 39 *P. aeruginosa* strains when grown on Trypticase soy agar rather than Mueller–Hinton agar. Such pronounced variation again occurred only with *P. aeruginosa* strains although a number of other Gram-negative bacteria were tested. In a subsequent report (Washington, Hermans & Martin, 1970) the concentrations of calcium and magnesium in the trypticase soy agar were found to be twice those in the Mueller–Hinton agar. Similarly, Gilbert, Kutscher, Ireland, Barnett & Sandford (1971) reported that the MIC of gentamicin for *P. aeruginosa* was increased when either the Ca^{2+} or Mg^{2+} contents of the medium were raised. On reviewing the available evidence they discounted some inhibition of the antibiotic *per se* (Wagman, Oden, Weinstein & Irwin, 1966) and from their own data it seemed unlikely that effects on medium tonicity were responsible. However, their suggestion that an increased uptake of cations by the bacteria may lead to a more stable cell wall seems unlikely in view of the findings of Brown & Melling (1969a,b) and Boggis (1971), who observed changes in antibiotic resistance related to phenotypic variation at calcium and magnesium concentrations a hundred times lower than those employed here. It would seem therefore that the results of Gilbert *et al.* (1971) may be related to the type of cation effects described by Newton (1954). In addition, recent work (Melling, Robinson & Ellwood, 1974) has shown that in continuous culture magnesium-limited (no calcium) cultures were more resistant to gentamicin than carbon-limited cultures, where the magnesium content was 10-fold greater.

Water washing of agar prior to use for determining MICs of polymyxin, neomycin, kanamycin and streptomycin reduced the MIC of all four antibiotics (Hanus, Sands & Bennett, 1967). This result was correlated with the removal of calcium and magnesium in the washing process. Variations in agar quality have also been correlated with the size of inhibition zones. Bechtle & Scherr (1958) found larger inhibition zones using ion agar, rather than conventional agar, to examine sensitivity to polymyxins and aminoglycosides. A similar potentiation occurred when agarose (a neutral polysaccharide extracted from agar) was employed (Kunin & Edmondson, 1968). Such variations are not unexpected since agar is composed of agarose and agaropectin. Agaropectin is sulphated and contains acid residues which can bind cations (Araki, 1959). Furthermore, agar may react with protein molecules (Brishammar, Hjerten & Hofsten, 1961) and basic molecules such as polymyxin and neomycin (Ford, Bergay, Brooks, Garrett, Alberti, Dyer & Carter, 1955) making a true evaluation difficult. Evidence that the antagonism of gentamicin by calcium and magnesium operates at the cell wall level was provided by Zimelis & Jackson (1973). They compared the antagonistic effects of cations on whole cells and spheroplasts and found that cations did not antagonize the action of gentamicin on spheroplasts. This is similar to the situation with polymyxin: Chen & Feingold (1972) observed that neither Ca^{2+} nor Mg^{2+} protected lipid spherules (prepared from bacterial phospholipids) from the release of trapped solutes caused by polymyxin. They also found that the phospholipid composition of the bacterial membrane was a determining factor in polymyxin sensitivity. It therefore appears that two sites, the cytoplasmic membrane and the cell wall, may be involved in polymyxin resistance. This is supported by the work of Teuber (1969) who reported that spheroplasts of *P. mirabilis* produced by use of penicillin G were as susceptible to polymyxin as other Gram-negative bacteria, although if allowed to reconvert to a bacillary form they again acquired polymyxin resistance. The author argued that the resistance of *Proteus* strains to polymyxin was due to the impermeability of the outer wall structures to the antibiotic. The involvement of the cell wall is also suggested by Sud & Feingold (1970). They analysed the total cell lipid of three types of *P. mirabilis*; (i) a resistant wild type (ii) a polymyxin sensitive mutant (iii) a wild type sensitized by growth in sulphonamide (Herman, 1959; Onozawa, Kumagai & Ishida 1967) and found no significant differences in their lipid compositions. In addition, the sensitive mutants and the sulphadiazine-treated organisms remained resistant to actinomycin D and erythromycin, thus suggesting that the lesion allowing polymyxin to pass through the cell wall does not result in generally increased permeability. Sud & Feingold (1972) reported increased sensitivity of *P. mirabilis* to surface-active agents after exposure to polymyxin. Spheroplast formation renders the organism sensitive to these agents (Taubeneck, 1962; see also Chapter 3, page 77). Brown & Wood (1972) showed that sensitivity to polymyxin correlated with the amount of phospholipid in wall fractions of *P. aeruginosa, Proteus vulgaris* and *Klebsiella aerogenes* and to a lesser extent correlated with wall cation. An involvement of the outer membrane is indicated by these results. These workers also showed that the affinity of polymyxin for phospholipid from *P. vulgaris* and *P. aeruginosa* was the same.

The composition of growth media with respect to NaCl has been found to affect the resistance of bacteria to antibiotics. Wick & Welles (1967) observed more than a 10-fold increase in the MIC of nembramycin for both *Staphylococcus aureus* and *Salmonella typhosa* on increasing the NaCl concentration from 0% to 5%. The addition of NaCl to nutrient broth was also found to raise the

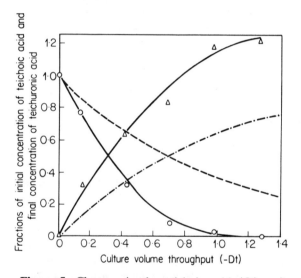

Figure 5. Changes in the teichoic acid (○) and teichuronic acid (△) contents of cell walls of *Bacillus subtilis* var *niger* following changeover from conditions of Mg^{2+}-limitation to phosphate-limitation in a chemostat culture. The regular broken line represents the theoretical washout rate assuming that teichoic acid synthesis ceased immediately the environment became depleted of inorganic phosphate. The irregular broken line represents the theoretical rate of increase in teichuronic acid, assuming that its synthesis started immediately the culture became phosphate-limited and continued at a rate proportional to the rate of synthesis of biomass. Reproduced with permission from D. C. Ellwood & D. W. Tempest, *Biochem. J.*, **118**, 367–373 (1969)

MIC of gentamicin for *P. aeruginosa, Serratia marcescens* and *E. coli* (Medeiros, O'Brian, Wacker & Yulug, 1971). No mechanism for this effect of NaCl was proposed, but it is significant that some Mg^{2+} is generally found loosely bound to the surface structures of bacteria (Strange & Shon, 1964) and this binding is competitively inhibited by Na^+. In Gram-positive organisms at least, the binding affinity of cell walls for Mg^{2+} was greater for Mg-limited cultures than for P-limited (Meers & Tempest, 1970). Under P-limited conditions an anionic wall polymer, teichuronic acid, is present whereas in Mg-limited bacteria this is completely replaced by the phosphorous-containing polymer teichoic acid (Ellwood & Tempest, 1969), Figure 5. However, the inclusion of 6% NaCl in the medium feeding a P-limited culture resulted in bacteria which contained no teichuronic acid, but only teichoic acid (Table 1)

Table 1. Effect of medium NaCl concentration on the anionic polymer content and composition of the walls of PO_4^{3-}-limited *Bacillus subtilis* var. *niger*. The organisms were grown in a chemostat culture with the temperature regulated at 35°, the pH controlled at 7·0 and the dilution rate at 0·3 hr^{-1}. (Reproduced with permission from D. C. Ellwood & D. W. Tempest, *Advan. Microb. Physiol,* **7,** 83–117, 1972).

Medium NaCl content (%, w/v)	Amount of wall (g/100 g)	Amount in walls (g/100 g dry weight)			
		Phosphorus	Hexose	Glucuronic acid	Galactos-amine
0	18·9	0·4	<2	24·0	17·0
2	22·3	0·7	10·4	19·7	17·0
4	19·1	3·3	16·7	6·1	3·0
6	16·1	4·3	18·8	<3	<3
		Teichoic acid		Teichuronic acid	

and the walls of these organisms had a higher affinity for Mg^{2+} than walls from bacteria grown in P-limited culture without NaCl (Ellwood & Tempest, 1972). Thus, the addition of NaCl in some respects simulates Mg-limitation. It seems a reasonable hypothesis therefore that a mechanism for Mg-binding should exist in Gram-negative bacteria. In view of the findings described above concerning the effect of Mg-limitation (Brown & Melling, 1969a,b; Melling, Robinson & Ellwood, 1974), and phosphate limitation (see below) on the resistance of *P. aeruginosa* to polymyxin it is further proposed that a phosphorous-containing wall constituent may be involved both in Mg-binding and in uptake of such antibiotics as polymyxin and gentamicin.

Anions

The anion which has been examined in relation to antibiotic exclusion is phosphate. Boggis (1971) found that batch-grown *P. aeruginosa* was more resistant to either EDTA or polymyxin as the phosphate content of the medium was reduced. The phosphorus content of cell walls of magnesium-depleted cells (resistant to EDTA and polymyxin) was about 75% of that in magnesium-plentiful cells and 50% of that in magnesium- and calcium-plentiful cells. However, the molar ratio of wall phosphorus to total calcium plus magnesium was reduced in the more sensitive bacteria.

In contrast, Tseng, Bryan & Van Den Elzen (1972) reported that the MIC of streptomycin to two strains of *P. aeruginosa* was reduced by some 50% in a trypticase soy broth in low phosphate (concentration unspecified) compared with high phosphate. In addition, the uptake of streptomycin was increased 12-fold by growth in low-phosphate medium. Unfortunately, no attempt was made to distinguish between the effects of phosphate concentration in the growth as opposed to the test situation. Recently, Melling, Robinson & Ellwood (1974), using continuous culture, observed that *P. aeruginosa* had a higher sensitivity to polymyxin B in phosphate-limited culture compared with magnesium-limited. There was, in addition, little change associated with varying the growth rate in phosphate-limited conditions; whereas in carbon-limited conditions a 30-fold difference in sensitivity existed between the slowest (D = 0·05) and fastest (D = 0·7) growth rates. These effects of phosphate limitation are of interest in view of the findings of Tamaki & Matsuhashi (1973) who found that *E. coli* mutants sensitive to novobiocin and spiromycin lacked phosphate and glucose in the polysaccharide portion of their LPS.

The differences between the results of the various workers are not readily explicable at the present time but may reflect the particular culture conditions used to achieve depletion of phosphate. Thus Boggis (1971) used phosphate-depleted cultures which were also glucose-depleted and a buffer system of 3,6-endomethylene-1,2,3,6-tetrahydrophthalic acid (EMTA).

Temperature

Few observations are available which clearly indicate an effect of growth temperature on the exclusion of antimicrobial agents from *P. aeruginosa*. Carson, Favero, Bond & Peterson (1972) reported that *P. aeruginosa* grown on trypticase soy agar showed increased resistance to acetic acid, chlorine dioxide, glutaraldehyde and a quaternary ammonium compound when grown at 25 °C, rather than 37 °C. Considering the mode of action of these agents, particularly glutaraldehyde, it seems unlikely that enzymatic inactivation or a change in target site would be involved. However, because of the sensitivity of this organism to temperature shock (see below, p. 59) such an effect may suffice to explain the observations if solutions of the agents at subgrowth temperatures were used.

The sensitivity of several strains of *P. aeruginosa* to serum and antibiotics was affected by growth temperature (Muschel, Ahl & Fisher, 1969). When grown at 41 °C instead of 37 °C an increased sensitivity to serum, polymyxin E, mitomycin C, erythromycin and actinomycin D was observed. Since polymyxins have never been shown to be subject to enzymic degradation then, for this agent at least, these results suggest some modification to the exclusion properties of the cell.

In view of the probable involvement of cell wall lipids, particularly phospholipids in the exclusion uptake of lethal agents (Newton, 1956; Ivanov, Markov, Golovinskii & Charisanova, 1964; Brown & Watkins, 1970; Brown & Wood, 1972) it does seem likely that variations in growth temperature should have some effect. The lipid composition of baterial cell walls has been found to vary with growth temperature with respect to both the degree of saturation of fatty acids (Farrell & Rose, 1967a,b) and the phospholipid composition (Bell, Mavis & Vagelos, 1972). A comparison of lipids from a variety of antibiotic-sensitive and resistant Gram-negative bacteria showed that there was a higher concentration of unsaturated acids and a lower concentration of cyclopropane acids in lipids from resistant strains (Dunnick & O'Leary, 1970).

Growth Phase

Although most work on antibiotic resistance of bacteria has been done using batch cultures, even in such cases the term 'growth phase' may not be a very meaningful expression. The resistance of logarithmic phase cultures has been studied either by the addition of some agent to a growing culture and monitoring subsequent effects, or by the determination of the MIC of some agent although the picture here is complicated by the use, in some cases, of non-replicating inocula. However, in complex media such as the various nutrient broths, even 'logarithmic' growth probably consists of a series of diauxies and the particular nutrient being consumed will vary as growth proceeds. Thus, standardization of the culture and the density at which an agent is added may prove critical. The term 'stationary phase' is also imprecise since, even when growth (cell division) has ceased, the metabolic state of a culture will vary with the length of time which has passed and therefore variations of resistance in relation to growth phase may be difficult to interpret.

In general, the resistance of bacteria to lethal agents is greatest for stationary-phase cultures and *P. aeruginosa* is no exception. Carson, Favero, Bond & Peterson (1972) reported that stationary-phase *P. aeruginosa* were more resistant to acetic acid than log. phase cultures.

Studies on the antibiotic resistance of *P. aeruginosa* grown in continuous culture (Melling, Robinson & Ellwood, 1974) may provide at least a partial explanation for the greater resistance of stationary-phase batch cultures over log. phase. It was found that for both carbon-limited and magnesium-limited cultures, the slower the growth rate, the greater was the resistance of *P. aeruginosa* to a number of agents including polymyxin, EDTA, carbenicillin, streptomycin and gentamicin. Batch culture studies have also shown variations in the lipid composition of bacteria with culture age (Knivett & Cullen, 1965; Crowfoot & Hunt, 1970) but correlation with antibiotic resistance is as yet lacking.

pH

It seems that the observed effects of growth medium pH on the resistance of *P. aeruginosa* and other organisms are more related to the degree of ionization of some agent or cell component than to any phenotypic variation. If this is the case then, although pH effects are often referred to in the context of the growth situation, 'growth' is clearly not always involved. A detailed account of the relationships between pH and activity of various antibacterial agents has been given by Albert (1965). The effects of pH on antibiotic activity were noticed soon after antibiotic therapy came into use. Gardner & Chain (1942) and Waksman, Bugie & Schatz (1944) observed that the basic antibiotics were considerably more active at pH 8·0 than at pH 6·0, while acidic antibiotics, such as penicillin (Florey, Gilliver, Jennings & Sanders, 1946) were more active at acid pH. A similar observation was made by Abraham & Duthie (1946) who found that the MIC of streptomycin against *P. aeruginosa* increased 2·5-fold with an increase in medium pH from 6·0 to 8·0. Eagle, Levy & Fleischman (1952) examined the effect of pH on the activity of penicillin, streptomycin, chloramphenicol and tetracycline. Penicillin showed decreased activity against *Micrococcus pyogenes* with increasing pH, but little change in activity occurred against *E. coli*. Streptomycin activity increased with pH against both organisms and tetracycline had an optimum pH of 7·7 for activity against *E. coli*, but showed little variation in activity against the Gram-positive organism. The activity of chloramphenicol also varied with pH, showing a minimum at pH 6.6. As this molecule is not ionizable this may reflect some change in the bacteria and such an effect may explain the differences in response to pH changes shown by *E. coli* and *M. pyogenes*.

The first indications of an increase in erythromycin activity with alkaline pH against the Gram-negative bacteria *E. coli*, *Proteus* species and *P. aeruginosa* were reported by Zager (1965) and Sylvester (1966). In a more detailed study Sabath *et al.* (1968) observed that the urine from healthy subjects taking erythromycin showed marked activity against *E. coli*, *Klebsiella pneumoniae*, *P. Mirabilis*, *P. aeruginosa* and *Serratia* species when the urine was rendered alkaline (pH 7·9–8·9) by concurrent administration of $NaHCO_3$ or acetazolamide. Little antibacterial activity was noted without such alkalization, when the urine pH was between 5·3 and 6·4, even though the erythromycin concentration in the urine was the same as in the first experiment. The fact that erythromycin, a weak base, shows a 1000-fold change in the total of material necessary to inhibit *E. coli* over the pH range 5·0 to 8·5, while there is no alteration in the amount of unionized material needed, may explain these findings. Garrett, Heman-Ackah & Perry (1970) studied this phenomenon in detail and confirmed that the erythromycin concentration necessary to achieve a standard effect was reduced dramatically as the pK_a value of 8·8 was approached. As this occurs there is an increasing proportion of unprotonated erythromycin available to enter the cell. Other possible explanations, since ionized molecules are not necessarily entirely devoid of biological activity, include a combination of factors such as ionization of cellular receptors, active transport mechanisms, competition between ionized antibiotics and H^+ or OH^- ions for cellular receptors (Albert, 1965). A reduction in the sensitivity of *Staph. aureus, Bacteroides fragilis* and *Haemophilus influenzae* to erythromycin and lincomycin was found on lowering the pH of the growth medium from 7·0 to 6·0 (Ingham, Selkon, Codd & Hale, 1970). Similar results were reported for the activities of erythromycin and of spiromycin on *Staph. pyogenes* (Garrod & Waterworth, 1956) and a *Streptococcus* (Haight & Finland, 1952). pH effects have been observed with other antibacterial agents. Bassett (1971) reported a decrease in the MIC of a combination of chlorhexidene and cetrimide against *P. vulgaris* and *P. multivorans* following a pH reduction from 7·2 to 6·0, although activity against *P. aeruginosa* was unchanged. Using an antibiotic disc method, Rosenblatt & Schoenknecht (1972) found that the sensitivity of *E. coli* to the aminoglycosides streptomycin, gentamicin and kanamycin as well as tetracycline and chloramphenicol increased with a pH change from 7·4 to 8·4. Inhibition zones were largest when incubated aerobically whilst the inclusion of 5% CO_2 caused a reduction in zone size due to a fall in pH. The MIC of tobramycin against *P. aeruginosa* changed from 1·56 mg/ml at pH 6·8 to 3·12 mg/ml at pH 7·4 (Dienstag & Neu, 1972), although a true picture is difficult to obtain due to changes in medium composition. Various test systems have been employed to determine the influence of pH on antibacterial activity, and recently Miller & Perkins (1973) assessed different methods used to determine the effect of pH on the activity of carbenicillin on *P. mirabilis*. Cylinder plate assays, growth-curve studies and scanning electron microscopy of treated bacteria all indicated that the greatest activity was at pH 7·2 and the least at pH 5·0. However, standard tube-dilution methods for determining MICs showed no significant differences at pH 5·0, 6·0, 7·0 and 8·0.

Phenotypic variation of bacteria in response to pH changes has been observed (Van Iterson & Op den Kamp, 1969) with respect to alterations in the phospholipid composition of the cell envelope of *B. subtilis* and this may imply alterations to the exclusion properties of the cell. However, the position concerning the effect of pH on bacterial resistance is not clear as often no attempt has been made to distinguish between phenotypic variation, physical effects on the cell and alterations of the agent.

Slime

It has been suggested that the extra-cellular slime produced by *P. aeruginosa* may be implicated in its resistance to chemotherapy, particularly *in vitro* (Brown & Richards, 1964) and in the toxicity and pathogenicity of this organism (Liu, Abe & Bates, 1961).

Slime production has been shown to depend upon various culture parameters including temperature, mineral salt and trace element concentration (Palumbo, 1972; Goto, Murakawa & Kuwahara, 1973) and the nature of the carbon source (Brown, Clamp & Foster, 1966; Brown, Foster & Clamp 1969).

However, Brown & Foster (1971) examined the resistance of slime-producing cultures (glucose grown) to both EDTA and polymyxin. They concluded that, at least *in vitro*, slime probably does not play a significant role in the resistance of *P. aeruginosa*. Nevertheless, slime production is relevant to resistance to *in vivo* body defences (Schwarzmann & Boring, 1971; Roe & Jones, 1974). The interaction between the environmental condition of the lung and mucoid strains of *P. aeruginosa* in cystic fibrosis is of great interest.

ENVIRONMENTAL CONDITIONS AFFECTING ENZYMATIC INACTIVATION

Enzymatic inactivation of antibiotics is one of the principal means by which micro-organisms are able to resist such agents. A number of antibiotic-inactivating enzymes have been identified in and isolated from *P. aeruginosa*: these include β-lactamases (Sabath, Jago & Abraham 1965; Sykes & Richmond, 1970; Fullbrook, Elson & Slocombe, 1970; Neu, 1970), dihydrostreptomycin phosphorylase (Kobayashi, Yamaguchi, Sato & Mitsuhashi, 1972), kanamycin, neomycin and streptomycin phosphorylases (Doi, Ogura, Tanaka & Umezawa, 1968). Therefore any alterations to the growth environment which affect the production, stability or activity of such enzymes are likely to modify bacterial resistance. Some environmental parameters involved will be discussed in relation to their effect on these factors.

Although there is evidence, as will be described, of variations in the content and activity of antibiotic-degrading enzymes under different growth conditions, direct evidence linking such variations with changes in antibiotic resistance is lacking. Nevertheless, the following observations are intended to focus attention on this area since this aspect of growth conditions may well be important in relation to antibiotic resistance *in vivo*.

Cations

Mg^{2+} ions have been found necessary for the activity of a kanamycin phosphorylating enzyme produced by *P. aeruginosa* (Doi, Kondo, Tanaka & Umezawa, 1969), although Mn^{2+}, Zn^{2+} and Co^{2+} could replace Mg^{2+} in this respect. Mg^{2+} is also essential for the activity of a dihydrostreptomycin phosphorylase from *P. aeruginosa* (Kobayashi, Yamaguchi, Sato & Mitsuhashi, 1972) and enzyme activity was eliminated by EDTA. The production of a cephalosporinase by *Bacillus cereus* (Kuwabarra, 1970) was reported to require Zn^{2+}, although it is probable that Zn^{2+} was involved in enzyme stability rather than being needed for enzyme formation.

It has been established that antibiotic resistance mediated by antibiotic-inactivating enzymes coded for by R-factors is transferable between different strains of *P. aeruginosa* (Stanisich & Holloway, 1971; Bryan, Van Den Elzen & Tseng, 1972) and between *P. aeruginosa* and *E. coli* (Sykes & Richmond, 1970; Fullbrook, Elson & Slocombe, 1970; Roe, Jones & Lowbury, 1971). From the work of Brinton (1971) it appears that transfer of R-factors requires filamentous surface appendages called sex pili. Some factors affecting pilus formation will be discussed below but, in the context of cations, Beard (1972) found that the inclusion of sodium chloride into the Difco nutrient broth for growth of *E. coli* significantly enhanced the formation of sex pili and hence the spread of drug resistance. The destruction of various microbial enzymes by an organism's own proteases has been observed for a number of different enzymes (Thurston, 1973) and at least one antibiotic-inactivating enzyme, a penicillinase. (Callow, Atkinson & Melling, 1973; Melling, Callow, Capel & Whitaker in preparation). Various cations have been found to be required for protease activity, and thus the level of activity of antibiotic inactivating enzymes may be affected indirectly by the cation content of the medium.

Temperature

A phosphorylase isolated from *P. aeruginosa* and acting on lividomycin showed a 20% loss of activity after 5 min at 37 °C and a 60% loss after the same time at 40 °C (Kobayashi, Yamaguchi & Mitsuhashi, 1972). A similar heat lability was found for a kanamycin phosphorylase also from *P. aeruginosa* (Doi, Kondo, Tanaka & Umezawa, 1969). The fertility of R-factors is expressed in only a small proportion of a population, unlike the fertility of F which ordinarily is always expressed (Meynell, Meynell & Datta, 1968; Watanabe & Fukasawa, 1961) and this has been attributed to synthesis of a cytoplasmic repressor. Furthermore, it has been shown that R-factor transfer is mediated by sex pili and that cells possessing these are sensitive to the male-specific phage MS 2 (Lawn, Meynell, Meynell & Datta, 1967) and that sex pilus formation is repressed by the cytoplasmic repressor (Meynell & Datta, 1967). Derepression of R-factor fertility may thus occur, either due to lack of repression or alteration in the site with which the repressor interacts (Frydman & Meynell, 1969; Meynell & Cooke, 1969; Hoar, 1970) and these authors have isolated mutants which exhibit both types of derepression. Phenotypic derepression is also possible and Silver & Cohen (1972) have shown that in one strain of *E. coli* there is a 300-fold reduction in R-factor transfer at 32 °C compared with 42 °C. They attributed this difference to the lability of the repressor substance at 42 °C. Observations concerning the antibiotic resistance of a culture may therefore depend upon the ability of an initially low concentration of R-factor containing bacteria to transmit R-factors throughout the culture.

As well as transmission of extra-chromosomal DNA, replication of such units is a critical factor. A methicillin-resistant *Staphylococcus aureus* grew more quickly than a methicillin-sensitive strain at lower temperatures (Annear, 1968; Hewitt, Coe & Parker, 1969). On screening a number of strains of *Staph. aureus* for methicillin resistance, Hewitt, Coe & Parker (1969) found that although at 30 °C 260 cultures showed evidence of resistance, only 201 of these were methicillin-resistant when grown at 37 °C. Annear (1968) reported a 30-fold reduction in the MIC of methicillin for methicillin-resistant *Staph. aureus* when grown at 43 °C rather than 31 °C. No such change occurred with methicillin-sensitive bacteria. These results may either be accounted for by the failure of plasmid replication to keep pace with cell division as observed by Ashevov (1966) or result from the temperature sensitivity of enzyme production (Knox & Collard, 1952) or a temperature-sensitive enzyme (Langridge, 1963). Recent observations (Melling, unpublished results) on β-lactamase production in *Bacillus cereus* support the first hypothesis. Repeated subculture of a *B. cereus* strain above 35 °C resulted in a gradual reduction from 100% of the bacteria being β-lactamase producers to less than 10%; whereas similar subculturing at 30 °C had no such effect even though samples taken at intervals were grown at 37 °C to eliminate the possibility that a temperature-sensitive enzyme or synthetic process was involved.

pH

The production of an R-factor mediated penicillinase in *E. coli* was found to be pH dependent (Melling & Ford, 1971). Maximum enzyme yields were at pH 7·0 and below this pH the reduced enzyme levels resulted from lower cell yields. However, the reduced enzyme levels above pH 7·0 have been shown to be caused by destruction of the penicillinase by a protease which is activated only above pH 6·5 (Melling, Callow, Capel & Whitaker in preparation). Clearly there are implications for the treatment of infection caused by penicillin-resistant bacteria since the ability to render, say, a patient's urine alkaline may be a useful adjunct to chemotherapy of bladder infections. A penicillinase-degrading enzyme capable of inactivating *Staph. aureus* penicillinase was reported by Iwai, Ohono, Takeshima, Yamaguchi, Omura & Hata (1973) to be produced by *Streptomyces gedanesis*. However, this situation differs from that in *E. coli* where it is the bacterial protease which is acting on the cell's own penicillinase, but these authors did propose that exogenous proteases could also be of therapeutic interest.

The activities of a number of antibiotic-inactivating enzymes from *P. aeruginosa* have been shown to be pH-dependent. A lividomycin phosphorylase was reported to have a pH optimum of 7·0 with less than 10% of peak activity below pH 6·0 or above pH 8·0 (Kobayashi, Yamaguchi & Mitsuhasni 1972). Conversely, Kobayashi, Yamaguchi, Sato & Mitsuhashi (1972) described a dihydrostreptomycin phosphorylase with a pH optimum of 9·5 which still retained 40% of peak activity at pH 6·0. A streptomycin adenylase from *E. coli* (Umezawa, Takasawa, Okanishi & Utahara, 1968) showed a very sharp pH optimum between 8·3 and 8·5. Doi, Ogura, Tanaka & Umezawa (1968) reported on the pH activity of extracts from *P. aeruginosa* which inactivated kanamycin and streptomycin. The extracts had sharp optima falling to around 20% of the maximum activity for a shift of a single pH unit. The optima were pH 7·5 for kanamycin inactivation and pH 8·5 for streptomycin inactivation.

As well as the stability of antibiotic-inactivating enzymes in relation to protease activity, some show purely pH-related effects. A kanamycin phosphorylase from *P. aeruginosa* was found to have maximum stability between pH 8·0 and pH 9·0 with considerable loss of stability outside this range (Doi, Kondo, Tanaka & Umezawa, 1969).

ENVIRONMENTAL CONDITIONS
INVOLVING THE TEST SITUATION

So far we have been concerned with various culture parameters and in general the discussion has been restricted to the culture conditions producing phenotypic variations involving bacterial resistance. It has become clear that bacterial resistance may be altered, in the absence of phenotypic variation, as a result of interactions between environmental factors and the organism or agent. Of necessity, this has already been mentioned in attempts to distinguish between such effects, and resistance changes associated with phenotypic variations. However, the discussion, which up to now has been confined to factors involved in the growth medium, would also apply to situations where the growth and test situations were so similar that some agent was applied to an otherwise unaltered culture. This has been achieved by the addition of such a small volume of agent relative to the culture volume that, essentially, there was no change in the temperature, pH or solute composition of the culture. Examples of this approach include the addition of small volumes of prewarmed antibiotic solutions to actively growing cultures (Brown & Garrett, 1964) and similar treatment for stationary-phase cultures (Brown & Melling, 1969a,b). In this section, therefore, it is intended to consider the effects of harvesting and handling procedures where a change in the bacterial environment occurs. Such environmental changes include both the test situation and subsequent treatments involved in recovery situations aimed at assessing the bacterial response to a particular agent. A critical appraisal of the effect of environmental parameters subsequent to the growth situation is, however, difficult. The growth conditions used by different workers vary widely and will affect the physiological state of the organism. A further factor which complicates the situation is the possible interaction between the various parameters of the test situation.

The Solute Composition of the Suspending Medium

Various physiological studies have indicated the existence of a selectively permeable barrier to the passage of solutes in bacteria. In Gram-positive bacteria it is the cytoplasmic membrane which functions in this respect (Mitchell & Moyle, 1956) but such a layer has also been identified in the wall of *E. coli* in addition to the cytoplasmic membrane (Payne & Gilvarg, 1968). As a consequence, bacteria transferred from one solution to another of different solute concentration, may undergo changes of size and shape (Mohr & Larsen,

1963) as well as lysis (Christian & Ingram, 1959) and loss of viability (Carlucci & Pramer, 1960). The importance of the magnitude of the change in tonicity is indicated by the results of Christian & Ingram (1959). When halphilic *Vibrio* cells were allowed to equilibrate in a medium having half the tonicity of the growth medium, the degree of dilution with distilled water necessary to achieve lysis was greater by some 50% compared with the degree of dilution to lyse bacteria which had been maintained in full-strength medium. Similarly, the rate of loss of viability shown by *E. coli* in the transition from sewage to sea-water was minimal at a sea-water concentration of 25% and increased as the sea-water concentration was either raised or lowered. Gossling (1958) also found that reducing the difference in ionic strengths between various suspending media lowered the lethal effect when bacteria were transferred from one to another.

The solute concentration *per se* has also been found to be important. Strange & Postgate (1964) observed that loss of viability of *Aerobacter aerogenes* subjected to cold shock, by sudden chilling from 37 ° to 0 °C, was enhanced by the inclusion of RNAase. However, increasing the ionic strength of the dilutent by the inclusion of increasing amounts of Na Cl resulted in a significant increase in viability. The authors proposed that, in the presence of Na Cl, adsorption of RNAase to the bacteria was reduced. An increase in the Na Cl concentration of the suspending medium from 0 to 2 M reduced the leakage of 260 nm absorbing material from *P. aeruginosa* (grown either in nutrient broth or broth +0·1% polysorbate 80) about 4-fold as shown in Figure 6 (Brown & Winsley, 1969). The survival of both *E. coli* and *Saccharomyces cerevisiae* was independent of the concentration of potassium phosphate buffer used as a suspending agent over the concentration range 0·001–0·5 M. With *Azotobacter agile*,

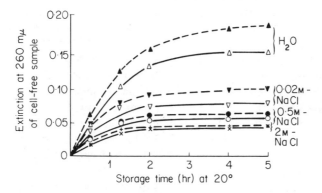

Figure 6. 260 mμ leakage during storage at 20° in water or aqueous sodium chloride solutions of washed pseudomonads grown in presence or absence of Polysorbate 80, ——, Organisms grown in broth; – – –, organisms grown in broth +0·1% Polysorbate 80. Reproduced with permission from M. R. W. Brown & B. E. Winsley, *J. gen. Microbiol.*, **56**, 99–107 (1969)

Pseudomonas spheroides and *P. fluorescens*, however, survival was linked to the buffer concentration (Gunter, 1954).

The nature, as well as the concentration, of the solutes comprising the suspending medium has important effects on survival of bateria. Cation effects which involve competition for sites on the bacteria between cations and antibiotics have already been discussed, but a direct interaction between the cations and the agent may also occur. In a review Weinberg (1957) cited examples of compounds which are neutralized by certain cations so that their antibiotic properties (not necessarily associated with their chelating activities) are lost. The tetracyclines were a good example. There is another class where the compounds act by depriving the cells of some essential cation and both izoniazid and α-picolinic acid act in this way. In both cases the effectiveness of the agents would be reduced as the particular cation concentration increased.

Divalent cations, particularly magnesium, have been found to exert a favourable effect on the survival of Gram-negative bacteria in addition to the specific interactions of such cations with various agents. The addition of magnesium significantly reduced the harmful effects of various buffer systems for storage of *P. fluorescens* (Gunter, 1954) and Gossling (1958) found that inclusion of magnesium reduced the loss of viability associated with osmotic shock. The survival of glycerol-limited *A. aerogenes* was improved by the inclusion of Mg^{2+}, Ca^{2+} or Fe^{2+} but Zn^{2+}, Mn^{2+}, Cu^{2+} and Co^{2+} had no effect (Postgate & Hunter, 1962). The effect of cold shock in reducing the viability of *A. aerogenes* (Strange, 1964) and *P. aeruginosa* (Farrell & Rose, 1968) was prevented by the addition of magnesium to the suspending medium. Similarly, Sato & Takahashi (1968) found that cold shock in *P. fluorescens* and *B. subtilis* could be prevented by the divalent cations in order of effectiveness $Mg^{2+} > Ca^{2+} > Mn^{2+}$. In contrast to these protective effects of magnesium is a report by Cheng, Costerton, Singh & Ingram (1973). *P. aeruginosa* which had been grown in a complex nutrient broth had all the detectable alkaline phosphatase and 28·6% of the lipopolysaccharide (LPS) removed as a result of washing with $0·2 \text{ M } MgCl_2$. Washing with $0·01 \text{ M } MgCl_2$, however, gave almost complete retention of alkaline phosphatase and LPS. It was not clear whether or not this was a specific effect of magnesium or of the high tonicity although washing with 50% sucrose removed only 50% of the alkaline phosphatase and 15·5% of the LPS. The presence of monovalent cations in suspending media also affects the survival of bacteria, although a number of the reported protective effects may well be the result of a non-specific maintenance of tonicity as described above.

Lysis of *P. aeruginosa* by an EDTA–lysozyme system was inhibited by sodium chloride (0·1–2%) (Shively & Hartsell, 1964). The effect of suspending both *Staph. aurons* and *Salmonella oranienburg* in solutions containing various cations and having the same water activity as the growth medium, was examined by Christian (1958, 1962). The retention of intracellular sodium was greatest after washing in water or glycerol while sucrose, sodium chloride, potassium chloride, ammonium chloride or magnesium chloride all allowed its release. Both potassium and 260 nm absorbing materials were largely retained in all solutions. It appeared that whilst sodium retention was dependent upon the composition of the washing solution the retention of potassium and 260 nm absorbing material was mainly affected by the water activity. Cations with small hydrated ionic radii (e.g. K^+ and NH_4^+) were most detrimental and non-electrolytes gave the greatest protection. In view of the results obtained by Strange & Shon (1964) Korngold & Kushner (1968) and De Voe & Oginsky (1969) it may be that the action of monovalent cations is due, at least in part, to the desorbtion of Mg^{2+} and other divalent cations from the cell surface.

As well as cations the presence of various metabolites affects bacterial survival. Peptone has been found to exert a protective action for a number of bacteria (Carlucci & Pramer, 1960; King & Hurst, 1963; Straka & Stokes, 1957; Weiler & Hartsell, 1969) and no deleterious action for this material has been noted. Individual amino acids increased the survival of *E. coli* in sea water (Carlucci & Pramer, 1960; Scarpino & Pramer, 1962) and the effect was correlated with the chelating ability of these materials. Chelating agents including EDTA improved the survival prospects of *Mycoplasma* cells (Butler & Knight, 1960). Conversely, cysteine increased the rate of lysis of *P. aeruginosa* in phosphate buffer (Bernheim, 1966) and other chelating agents lowered the resistance of protoplasts to osmotic shock (Indge, 1968).

The effect of adding various carbohydrates to suspending media has been examined. Glucose reduced the death rate of *E. coli* in sea water (Carlucci & Pramer, 1960) and also reduced the lethal effects of changes from one suspending medium to another (Gossling, 1958). The loss of nucleic acids from a *Lactobacillus* was reduced in the presence of glucose for bacteria grown in a 'complete' medium but glucose had no effect when the bacteria were grown in the absence of vitamin B_6 (Holden, 1958). The use of sucrose solutions for washing *Salmonella* caused less change in the intracellular levels of sodium potassium and 260 nm absorbing substances than salt solutions of the same water activity (Christian, 1958). However, sucrose was less effective than divalent cations in preventing cold shock in *B. subtilis* and *P. fluorescens* (Sato & Takahashi, 1968) although it did protect PPLOs from losing viability when subjected to osmotic shock, as did glycerol (Smith & Sasaki, 1958). A specific effect of carbohydrates on the viability of *A. aerogenes* grown in a chemostat and stored at growth temperatures was noted (Strange & Dark, 1965). In a non-nutrient buffer addition of the growth-limiting carbohydrate resulted in loss of viability. Metabolism of the added substrate was needed to obtain this effect of substrate-accelerated death. A lesser effect was observed with some intermediate metabolites such as pyruvate, citrate and malate.

Various complex organic materials have been found to exert a protective effect on bacteria. Volatile solids from sewage reduced the death rate of *E. coli* in sea water (Carlucci & Pramer, 1960). Pseudomonads were protected by scab tissue from burned patients (Hurst & Sutter, 1966), corn steep liquor, gelatin mucin and defibrinated rabbit blood (Stephens, 1957). The inclusion of the non-ionic surfactant polysorbate 80 in suspending media for *P. aeruginosa* resulted in an immediate increase in the susceptibility of this organism to changes in pH, temperature or medium tonicity, although polysorbate 80 itself was non-toxic (Brown & Winsley, 1969). The enhancement of the effect of polymyxin B on this organism was also observed (Brown & Winsley, 1971) and it was suggested that polysorbate 80 altered the outer lipid structure of the envelope of *P. aeruginosa*, thus affecting the permeability barrier of the cell.

The pH of the Suspending Medium

The effects of pH on the interactions between antimicrobial agents and bacteria have already been discussed above and it remains to consider this parameter in relation to the viability *per se* of bacterial suspensions subsequent to the culture stage. It was shown by Brown & Winsley (1969) that although the pH of the suspending medium for *P. aeruginosa* over the range 5·7–9·5 had little effect on leakage of 260 nm absorbing material, the magnitude of a sudden pH change did correlate with a loss of viability. Other workers have, however, reported particular pH values as being optimal for the maintenance of viability. These include pH 8·5 for *Strep. lactis* and *Strep. cremoris* (Cowell, Koburger & Weese, 1966); pH 7·0 for *Strep. lactis* (Thomas & Blatt, 1968); pH 7·0 for chilled *Aerobacter aerogenes* (Strange & Postgate, 1964). In this latter case, variations from neutral were more significant for cells chilled to 0 °C compared with bacteria chilled only to 20 °C.

The pH of suspending media allowing survival may vary according to the other environmental conditions pertaining. Gossling (1958) reported that pH values of either 6·2 or 8·0 were optimal for the survival of *E. coli* during a change of suspending medium from phosphate buffer to Ringer solution or *vice versa*, while pH 5·0 proved best for survival of *E. coli* isolated from sea water (Carlucci & Cramer, 1960). A pH of 6·0 allowed maximum retention of potassium in *Salmonella oranienburg* after washing in water, sucrose or ammonium chloride solutions (Christian, 1958).

The Temperature of the Suspending Medium

The effect of high temperatures (above the growth temperature) will not be considered and a recent review (Brown & Melling, 1971) of the inhibition and destruction of micro-organisms by heat covers some aspects of high temperatures. A reduction in the temperature of bacterial suspensions can result in either enhanced stability or loss of viability, depending upon the rate of temperature change as well as the composition of the suspending medium. Provided that the temperature reduction is gradual, there is evidence that the viability of bacterial suspensions was maintained better at lower temperatures, although there are exceptions to this generalization. *E. coli* and *P. aeruginosa* showed a slight increase in survival when stored at 10 °C, rather than room temperature for a month (Cook & Wills, 1956). Storage at 37 °C greatly reduced the viability, while the sensitivity to phenol was increased as the storage temperature increased. *P. aeruginosa* grown in nutrient broth and diluted in water survived equally well at temperatures over the range 6–37 °C, but lost viability on storage at −10 °C (Emmanouilidou-Arseni & Koumentakou, 1964). Whereas *P. aeruginosa*, grown in a salts–glucose medium and stored in either water, fresh medium, saline or magnesium solution at 37°, 20° or 4 °C, retained viability best at 20 °C. Similarly, Ballantyne (1930) found that both *E. coli* and *S. typhi* survived better at room temperature than at 37°, 8° or 0 °C when stored in water or saline solution.

As well as affecting the viability of stored bacterial suspensions, the temperature of the suspending medium may modify the interactions between the organism and some agent. Leive & Kollin (1967) reported that washing *E. coli* with Tris at 4°C caused loss of acid soluble u.v. absorbing material. This did not occur if sodium chloride solution was used at the same temperature, nor if the bacteria were washed with Tris at either 24° or 37°C. Conversely, damage to *E. coli* by colicin K (Plate, 1973) was greatly reduced at 10 °C compared with that arising at higher temperatures. The author proposed that this effect of temperature may have resulted from changes in the physical properties of the cell membrane. It has been shown (Chapman, 1968; Chapman & Leslie, 1970) that phospholipids undergo a phase transition at a certain temperature and below this they exist in a packed state with their fatty acyl chains in a restricted and ordered state. Above the endothermic transition temperature a looser, more random conformation exists. The transition temperature for any class of phospholipids depends upon a number of factors, including the degree of saturation of the fatty acyl chains and whether the fatty acids are in the *cis-* or *trans*-configuration.

A lethal effect of chilling on Gram-negative bacteria, called cold shock, has been observed by several workers (Sherman & Albus, 1923; Hegarty & Weeks, 1940; Gorrill & McNeil, 1960). A rapid temperature reduction is an essential feature of cold shock and various factors can modify the bacterial response to this stress. Meynell (1958) reported that 0·3 M sucrose could protect *E. coli* from cold shock and that stationary-phase cultures of this organism were not susceptible. Similarly, Gorrill & McNeil (1960) found that early log-phase cultures of *P. aeruginosa* grown at 37 °C were affected by cold shock whereas older cultures were not, and only dilution in solutions below 18 °C was effective. However, MacKelvie, Gronlund & Campbell (1968) observed an increase in sensitivity with culture age for *P. aeruginosa*. Brown & Winsley (1969) also observed loss of viability and release of 260 nm absorbing materials when *P. aeruginosa* suspensions were chilled rapidly. The magnitude of the effect was related to such colligative properties of the suspending medium as salt concentration and pH. The inclusion of polysorbate 80 increased the susceptibility to cold shock. These findings support the view that the lethal effect of sudden chilling may be due to interference with permeability control mechanisms which results in leakage of normal endocellular constituents (Strange & Dark, 1962; Strange & Ness, 1963) and allows penetration of substances into cold-shocked bacteria to a greater extent than into normal organisms (Strange & Postgate, 1964).

SOME CONCLUSIONS

It is clear from the information which has been presented that no absolute measure of microbial resistance is possible and even comparisons between different bacteria must be related to the environmental conditions. Although a number of organisms other than *P. aeruginosa* have been considered, particularly in relation to the exclusion of antibacterial agents, the intention was to examine the phenomenon of Gram-negative resistance, with *P. aeruginosa* exemplifying perhaps one extreme. In this respect the various chemical antibacterials differ significantly from stresses imposed by physical agents such as heat, in that organisms are able, by modification of their cellular composition, to exclude or degrade the chemical. This is not possible in respect of physical agents.

As well as providing information about the mode of action of various agents, the variations in bacterial resistance with environmental changes emphasize the problems of *in vitro* assessment of antibiotics and, indeed, the measure of agreement between such tests and the final *in vivo* effectiveness may vary considerably. It is arguable that effective agents may have been overlooked as a result of this situation. Methods of antibiotic testing which rely upon the determination of drug activity in the presence of EDTA (Russell & Morris, 1973) may also be misleading since if EDTA were present in excess no free Mg^{2+} would be available for bacterial growth and if EDTA were not in excess then EDTA-cell interaction would not be likely. Any effects observed may be due to a lowering of the medium cation content, thus affecting the type of antibiotic/cation cell interaction described above. Finally, it seems possible that greater use may be made of some of the phenotypic variations of which bacteria are capable in devising appropriate therapeutic regimes. Variations in pH (referred to above), and perhaps salt concentrations, may be of value in potentiating the actions of some antibiotics used for urinary tract infections. A report of a lowering of the levels of both Ca^{2+} and Mg^{2+} in the serum of burned patients (Broughton, Anderson & Bowden, 1968) may be relevant in relation to the development of polymyxin resistance in *P. aeruginosa* infections of burned areas and to the effectiveness of topical applications of silver nitrate solution in reducing the incidence of such infections (Lowbury, 1967). In point of fact there has been virtually no work investigating the effect of the *in vivo* environment on bacterial resistance. It seems highly likely that special *in vivo* environmental circumstances such as pH, aeration or specific nutrient depletion would affect drug resistance. Furthermore, environmental conditions causing resistance variations in the surface characteristics of the bacteria may well alter the efficacy of the body defence mechanisms.

REFERENCES

Abraham, E. P. & Duthie, E. S. (1946). Effect of pH of the medium on activity of streptomycin and penicillin. *Lancet*, **i**, 455–459.

Acred, P., Brown, D. M., Knudsen, E. T., Rolinson, G. N. & Sutherland, R. (1967). New semisynthetic penicillin active against *Pseudomonas pyocyanea*. *Nature*, **215**, 25–30.

Albert, A. (1965). *Selective toxicity*, Methuen & Co., London.

Annear, D. I. (1968). The effect of temperature on resistance of *Staphylococcus aureus* to methicillin and some other antibiotics. *The Medical Journal of Australia*, **1**, 444–446.

Araki, C. (1959). Seaweed polysaccharides. *Proceedings of the 4th International Congress of Biochemistry, Vienna*, **1**, 15–30.

Ashevov, E. H. (1966). Loss of antibiotic resistance in *Staphylococcus aureus* resulting from growth at high temperature. *Journal of General Microbiology*, **42**, 403–410.

Ayliffe, G. A. J., Lowbury, E. J. L. & Roe, E. (1972). Transferable Carbenicillin Resistance in *Pseudomonas aeruginosa*. *Nature New Biology*, **235**, 141.

Ballantyne, E. N. (1930). On certain factors influencing the survival of bacteria in water and in saline solutions. *Journal of Bacteriology*, **19**, 303–320.

Bass, G. K. & Stuart, L. S. (1968). Methods of testing disinfectants. In *Disinfection, sterilisation and preservation*, (Eds. C. A. Laurence & S. S. Black), Lea and Febiger, Philadelphia, p. 133–158.

Bassett, D. C. (1971). The effect of pH on the multiplication of *Pseudomonas* in chlorhexidine and cetrimide. *Journal of Clinical Pathology*, **24**, 708–711.

Beard, J. P. (1972). Studies on the sex pili specified by antibiotic resistance factors in *Escherichia coli*. Ph.D. Thesis, University of Bristol, England.

Bechtle, R. M. & Scherr, G. H. (1958). New agar for antimicrobial sensitivity testing *in vitro*. *Antibiotics and Chemotherapy*, **8**, 599–606.

Bell, R. M., Mavis, R. D. & Vagelos, P. R. (1972). Altered phospholipid metabolism in a temperature sensitive mutant of *Escherichia coli* $CR_{34}T_{46}$. *Biochimica Biophysica Acta*, **270**, 504–512.

Bernheim, F. (1966). The effect of mercuric chloride and certain sulfhydryl compounds on the changes in optical density of suspensions of *Pseudomonas aeruginosa* in sodium, potassium and sodium-potassium buffers. *Biochemical Pharmacology*, **15**, 1105–1110.

Bodey, G. P. & Terrell, L. M. (1968). *In vitro* activity of carbenicillin against Gram-negative bacilli. *Journal of Bacteriology*, **95**, 1587–1590.

Boggis, E. (1971). The effect of metal cations and phosphate upon EDTA and polymyxin mediated lysis of *Pseudomonas aeruginosa*. Ph.D. Thesis, University of Bath.

Brinton, C. C. Jr. (1971). The properties of sex pili, the vital nature of 'conjugal' genetic transfer systems, and some possible approaches to the control of bacterial drug resistance. *Critical Reviews of Microbiology*, **1**, 105–160.

Brishammar, S. Hjerten, S. & Hofsten, B. V. (1961). Immunological precipitates in agarose gels. *Biochimica Biophysica Acta*, **53**, 518–521.

Broughton, A., Anderson, I. R. M. & Bowden, C. H. (1968). Magnesium-deficiency syndrome in burns. *Lancet*, **ii**, 1156–1158.

Brown, M. R. W. (1971). Inhibition and destruction of *Pseudomonas aeruginosa*. In *Inhibition and Destruction of the Microbial Cell*, (Ed. W. B. Hugo), Academic Press, London, p. 307–367.

Brown, M. R. W. & Anderson, R. A. (1968). The bactericidal effect of silver ions on *Pseudomonas aeruginosa*. *Journal at Pharmacy and Pharmacology*, **20**, (Suppl.) 15–35.

Brown, M. R. W. & Foster, J. H. (1971). Effect of slime on the sensitivity of *Pseudomonas aeruginosa* to EDTA and polymyxin. *Journal of Pharmacy and Pharmacology*, **23**, Supplement 236S.

Brown, M. R. W., Clamp, J. R. & Foster, J. H. S. (1966). The presence of hyaluronic acid in the extracellular slime of *Pseudomonas aeruginosa. Journal of General Microbiology*, **45**, v.

Brown, M. R. W., Foster, J. H. S. & Clamp, J. R. (1969). Composition of *Pseudomonas aeruginosa* slime. *Biochemical Journal*, **112**, 521–525.

Brown, M. R. W. & Garrett, E. R. (1964). Kinetics and mechanisms of action of antibiotics on microorganisms I. Reproducibility of *Escherichia coli* growth curves and dependence upon tetracycline concentration. *Journal of Pharmaceutical Sciences*, **53**, 179–183.

Brown, M. R. W. & Hodges, N. A. (1974). Growth and sporulation characteristics of *Bacillus megaterium* under different conditions of nutrient limitation. *J. Pharm. Pharmac*, **26**, 217–227.

Brown, M. R. W. & Melling, J. (1969a). Loss of sensitivity to EDTA by *Pseudomonas aeruginosa* grown under conditions of Mg-limitation. *Journal of General Microbiology*, **54**, 439–444.

Brown, M. R. W. & Melling, J. (1969b). Role of divalent cations in the action of polymyxin B and EDTA on *Pseudomonas aeruginosa. Journal of General Microbiology*, **59**, 263–274.

Brown, M. R. W. & Melling, J. (1971). Inhibition and destruction of microorganisms by heat. In *Inhibition and Destruction of the Microbial Cell*, (Ed. W. B. Hugo), Academic Press, London, pp. 1–37.

Brown, M. R. W. & Richards, R. M. E. (1964). *Pharmaceutical Journal*, **16**, 517.

Brown, M. R. W. & Richards, R. M. E. (1965). Effect of ethylenediaminetetra acetate on the resistance of *Pseudomonas aeruginosa* to antibacterial agents. *Nature*, **207**, 1391–1393.

Brown, M. R. W. & Watkins, W. M. (1970). Low magnesium and phospholipid content of cell walls of *Pseudomonas aeruginosa* resistant to polymyxin. *Nature*, **227**, 1360–1361.

Brown, M. R. W. & Winsley, B. E. (1969). Effect of polysorbate 80 on cell leakage and viability of *Pseudomonas aeruginosa* exposed to rapid changes of pH, temperature and tonicity. *Journal of General Microbiology*, **56**, 99–107.

Brown, M. R. W. & Winsley, B. E. (1971). Synergism between polymyxin and polysorbate 80 against *Pseudomonas aeruginosa. Journal of General Microbiology*, **68**, 367–373.

Brown, M. R. W. & Wood, S. M. (1972). Relation between cation and lipid content of cell walls of *Pseudomonas aeruginosa, Proteus vulgaris* and *Klebsiella aerogenes* and their sensitivity to polymyxin B and other antibacterial agents. *J. Pharm. Pharmac.*, **24**, 215–218.

Brumfitt, N. Percival, A. & Leigh, D. A. (1967). Clinical and laboratory studies with carbenicillin. A new penicillin active against *Pseudomonas pyocyanea. Lancet*, **i**, 1289–1293.

Bryan, L. E., Van Den Elzen, H. M. & Tseng, J. T. (1972). Transferable drug resistance in *Pseudomonas aeruginosa. Antimicrobial Agents and Chemotherapy*, **1**, 22–29.

Butler, M. & Knight, B. C. T. J. (1960). The survival of washed suspensions of mycoplasma. *Journal of General Microbiology*, **22**, 470–477.

Callow, D. S., Atkinson, A. & Melling, J. (1973). Interference by bacterial proteases in enzyme production and purification. FEBS meeting Dublin 1973 Abstract No. 54.

Carlucci, A. F. & Pramer, D. (1960). An evaluation of factors affecting the survival of *Escherichia coli* in sea water. II Salinity, pH and nutrients. *Applied Microbiology*, **8**, 247–250.

Carson, L. S., Favero, M. S., Bond, W. W. & Peterson, N. J. (1972). Factors affecting comparative resistance of naturally occurring and sub-cultured *Pseudomonas aeruginosa* to disinfectants. *Applied Microbiology*, **23**, 863–869.

Chabner, B. A. & Bertino, J. R. (1972). Activation and inhibition of carboxypeptidase G, by divalent ions. *Biochemica Biophysica Acta*, **276**, 234–240.

Chapman, D. (1968). Physical studies of biological membranes and their constituents. In *Membrane models and the formation of biological membranes*, (Eds. L. Bolis & B. A. Pethica), North-Holland Publishing Co., Amsterdam, p. 6–18.

Chapman, D. & Leslie, (1970). Structure and function of phospholipids in membranes. In *Membranes of Mitochondria and Chloroplasts*, (Ed. E. Racker), Van Nostrand Reinhold Co., New York, p. 91–126.

Chapman, D., Owens, N. F. & Walker, D. A. (1966). Physical studies of phospholipids, II. Monolayer studies of some synthetic 2,3-diacyl-DL phosphatidylethanolamines and phosphatidylcholines containing *trans* double bonds. *Biochemica Biophysica Acta*, **120**, 148–155.

Chen, C. H. & Feingold, D. S. (1972). Locus of divalent cation inhibition of the bactericidal action of polymixin B. *Antimicrobial Agents and Chemotherapy.*, **2**, 331–335.

Cheng, K. J., Costerton, J. W., Singh, A. P., & Ingram, J. M. (1973). Susceptibility of whole cells and spheroplasts of *Pseudomonas aeruginosa* to actinomycin D. *Antimicrobial Agents and Chemotherapy*, **3**, 399–406.

Christian, J. H. B. (1958). Effects of washing treatments on the composition of *Salmonella oranienburg*. *Australian Journal of Biological Sciences*, **11**, 538–547.

Christian, J. H. B. (1962). The effects of washing treatments on the composition of *Staphylococcus aureus*. *Australian Journal of Biological Science*, **15**, 324–332.

Christian, J. H. B. & Ingram, M. (1959). Lysis of *Vibrio costicolus* by osmotic shock. *Journal of General Microbiology*, **20**, 32–42.

Cook, A. M. & Wills, B. A. (1956). Reproducibility of extinction time estimates. I. Variations in resistance of test organisms and viability of test suspensions. *Journal of Pharmacy and Pharmacology*, **8**, 266–276.

Cowell, G. R., Koburger, J. A. & Weese, S. J. (1966). Storage of *Lactic streptococci*. I. Effect of pH on survival and enodogenous metabolism in phosphate buffer. *Journal of Dairy Science*, **49**, 365–369.

Crowfoot, P. D. & Hunt, A. L. (1970). The effect of oxygen tension on methylene hexadecanoic acid formation in *Pseudomonas fluorescens* and *E. coli*. *Biochimica et Biophysica Acta*, **202**, 550–552.

Darrell, J. H. & Waterworth, P. M. (1967). Dosage of gentamicin for *Pseudomonas* infections. *British Medical Journal*, **2**, 535–537.

Davis, S. D. & Ianetta, A. (1972a). Influence of serum and calcium on the bactericidal activity of gentamicin and carbenicillin on *Pseudomonas aeruginosa*. *Applied Microbiology*, **23**, 775–779.

Davis, S. D. & Iannetta, A. (1972b). Antagonistic effect of calcium in serum on the activity of tobramycin against *Pseudomonas*. *Antimicrobial Agents and Chemotherapy*, **1**, 466–469.

Davis, S. D., Ianetta, A. & Wedgwood, R. J. (1971a). Paradoxical synergism and antagonism between serum and the antibacterial activity of colistin. *Journal of Infectious Diseases*, **123**, 392–398.

Davis, S. D., Ianetta, A. & Wedgwood, R. J. (1971b). Activity of colistin against *Pseudomonas aeruginosa*: inhibition by calcium. *Journal of Infectious Diseases*, **124**, 610–612.

De Voe, I. W. & Oginsky, E. L. (1969). Cation interactions and biochemical composition of the cell envelope of a marine bacterium. *Journal of Bacteriology*, **98**, 1368–1377.

Dienstag, J. & Neu, H. C. (1972). *In vitro* studies of Tobramycin, an aminoglycoside antibiotic. *Antimicrobial Agents and Chemotherapy*, **1**, 41–45.

Doi, O. Kondo, S., Tanaka, N. & Umezawa, H. (1969). Purification and properties of kanamycin phosphorylating enzyme from *Pseudomonas aeruginosa*. *Journal of Antibiotics*, **XXII**, 273–282.

Doi, O., Ogura, M., Tanaka, N. & Umezawa, H. (1968). Inactivation of kanamycin, neomycin and streptomycin by enzymes obtained in cells of *Pseudomonas aeruginosa*. *Journal of Applied Microbiology*, **16**, 1276–1281.

Dunnick, J. K. & O'Leary, W. M. (1970). Correlation of bacterial lipid composition with antibiotic resistance. *Journal of Bacteriology*, **101**, 892–900.

Eagle, H., Levy, M. & Fleischman, R. (1952). The effect of the pH of the medium on the antibacterial action of penicillin, streptomycin, chloramphenicol, terramycin and Bacitracin. *Antibiotics and chemotherapy*, **2**, 563–575.

Ellwood, D. C. & Tempest, D. W. (1969). Controlk of teichoic and teichurunic acid in the walls of *Bacillus subtilis var. niger* grown in a chemostat. *Biochemical Journal*, **118**, 367–373.

Ellwood, D. C. & Tempest, D. W. (1972). Environmental effects on bacterial walls. *Advances in Microbial Physiology*, **7**, 83–117.

Emmanouilidou-Arseni, A. & Koumentakou, I. (1964). Viability of *Pseudomonas aeruginosa*. *Journal of Bacteriology*, **87**, 1253.

Farrell, J. & Rose, A. H. (1967a). Temperature effects on micro-organisms. In *Thermobiology*, (Ed. A. H. Rose), Academic Press, London, pp. 147–218.

Farrell, J. & Rose, A. H. (1967b). Temperature effects on micro-organisms. *Annual Review of Microbiology*, **21**, 101–120.

Farrell, J. & Rose, A. H. (1968). Cold shock in a mesophilic and a psychrophilic pseudomonad. *Journal of General Microbiology*, **50**, 429–439.

Farwell, J. A. & Brown, M. R. W. (1971). Effect of inoculum history on the inhibition and destruction of the microbial cell. In *Inhibition and destruction of the microbial cell*, (Ed. W. B. Hugo), Academic Press, London.

Feingold, D. S. & Oski, F. (1965). Pseudomonas infection. Treatment with immune human plasma. *Archives of International Medicine*, **116**, 326–328.

Florey, H. N., Gilliver, K., Jennings, M. A. & Sanders, A. G. (1946). Mycophendic acid: an antibiotic from *Penicillium breviecompactum* dierckx. *Lancet*, **i**, 46–49.

Ford, J. H., Bergy, M. E., Brooks, A. A., Garrett, E. R., Alberti, J., Dyer, J. R. & Carter, H. E. (1955). Further characterization of neomycin B and neomycin C. *Journal of the American Chemical Society*, **77**, 5311–5312.

Frydman, A. & Meynell, E. (1969). Interaction between de-repressed F-like R factors and wild type colicin B factors: superinfection immunity and repressor susceptibility. *Genetical Research, Cambridge*, **14**, 315–332.

Fullbrook, P. D., Elson, S. W. & Slocombe, B. (1970). R-factor mediated β-lactamase in *P. aeruginosa*. *Nature*, **226**, 1054–1056.

Gardner, A. D. & Chain, E. (1942). Proactinomycin: a 'bacteriostatic' produced by a species of Proactinomyces. *British Journal of Experimental Pathology*, **23**, 123–127.

Garrett, E. R., Heman-Ackah, S. H. & Perry, G. L. (1970). Kinetics and mechanisms of action of drugs on microorganisms. XI. Effects of erythromycin and its supposed antagonism with lincomycin on the microbial growth of *Escherichia coli*. *J. Pharm. Sci.*, **59**, 1448–1456.

Garrod, L. P. & Waterworth, P. M. (1956). Behaviour *in vitro* of some new anti-staphylococcal antibiotics. *British Medical Journal*, **II**, 61–65.

Garrod, L. P. & Waterworth, P. M. (1969). Effect of medium composition on the apparent sensitivity of *Pseudomonas aeruginosa* to gentamicin. *Journal of Clinical Pathology*, **22**, 534–538.

Gilbert, D. N., Kutscher, E., Ireland, P., Barnett, J. A. & Sanford, J. P. (1971). Effect of the concentration of magnesium and calcium on the *In vitro* susceptibility of

Pseudomonas aeruginosa to gentamicin. *The Journal of Infectious Diseases,* **124**, supplement 537–545.

Gossling, B. S. (1958). The loss of viability of bacteria in suspension due to changing the ionic environment. *Journal of Applied Bacteriology,* **21**, 220–243.

Gorrill, R. H. & McNeil, E. M. (1960). The effect of cold diluent on the viable count of *Pseudomonas pyocyanea. Journal of General Microbiology,* **22**, 437–442.

Goto, S., Murakawa, T. & Kuwahara, S. (1973). Slime production by *Pseudomonas aeruginosa* II. A new synthetic medium and cultural conditions suitable for slime production by *Pseudomonas aeruginosa. Japanese Journal of Microbiology,* **17**, 45–51.

Gray, G. W. & Wilkinson, S. G. (1965). The effect of ethylenediamine tetraacetic acid on the cell walls of some Gram-negative bacteria. *Journal of General Microbiology,* **39**, 385–399.

Gunter, S. E. (1954). Factors determining the viability of selected microorganisms in inorganic media. *Journal of Bacteriology,* **67**, 628–634.

Haight, T. H. & Finland, M. (1952). The antibacterial action of erythromycin. *Proceedings of the Society of Experimental Biology and Medicine,* **81**, 175–183.

Hanus, F. J., Sands, J. G. & Bennett, E. O. (1967). Antibiotic activity in the presence of agar. *Applied Microbiology,* **15**, 31–34.

Hegarty, C. P. & Weeks, O. B. (1940). Sensitivity of *Escherichia coli* to cold shock during the logarithmic growth phase. *Journal of Bacteriology,* **39**, 475–484.

Hepding, L. (1967). Chemotherapy of experimental *Pseudomonas* Infections. *Proceedings of Fifth International Congress of Chemotherapy,* **1**, 215–220.

Herbert, D. (1961). The chemical composition of micro-organisms as a function of their environment. *Symposium of the Society for General Microbiology,* **11**, 391–416.

Herman, L. G. (1959). Antibiotic sensitivity using pretreated plates. II. A demonstration of inhibitory activity with a low level combination of a sulphonamide and polymyxin B against *Proteus* species. *Antibiotics Annual,* **1958–1959**, 836–839.

Hewitt, J. A., Coe, A. N. & Parker, M. T. (1969). The detection of methicillin resistance in *Staph. aureus. Journal of Medical Microbiology,* **2**, 443–456.

Hoar, D. I. (1970). Fertility regulation in F-like resistance transfer factors. *Journal of Bacteriology,* **101**, 916–920.

Holden, J. T. (1958). Degradation of intracellular nucleic acid and leakage of fragments. *Biochimica et Biophysica Acta,* **29**, 667–668.

Hurst, V. & Sutter, V. L. (1966). Survival of *Pseudomonas aeruginosa* in the hospital environment. *Journal of Infectious Diseases,* **116**, 151–154.

Indge, K. J. (1968). The effects of various anions and cations on the lysis of yeast protoplasts by osmotic shock. *Journal of General Microbiology,* **51**, 425–432.

Ingham, H. R., Selkon, J. B., Codd, A. A. & Hale, J. H. (1970). The effect of carbon dioxide on the sensitivity of *Bacteroides fragilis* to certain antibiotics *in vitro. Journal of Clinical Pathology,* **23**, 254–258.

Ivanov, von W., Markov, K. I., Golowinskii, E. & Charisanova, T. (1964). The importance of surface lipids for some biological properties of a *Pseudomonas aeruginosa* strain. *Z. Naturforschg.,* **196**, 604–606.

Iwai, Y., Ohono, H., Takeshima, H., Yamaguchi, N., Omura, S. & Hata, T. (1973). Screening and Isolation of a Penicillinase Inhibitor KA-107. *Antimicrobial Agents and Chemotherapy,* **4**, 222–225.

Jacob, F. & Monod, J. (1961). Genetic regulatory mechanism in the synthesis of proteins. *Journal of Molecular Biology,* **3**, 318–356.

Jones, R. J. & Lowbury, E. J. L. (1967). Prophylaxis and therapy for *Pseudomonas aeruginosa* infection with carbenicillin and with gentamicin. *British Medical Journal,* **3**, 79–82.

King, W. L. & Hurst, A. (1963). A note on the survival of some bacteria in different diluents. *Journal of Applied Bacteriology,* **26**, 504–506.

Knivett, V. A. & Cullen, J. (1965). Some factors affecting cyclopropane acid formation in E. coli. Biochemical Journal, 96, 771–776.

Knox, R. & Collard, P. (1952). The effect of temperature on the sensitivity of Bacillus cereus to penicillin. Journal of General Microbiology, 6, 369–373.

Kobayashi, F., Yamaguchi, M. & Mitsuhashi, S. (1971). Phosphorylated inactivation of aminoglycoside antibiotics by Pseudomonas aeruginosa. Japanese Journal of Microbiology, 15, 265–272.

Kobayashi, F., Yamaguchi, M. & Mitsuhashi, S. (1972). Activity of Lividomycin against Pseudomonas aeruginosa. Its inactivation by phosphorylation induced by resistant strains. Antimicrobial Agents and Chemotherapy, 1, 17–21.

Kobayashi, F., Yamaguchi, M., Sato, J. & Mitsuhashi, S. (1972). Purification and properties of dihydrostreptomycin phosphorylating enzyme from Pseudomonas aeruginosa. Japanese Journal of Microbiology, 16, 15–19.

Korngold, R. R. & Kushner, O. J. (1968). Responses of a psychrophilic marine bacterium to changes in its ionic environment. Canadian Journal of Microbiology, 14, 253–263.

Kunin, C. M. & Edmondson, W. P. (1968). Inhibitor of antibiotics in bacteriologic agar. Proceedings of the Society of Experimental Biology and Medicine, 129, 118–122.

Kuwabarra, S. (1970). Purification and properties of two extracellular β-lactamases from Bacillus cereus 569/H. Biochemical Journal, 118, 457–465.

Langridge, J. (1963). Biochemical aspects of temperature response. Annual Reviews of Plant Physiology, 14, 441–462.

Lawn, A. M., Meynell, E., Meynell, G. G. & Datta, N. (1967). Sex pili and the classification of sex factors in the Enterobacteriaceae. Nature, 216, 343–346.

Leive, L. & Kollin, V. (1967). Controlling EDTA treatment to produce permeable Escherichia coli with normal metabolic process. Biochemical and Biophysical Research Communications, 28, 229–236.

Leive, L., Shovlin, V. K. & Mergenhagen, Ş. E. (1968). Physical and immunological properties of lipopolysaccharide released from Escherichia coli by ethylenediamine tetraacetic acid. Journal of Biological Chemistry, 243, 6384–6391.

Liu, P. V., Abe, Y. & Bates, J. L. (1961). The roles of various fractions of Pseudomonas aeruginosa in its pathogenesis. Journal of Infectious Diseases, 108, 218–228.

Lowbury, E. J. L. (1967). British Journal of Plastic Surgery, 20, 211–217.

Lowbury, E. J. L. & Jackson, D. M. (1968). Local chemoprophylaxis for burns with gentamicin and other agents. Lancet, i, 654–657.

MacKelvie, R. M., Grunlund, A. F. & Campbell, J. J. R. (1968). Influence of cold-shock on the endogenous metabolism of Pseudomonas aeruginosa. Canadian Journal of Microbiology, 14, 633–638.

Magasanik, B. (1961). Catabolite repression. Cold Spring Harbour Symposium on quantitative Biology, 26, 249–256.

Masukawa, H. (1969). Localization of sensitivity to kanamycin and streptomycin in 305 ribosomal proteins of Escherichia coli. The Journal of Antibiotics, XXII, 612–623.

Medeiros, A. A., O'Brian, T. F., Wacker, W. E. C. & Yulug, N. F. (1971). Effect of salt concentration on the apparent in vitro susceptibility of Pseudomonas and other Gram-negative bacilli to gentamicin. Journal of Infectious Diseases, 124, Supplement, S59.

Meers, J. L. & Tempest, D. W. (1970). The influence of growth-limiting substrate and media NaCl concentration on the synthesis of magnesium-binding sites in the walls of Bacillus subtilis var. niger. Journal of General Microbiology, 63, 325–331.

Melling, J. & Ford, J. W. S. (1971). Large-scale production and purification of a penicillinase from Escherichia coli. Journal of General Microbiology, 65, iv.

Melling, J., Robinson, A. & Ellwood, D. C. (1974). Effect of growth environment in a chemostat on the sensitivity of Pseudomonas aeruginosa to polymyxin B sulphate. Proceedings of the Society for General Microbiology, 1, 61.

Meynell, E. & Cooke, M. (1969). Repressor-minus and operator-constitutive de-repressed mutants of F-like R factors: their effect on chromosomal transfer by HfrC. *Genetical Research, Cambridge*, **14**, 309–313.

Meynell, E. & Datta, N. (1967). Mutant drug resistant factors of high transmissibility. *Nature*, **214**, 885–887.

Meynell, E., Meynell, G. G. & Datta, N. (1968). Phylogenetic relationships of drug-resistance factors and other transmissible bacterial plasmids. *Bacteriological Reviews*, **32**, 55–83.

Meynell, G. G. (1958). The effect of sudden chilling on *Escherichia coli*. *Journal of General Microbiology*, **19**, 380–389.

Miller, M. A. & Perkins, R. L. (1973). Effect of pH on *in vitro* activity of carbenicillin against *Proteus vulgaris*. *Journal of Infectious Diseases*, **127**, 689–693.

Mitchell, P. & Moyle, J. (1956). Osmotic function and structure in bacteria. In *Bacterial Anatomy*, 6th Symposium of the Society of General Microbiology pp. 150–180.

Mohr, V. & Larsen, H. (1963). On the structural transformations and lysis of *Halobacterium salinarium* in hypotonic and isotonic solutions. *Journal of General Microbiology*, **31**, 267–280.

Monod, J., Changeux, J. P. & Jacob, F. (1963). Allosteric proteins and cellular control systems. *Journal of Molecular Biology*, **6**, 306–329.

Muschel, L. H., Ahl, L. A. & Fisher, M. W. (1969). Sensitivity of *Pseudomonas aeruginosa* to normal serum and polymyxin. *Journal of bacteriology*, **98**, 453–457.

Neu, H. C. (1970). Update: bacterial resistance to antimicrobial agents. *Medical Times*, **98**, 131–138.

Newton, B. A. (1954). Site of action of polymyxin on *Pseudomonas aeruginosa*: antagonism by cations. *Journal of General Microbiology*, **10**, 491–499.

Newton, B. A. (1956). The properties and mode of action of polymyxins. *Bacteriological Reviews*, **20**, 14–27.

Nishiura, T., Kawada, Y. Tahara, M., Mizutani, H. & Miyamura, R. (1967). Oral administration of sodium colistinmethane-sulphonate on urinary tract infections. *Journal of Antibiotics*, **20**, 377–379.

Olesen, S. & Madsen, P. O. (1967). Intravenous administration of sodium colismethate in urinary tract infections. *Current Therapeutic Research*, **9**, 283–287.

Onozawa, Y., Kumagai, K. & Ishida, N. (1967). Mode of synergism between colistin and sulfisomezole in inhibiting the growth of proteus organism. *Japanese Journal of Microbiology*, **11**, 221–227.

Palumbo, S. A. (1972). Role of iron and sulphur in pigment and slime formation by *Pseudomonas aeruginosa*. *Journal of Bacteriology*, **III**, 430–436.

Payne, J. W. & Gilvarg, C. (1968). Size restriction on peptide utilization in *Escherichia coli*. *Journal of Biological chemistry*, **243**, 6291–6294.

Plate, C. A. (1973). Effects of temperature and of fatty acid substitution on Colicin K action. *Antimicrobial Agents and Chemotherapy*, **4**, 16–24.

Postgate, J. R. & Hunter, J. R. (1962). The survival of starved bacteria. *Journal of General Microbiology*, **29**, 233–263.

Robinson, A. & Tempest, D. W. (1973). Phenotypic variability of the envelope proteins of *Klebsiella aerogenes*. *J. gen. Microbiol.*, **78**, 361–370.

Roe, E. A. & Jones, R. J. (1974). Intracellular killing of different strains of *Pseudomonas aeruginosa* by human leucocytes. *British Journal of Experimental Pathology*, **55**, 336–343.

Roe, E., Jones, R. J. & Lowbury, E. J. L. (1971). Transfer of antibiotic resistance between *Pseudomonas aeruginosa, Escherichia coli,* and other Gram-negative bacilli in burns. *Lancet*, **i**, 149–152.

Rogers, S. W., Gilleland, H. E. & Eagon, R. G. (1969). Characterisation of a protein-lipopolysaccharide complex released from cell walls of *Pseudomonas aeruginosa* by ethylenediamine-tetraacetic acid. *Canadian Journal of Microbiology*, **15**, 743–748.

Rosenblatt, J. E. & Schoenknecht, F. (1972). Effect of several components of anaerobic incubation on antibiotic susceptibility results. *Antimicrobial Agents and Chemotherapy*, **1**, 433–440.

Russell, A. D. & Morris, (1973). Methods for assessing damage to bacteria induced by chemical and physical agents. In *Methods in Microbiology*, (Eds. J. R. Norris & D. W. Ribbons), Academic Press, London, pp. 95–182.

Sabath, L. D., Gerstein, D. A., Loder, P. B. & Finland, M. (1968). Excretion of erythromycin and its enhanced activity in urine against Gram-negative bacteria with alkalinization. *Journal of Laboratory and Clinical Medicine*, **72**, 916–923.

Sabath, L. D., Jago, M. & Abraham, E. P. (1965). Cephalosporinase and penicillinase activities of a β-lactamase from *Pseudomonas pyocyanea*. *Biochemical Journal*, **96**, 739–752.

Sato, M. & Takahashi, H. (1968). Two critical temperature zones in the cold shock of *Bacillus subtilis* and *Pseudomonas fluorescens*. *Agricultural and Biological chemistry*, **32**, 259–260.

Scarpino, P. V. & Pramer, D. (1962). Evaluation of factors affecting the survival of *Escherichia coli* in sea water. VI. Cysteine. *Applied Microbiology*, **10**, 436–440.

Schwarzmann, S. and Boring, J. R. (1971). Antiphagocytic effect of slime from a mucoid strain of *Pseudomonas aeruginosa*. Slime inhibited phagocytosis with *E. coli, Staph. aureus* and especially *P. aeruginosa*. *Infection and Immunity*, **3**, 762–767.

Sherman, J. M. & Albus, W. R. (1923). Physiological youth in bacteria. *Journal of Bacteriology*, **8**, 127–139.

Shively, J. M. & Hartsell, S. E. (1964). Bacteriolysis of the pseudomonads II. Chemical treatment affecting the lytic response. *Canadian Journal of Microbiology*, **10**, 911–915.

Silver, R. P. & Cohen, S. N. (1972). Nonchromosomal antibiotic resistance in bacteria. V. Isolation and characterisation of R-factor mutants exhibiting temperature sensitive repression of fertility. *Journal of Bacteriology*, **110**, 1082–1088.

Smith, C. B. & Finland, M. (1968). Carbenicillin: activity *in vitro* and absorption and excretion in normal young men. *Applied Microbiology*, **16**, 1753–1760.

Smith, D. D., Sasaki, S. (1958). Stability of pleuropneumonia-like organisms to some physical factors. *Applied Microbiology*, **6**, 184–189.

Spotts, C. R. & Stainer, R. T. (1961). Mechanism of streptomycin action on bacteria: a unitary hypothesis. *Nature*, **192**, 633–637.

Stanisich, V. A. & Holloway, B. W. (1971). Chromosome transfer in *Pseudomonas aeruginosa* mediated by R-factors. *Genetics Research*, **17**, 169–172.

Stephens, J. M. (1957). Survival of *Pseudomonas aeruginosa* (Schroeter) Migula suspended in various solutions and dried in air. *Canadian Journal of Microbiology*, **3**, 995–1000.

Straka, R. P. & Stokes, J. L. (1957). Rapid destruction of bacteria in commonly used diluents and its elimination. *Applied Microbiology*, **5**, 21–25.

Strange, R. E. (1964). Effect of magnesium on permeability control in chilled bacteria. *Nature, London*, **203**, 1304–1305.

Strange, R. E. & Dark, F. A. (1962). Effect of chilling on *Aerobacter aerogenes* in aqueous suspension. *Journal of General Microbiology*, **29**, 719–730.

Strange, R. E. & Dark, F. A. (1965). Substrate-accelerated death of *Aerobacter aerogenes*. *Journal of General Microbiology*, **39**, 215–228.

Strange, R. E. & Ness, A. G. (1963). Effect of chilling on bacteria in aqueous suspension. *Nature, London*, **197**, 819.

Strange, R. E. & Postgate, J. R. (1964). Penetration of substances into cold-shocked bacteria. *Journal of General Microbiology*, **36**, 393–403.

Strange, R. E. & Shon, M. (1964). Effects of thermal stress on viability and ribonucleic acid of *Aerobacter aerogenes* in aqueous suspension. *Journal of General Microbiology*, **34**, 99–114.

Sud, I. J. & Feingold, D. S. (1970). Mechanism of Polymixin B resistance in *Proteus mirabilis. Journal of Bacteriology*, **104**, 289–294.

Sud, I. J. & Feingold, D. S. (1972). Effect of polymixin B on antibiotic resistant. *Proteus mirabilis. Antimicrobial Agents and Chemotherapy*, **1**, 417–421.

Sykes, R. B. & Richmond, M. H. (1970). Intergeneric transfer of a β-lactamase gene between *P. aeruginosa* and *E. coli. Nature*, **226**, 932–954.

Sylvester, J. C. (1966). Microbiological records, Abbott Laboratories quoted in Erythromycin, North Chicago, Ill., Abbott Laboratories, p. 14.

Tamaki, S. & Matsuhashi, M. (1973). Increase in sensitivity to antibiotics and lysozyme on deletion of lipopolysacchardides in *Escherichia coli* strains. *Journal of Bacteriology*, **114**, 453–454.

Tanaka, N. (1970). Biochemical studies on gentamicin resistance. *Journal of Antibiotics*, **23**, 469–471.

Taubeneck, U. (1962). Susceptibility of *Proteus mirabilis* and its stable L forms to erythromycin and other macrolides. *Nature*, **196**, 195–196.

Teuber, M. (1969). Susceptibility to Polymixin B of Penicillin G induced *Proteus mirabilis* L forms and spheroplasts. *Journal of Bacteriology*, **98**, 347–350.

Thomas, T. D. & Blatt, R. D. (1968). Survival of *Streptococcus lactis* in starvation conditions. *Journal of General Microbiology*, **50**, 367–382.

Thurston, C. F. (1972). Disappearing enzymes. *Process Biochemistry*, **7**(8), 18–21

Tseng, J. T., Bryan, L. E. & Van Den Elzen, H. M. (1972). Mechanisms and spectrum of streptomycin resistance in a natural population of *Pseudomonas aeruginosa. Antimicrobial Agents and Chemotherapy*, **2**, 136–141.

Umezawa, H., Takasawa, S., Okanishi, M. & Utahara, R. (1968). Adenylstreptomycin, a product of streptomycin inactivated by *E. coli* carrying R-factor. *The Journal of Antibiotics*, **XXI**, 81–82.

Van Iterson, W. & Op Den Kamp, J. A. F. (1969). Bacterial shaped gymnoplasts (protoplasts) of *Bacillus subtilis. Journal of Bacteriology*, **99**, 304–315.

Van Rooyen, C. E., Ross, J. F., Bethune, G. W. & MacDonald, A. D. (1967). Bacteriological observations on carbenicillin in the control of *Pseudomonas aeruginosa* infections in burns. *Canadian Medical Association Journal*, **97**, 1227–1229.

Wagman, G. H., Oden, E. M., Weinstein, N. J. & Irwin, S. (1966). Effect of calcium on the toxicity of gentamicin. *Antimicrobial Agents and Chemotherapy*, **6**, 175–181.

Waitz, J. A. & Weinstein, M. J. (1969). Recent microbiological studies with gentamicin. *Journal of Infectious Diseases*, **119**, 355–366.

Waksman, S. A., Bugie, E. & Schatz, A. (1944). Isolation of antibiotic substances from soil microorganisms with special reference to streptothricin and streptomycin. *Mayo Clinic Proceedings*, **19**, 537–548.

Washington, J. A. (1969). Antimicrobial susceptibility of *Enterobacteriaceae* and non fermenting Gram-negative bacilli. *Mayo Clinic Proceedings*, **44**, 811–824.

Washington, J. A., Hermans, P. E. & Martin, W. J. (1970). *In vitro* susceptibility of *Staphylococci* and *Streptococci* and influence of agar medium on minimum inhibitory concentration. *Mayo Clinic Proceedings*, **45**, 527-539.

Washington, J. A., Yu, P. K. W. & Martin, W. J. (1970). *In vitro* antibacterial activity of minocycline and effect of agar medium utilised in its susceptibility testing. *Applied Microbiology*, **19**, 259–263.

Washington, J. A., Ritts, R. E. & Martin, W. J. (1970). *In vitro* susceptibility of Gram-negative bacilli to gentamicin. *Mayo Clinic Proceedings*, **45**, 146–149.

Watanabe, T. & Fukasawa, T. (1961). Episome-mediated transfer of drug resistance in *Enterobacteriaceae*. I. Transfer of resistance factors by conjugation. *Journal of Bacteriology*, **81**, 669–678.

Weiler, W. A. & Hartsell, S. E. (1969). Diluent composition and the recovery of *Escherichia coli. Applied Microbiology,* **18,** 956–957.

Weinberg, E. D. (1957). The mutual effects of antimicrobial compounds and metallic cations. *Bacteriological Reviews,* **21,** 46–48.

Weinstein, M. J., Drube, C. G., Moss, E. L. & Waitz, J. A. (1971). Microbiologic studies related to bacterial resistance to gentamicin. *Journal of Infectious Diseases,* **124,** 511–517.

Weisner, R., Asscher, A. W. & Wimpenny, J. (1968). *In vitro* reversal of antibiotic resistance by ethylenediamine tetraacetic acid. *Nature,* **219,** 1365–1366.

Wick, W. E. & Welles, J. S. (1967). Nebramycin, a new broad-spectrum antibiotic complex. IV. *In vitro* and *in vivo* laboratory evaluation. *Antimicrobial Agents and Chemotherapy,* **7,** 341–348.

Wilson, L. A. (1970). Chelation in experimental *Pseudomonas* keratinitis. *British Journal of Ophthalmology,* **54,** 587–593.

Zagar, Z. (1965). Sensitivity of *E. Coli, P. aeruginosa* and *B. proteus* to erythromycin in various pH culture media. *Chemotherapia,* **6,** 82–89.

Zimelis, V. M. & Jackson, G. G. (1973). Activity of aminoglycoside antibiotics against *Pseudomonas aeruginosa:* specificity and site of calcium and magnesium antagonism. *The Journal of Infectious Diseases,* **127,** 663–669.

CHAPTER 3

The Role of the Cell Envelope in Resistance

M. R. W. BROWN

INTRODUCTION

All compounds, whether toxic or nutrient, which have an effect upon bacteria must go through some or all of the following steps before achieving any specific activity: namely interaction with and penetration through the various layers of the cell envelope and the achievement of an effective concentration at the site of action. The site of antibacterial action may well be part of the envelope itself.

The envelope of bacteria is a remarkably plastic and variable structure. The occurrence of envelope variants as a result of genetic change (see Chapter 1) as well as the ready variation in structure and composition in response to environmental change (Ellwood & Tempest, 1972; Holme, 1972; Robinson & Tempest, 1973) all confer survival advantages.

The dependence of envelope composition on environmental conditions makes any absolute statement about composition quite impossible. The most that can be achieved at present would seem to be an indication of the spectrum of the variation due to specific environmental factors or combinations of factors. It is now clear in retrospect that the role of environment in determining structure has been grossly underestimated, especially the influence of specific nutrient limitation. What has clouded the issue has been the very widespread use of oxygen-depleted cultures grown in complex nutrient broth. So many workers for so long have used 'overnight' broth cultures, especially in drug resistance studies, that to some extent such cultures have come to be regarded as normal. The concept of the 'normal' bacterium can be dangerously misleading unless there is embedded in it the idea of a potentially wide spectrum of variation through phenotypic or genotypic influences. Nevertheless, comparisons *between* such cultures are, of course, often helpful. Another misleading influence has been the belief that the use of simple salts media necessarily defines a culture of bacteria. It is commonly the case that the nature of the growth-limiting nutrient is not known. Furthermore, it would appear not to have been considered. The determination of which nutrient is depleted first, and at what population size, requires empirical study. It may be that a culture enters a stationary phase under the influence of lack of more than one essential nutrient. It could also be that, where such measurements have not been made, a small variation in contamination of medium constituents might tilt the balance so that one essential nutrient is depleted first rather than another. Chapter 2 considers these factors in some detail.

As indicated in the preface, a basic question would seem to be the following: what are the mechanisms by which *Pseudomonas aeruginosa* has achieved its notorious and pre-eminent position as a drug-resistant pathogen and spoilage organism? An attractive pastime while reviewing the literature is to speculate on which of the main mechanisms of bacterial resistance are the most important for *P. aeruginosa*. Broadly speaking, drug resistance arises in two general ways. The first way is that the cell changes and becomes less vulnerable and the second is that the cell changes the drug to an inactive form. More specifically, based on Gale *et al.*, 1972:

(1) The target is either altered or its physiological importance reduced.
(2) Access by the drug to the target is reduced so that it is excluded.
(3) Drug-degrading enzymes are produced.

A previous comprehensive review concluded that it was difficult to consider the nature of the resistance of *P. aeruginosa* without also considering resistance of Gram-negative bacteria in general (Brown, 1971). This is still the case and it would now seem that the mechanisms of resistance for Gram-negative bacteria in general and for *P. aeruginosa* in particular are related in some degree to the very features of the cell involved in the Gram stain, namely in the envelope (Salton, 1963, 1964; Costerton, 1970; Smith, 1971; Gustafsson, Nordström & Normark, 1973).

In this chapter it is proposed to take a wide look at the role of the cell envelope in the resistance of *P. aeruginosa*, although most attention will be paid to drug resistance by exclusion. Of special interest is the activity of ethylenediaminetetraacetic acid (EDTA), polymyxin and some non-ionic surfactants. In sub-inhibitory concentrations these compounds reduce the resistance of some Gram-negative bacteria to a variety of antibacterial agents. This sensitizing effect is most pronounced with *P. aeruginosa* and a study of the mode of action of these agents is obviously relevant to an understanding of the notorious resistance of this organism. The structure of the envelope of *P. aeruginosa* is dealt with extensively in the related volume to this book (Meadow, 1974) and aspects specially related to resistance also occur elsewhere in this volume (Chapters 4 and 5). Several chapters in the book refer to the involvement of the envelope in resistance from one aspect or other. Consequently, the present purpose is to take a relatively broad view of the role of the envelope in the resistance of *P. aeruginosa*, especially by a mechanism of exclusion.

MODIFICATION OF TARGET

In the general terms of the above classification of mechanisms of resistance, the Gram-negative wall might perhaps be considered as a modified Gram-positive wall. Thus the peptidoglycan in Gram-negative species is somewhat different and also is less physiologically important to the bacterium than it is in Gram-positive species. The role of the peptidoglycan in maintaining cell rigidity is important in mechanisms of antibacterial activity. The peptidoglycan comprises only about 15% of the wall or less (Rogers, 1965), in contrast to Gram-positive species where it comprises about 50–60% and in some cases 80–90% of the wall (Perkins & Rogers, 1959). There is also, in general, greater cross-linkage between the polysaccharide chains of mainly *N*-acetyl-glucosamine and *N*-acetylmuramic acid comprising the peptidoglycan polymer in Gram-positive as compared to Gram-negative walls. Also, Gram-positive envelopes are about double or more the thickness of Gram-negative (see Table 4, Salton, 1964). These structural differences match the greater hydrostatic pressure in the former, namely 20 atm. compared to about 4 in Gram-negative bacteria. Bearing in mind the role of environment in affecting envelope composition, there is nevertheless some evidence that *P. aeruginosa* may have less peptidoglycan per bacterium than is characteristically the case in other Gram-negative species (Meadow, 1974). There is now clear evidence that macromolecular components in addition to the peptidoglycan sacculus contribute to wall rigidity and cell shape in Gram-negative bacteria (Salton, 1964). It would seem that the wall outer membrane affords significant structural support (Henning, Höhn & Sonntag, 1973).

Some early and indirect evidence implying target modification came from Hamilton-Miller (1965) who studied the modes of resistance of 12 penicillinase-producing strains of *Klebsiella* (see also Smith, Hamilton-Miller & Knox, 1969). He concluded that penicillinase was responsible for the observed resistance of only 2 of the 12 strains. The primary reason for the resistance of the other 10 strains was neither their possession of penicillinase nor their permeability barrier, but presumably an innate lack of sensitivity of the cell wall synthesizing complex to inhibition by penicillins. One can speculate, with hindsight, that it may also have been possible that components other than the peptidoglycan contributed to cell stability after penicillin induced damage.

The evidence for *P. aeruginosa* that components other than peptidoglycan may contribute to cell rigidity has come mainly from Eagon and his colleagues (see Chapter 4). Although lysozyme alone did not cause lysis or death, there was an effect and cell surface deformities occurred (Eagon & Carson, 1965; Asbell & Eagon, 1966a,b). Carson & Eagon (1966) reported that lysozyme alone did attack the peptidoglycan which was not solely responsible for wall rigidity. Further support for these findings came from Cox & Eagon (1968) with evidence about the role of cations in maintaining the structural integrity of the outer wall layers. Clarke, Gray & Reaveley (1967) found a difference in shape between the more elongated peptidoglycan sacculus and the cell wall. This supported the idea that the former was not exclusively responsible for the shape of the wall or the whole cell. Consequently, although exclusion and inactivation are important in resistance to, for example, β-lactam antibiotics, nevertheless the diminished importance of the peptidoglycan would seem likely to contribute to the overall resistance pattern to anti-peptidoglycan agents.

The outer membrane of *P. aeruginosa* and other Gram-negative bacteria is readily modified by genetic and environmental influences. Sensitivity by the cell to numerous chemical agents is profoundly affected by the affinity for outer membrane components. This interaction often damages the outer membrane and hence the cell, even when another site is the more critical, sensitive target. Structural modifications caused by environmental or genetic influences alter this pattern of sensitivity and may also eliminate sensitivity to an agent which characteristically has the outer membrane as its main target. This is illustrated by the change in resistance both to EDTA and to polymyxin B and in ultrastructure of *P. aeruginosa* when grown in magnesium-depleted media (Brown & Melling, 1969a,b; Gilleland, Stinnett & Eagon, 1974). The effects on resistance of changes in the outer membrane will be dealt with in detail later, in the section on exclusion.

DRUG-DEGRADING ENZYMES

In terms of antibiotic inactivation the characteristic properties of the Gram-negative envelope are also important. The cell-bound antibiotic-degrading enzyme confers an advantage on the cell compared to the extracellular Gram-positive counterpart (Percival, Brumfitt & de Louvois, 1963). This is discussed fully in Chapter 1 (see also Richmond & Sykes, 1973) but deserves a brief comment in the present context. It seems likely that the β-lactamases of most Gram-negative species, including *P. aeruginosa*, are acting in the periplasmic space beneath the outer membrane which only slowly allows the substrate through. Thus the cell-bound enzyme is much less liable to dilution than the extracellular enzyme, and is also acting on a substrate with restricted access in many cases so that less enzyme is necessary. Furthermore, the population effect involved in extracellular antibiotic inactivation is not apparent as a consequence.

EXCLUSION

General Evidence for Exclusion

There is now considerable evidence that resistance of bacteria to many chemical antibacterial agents may sometimes be due to the inability of an otherwise active agent to achieve an effective concentration at its site(s) of action. The envelope plays a crucial role in resistance by such an exclusion mechanism. The evidence is abundant for Gram-negative bacteria (Franklin, 1973) including and perhaps especially *Pseudomonas aeruginosa* (Brown, 1971; 1972).

Basis for Gram-Reaction Discrimination

Before looking in detail at the evidence for exclusion as a mechanism of drug resistance it would seem appropriate to consider the mechanism of the Gram-staining reaction. Recent work suggests that the two may be related. Salton (1964) reviewed the early evidence relating the nature of the cell wall and the Gram-stain. With reservations, he concluded that the most likely hypothesis was that of Burke & Barnes (1929), according to which Gram differentiation is due to trapping of the crystal violet–iodine complex within the cells of Gram-positive bacteria, probably by a barrier in the form of the dehydrated, mordanted wall. He suggested that the solubility of the surface lipids of the gram-negative bacteria may also contribute to the ease with which the differentiating solvent extracts the crystal violet–iodine from the cell. It would now seem possible that, for Gram-negative bacteria, the dye does not characteristically penetrate into the cytoplasm. Indirect evidence of dye/envelope interaction was obtained by Brown & Winsley (1969). They studied the effect of the non-ionic surfactant polysorbate 80 on the permeability of *P. aeruginosa* by (a) measuring effects on the penetration of the dye 1-anilinonaphthylamine-8-sulphonic acid (ANS) and (b) the effect of polysorbate 80 on the optical effect. The ability of bacteria to alter their light-scattering properties with changes in environmental osmotic pressure may be regarded as a measure of the integrity of the osmotic barrier (Mager, Kuczynski, Schatzberg & Avi-Dor, 1956; Postgate & Hunter, 1962). Polysorbate 80 was found not to alter the pronounced optical effect of the bacteria at various NaCl concentrations. On the other hand the fluorescence of the bacteria, and therefore the amount of dye/protein conjugate, increased with polysorbate concentration in the growth medium up to 0·125%. It seemed very unlikely that polysorbate would allow entry into the cytoplasm of the bacterium of ANS but cause no change in the optical effect. The hypothesis proposed was that polysorbate enhanced dye/protein conjugation at an external site rather than in the cytoplasm. Since the work of Newton (1954), who used a similar dye to explore permeability changes in *P. aeruginosa*, many workers have assumed that fluorescence of such dyes due to protein conjugation demonstrated penetration into the cell cytoplasm. In the light of our current knowledge of Gram-negative envelopes this conclusion may not always be justified.

Direct evidence that the outer parts of the bacterial envelope constitute a barrier to the penetration of gentian violet came from the important work of Gustafsson, Nordström & Normark (1973). They used wild-type strains of *E. coli* K-12 together with envelope mutants derived from *E. coli* K-12. The uptake of gentian violet could be divided into at least two processes. Type I occurred instantaneously even at 0 °C, was independent of energy metabolism and was the same for all mutants tested as well as for the parent strain. The dye taken up by Type I kinetics is solely located in the envelope. It is significant that Wistreich & Bartholomew (1969) found that Gram-positive and Gram-negative envelopes showed similar binding of crystal violet. In contrast, Type II uptake occurred gradually only at higher temperatures and was affected by agents known to block energy metabolism. It represents a transport into the cytoplasm, where the main part of the dye is bound to the ribosomal fraction. Resistance to gentian violet was found to be inversely correlated with the rate of penetration into the cytoplasm. Gustafsson *et al.* (1973) concluded that constituents of the outer membrane, lipopolysaccharide and phospholipid were important components of the barrier function of the envelope. They also suggested that the peptidoglycan may either be a component of the barrier or may indirectly affect the integrity of the outer membrane.

This recent work would suggest that for Gram-negative bacteria the Gram-stain is characteristically excluded from the cytoplasm, being retained outside the penetration barrier. Thus the stain is relatively accessible to solvent extraction.

Ratio Between Cell and Enzyme Inhibition

In many cases considerably lower concentrations of antibiotics are required for enzyme inhibition in cell free systems than are required for inhibition of cell growth. Much less actinomycin D was required for inhibition of the deoxyribonucleic acid-dependent ribonucleic acid polymerase in *E. coli* than was needed for inhibition of growth (Hurwitz, Furth, Malamy & Alexander, 1962). A similar situation has been shown with several antibiotics inhibiting cell wall synthesis: ristocetin and vancomycin (Anderson, Matsuhashi, Haskin & Strominger, 1967), bacitracin (Siewert & Strominger, 1967), penicillins (Izaki, Matsuhashi & Strominger, 1968) and enduracidin (Matsuhashi, O'Hara & Yoshiyama, 1970). Gram-positive bacteria accumulate 100-fold more erythromycin than Gram-negative bacteria. On the other hand, cell-free protein synthesizing preparations from both *E. coli* and *Staph. aureus* were rapidly sensitive to erythromycin (Mao & Putterman, 1968).

Crypticity

A quantitative indication of the ease of penetration of antibiotics through the envelope is given by crypticity studies. The procedure is to compare the rate of enzymatic destruction of an antibiotic using broken cell preparations with that obtained by equal numbers of whole cells. Relatively unimpeded access by the antibiotic to the periplasmic space is indicated by a crypticity value of 1·0. The term 'crypticity' now seems to be widely used, although 'permeability factor' was used by Hamilton-Miller (1965) to describe the same ratio. Relatively high crypticity values have been obtained with various Gram-negative bacteria including *P. aeruginosa* for penicillins and with *P. aeruginosa* for cephaloridine (Richmond & Sykes, 1973).

Percival, Brumfitt & de Louvois (1963) speculated for Gram-negative bacteria on the possible cooperative interaction between lack of access *per se* and the production of antibiotic inactivating enzymes in resistance to penicillins. The interaction between different resistance mechanisms is illustrated in a special way by the transfer of resistance between various Gram-negative bacteria including *P. aeruginosa*. Roe, Jones & Lowbury (1971) found that a strain of *P. aeruginosa* acquired intrinsic resistance without carbenicillinase production from a donor strain of resistant, carbenicillinase—producing *E. coli*. When this strain of *P. aeruginosa* was used as a donor, the *E. Coli* to which it transferred resistance also acquired the property of producing carbenicillinase. Much elegant quantitative work has been done recently by Richmond and co-workers in this area and the subject is reviewed in detail in Chapter 1.

Drug Sensitivity in the Absence of the Wall

Studies of several species, including *P. aeruginosa*, using cells, protoplasts and spheroplasts have indicated that drug resistance in many cases was due to non-penetration. Tulasne & Minck (1952) reported that *P. vulgaris* and *P. morganii* L-forms showed enhanced sensitivity to membrane active agents. Taubeneck (1962) found that L-forms of *Proteus mirabilis*, but not whole cells, were especially sensitive to macrolide antibiotics. With *E. coli*, Mach & Tatum (1963) found that spheroplasts were more sensitive to erythromycin than whole cells. Similarly, the involvement of the wall has been shown in the resistance of *Cholera vibrio* to polymyxin. Protoplasts of sensitive and resistant strains showed similar sensitivites (Biswas & Mukerjee, 1967). The conversion of a polymyxin B-resistant strain of *P. mirabilis* into L-forms and spheroplasts by penicillin G resulted in a 400-fold increase in polymyxin B susceptibility (Teuber, 1969). Montgomerie, Kalmanson & Guze (1966) and Teuber (1969) have pointed out the need to consider the possible sensitizing effects on the cytoplasmic membrane of the spheroplasting process itself. Hamilton (1968, 1970) studied quantitatively the effects of several membrane active agents on whole cells, protoplasts and spheroplasts of a variety of Gram-positive and Gram-negative bacteria including *P. aeruginosa*. He measured drug uptake, lysis and leakage. It was found that the naked membranes from both sensitive and non-sensitive species were equally sensitive to the specific ion permeability effects found with the several agents used. He found that the wall acted as a barrier which could be either adsorbing or non-adsorbing.

These results are compatible with the hypothesis (Hamilton, 1968) that resistance to membrane active agents is due to the agent not penetrating through the wall. MacAlister, Costerton & Cheng (1972) removed the outer wall layers (not the peptidoglycan) of a marine pseudomonad and showed enhanced penetration by actinomycin D. These authors were among the first who specifically referred to the role of the outer double track layer and lipopolysaccharide in constituting an antibiotic-excluding barrier. The presence of the peptidoglycan layer in the mureinoplasts studied indicated that neither this layer nor the cytoplasmic membrane played any significant role in excluding actinomycin D under the conditions used. These results strongly support the idea that in many significant cases (but not all: see Spicer & Spooner, 1974) the wall or wall component(s) offer a penetration barrier to drugs reaching the cytoplasmic membrane. It would now seem likely that the wall outer membrane largely constitutes this barrier. The barrier may involve either the absence or depletion of a specific drug-binding wall component.

Lipid Content and Resistance

There is much early evidence that ease of uptake and penetration in Gram-positive resistance is related to lipid content, especially readily extractable (chloroform-methanol) lipid (REL). Much of this evidence largely related overall *cell* REL to drug resistance (Vaczi, 1966; Hugo & Stretton, 1966; Hugo, 1967; see especially the recent review by Vaczi, 1973). It would seem likely that quantitative and qualitative changes in membrane REL, with the possibility of changed membrane structure, would affect drug/lipid interaction, leading to altered ease of penetration. The location of this altered lipid in Gram-positive studies has not always been reported, although association with the outer layers of the envelope has been shown in some cases, e.g. tetracyline resistance *Staph. pyogenes* (Hill, James & Maxted, 1963; Norrington & James, 1970). It seems highly likely that such lipid changes reflect alterations in the cytoplasmic membrane. Changes in cell shape, with differing surface/volume ratios, may affect cell lipid content. Nevertheless, the large cell lipid changes reported in the literature probably reflect radical changes in membrane structure.

In the case of Gram-negative bacteria, the interpretation of analyses of readily extractable lipid is more complex. In addition to possible changes in the structure and composition of the cytoplasmic membrane, alterations in cell REL (Anderes, Sandine & Elliker, 1971) may also reflect changes in the wall outer membrane. Furthermore, the involvement of lipopolysaccharide and also lipoprotein in the outer membrane further complicates the situation (see Chapter 5 and also Meadow, 1974). Thus the outer membrane in the case of *P. aeruginosa* and other Gram-negative species allows an enhanced degree of specificity in determining access by external compounds. The effect of gross changes in outer membrane lipid from *P. aeruginosa* is indicated by the work of Ivanov, Markov, Golowinsky & Charisanova (1964). They extracted *P. aeruginosa* with petroleum ether without altering viability, but found that sensitivity to a variety of agents was enhanced. Similarly, by means of electrophoretic mobility studies involving *P. aeruginosa* treated with sodium dodecyl sulphate, Pechey & James (1973) found a linear relationship between gentamicin MIC and surface lipid. The nature of the surface lipid was not determined and may possibly have been LPS.

The role of lipid in resistance might be regarded as two related parts. Firstly, different drugs have high affinity for specific lipids, e.g. phospholipid and lipopolysaccharide. This affinity has been proposed, as will be indicated below, both as a mechanism of exclusion and as an aid to penetration. Secondly, lipid plays an essential part in the overall structure of the two envelope membranes. It is in this structural context that the involvement of lipid in resistance will be considered in more detail in the next section. In summary, the highly complex role of lipid in Gram-negative resistance, notably *P. aeruginosa*, consists mainly in contributing to the composition and structure of the inner cytoplasmic membrane and especially the adaptable outer wall membrane. Thus lipid plays a part, directly or indirectly, in all three mechanisms of resistance outlined at the beginning of this chapter. The special nature, if any, of *P. aeruginosa* lipids will be considered in the next section on specific envelope layers.

ROLE OF ENVELOPE LAYERS

There have recently been several excellent reviews. Schnaitman (1971b) proposed a model (p. 4) for the *E. coli* wall, including the outer membrane, based partly on results of various extraction procedures. Recently, Costerton, Ingram & Cheng (1974) have comprehensively reviewed the structure and function of the envelope of Gram-negative bacteria in general and Leive (1974) has considered the barrier function of the Gram-negative envelope with particular respect to EDTA-induced damage. Meadow (1974) has reviewed the *P. aeruginosa* envelope in particular. Elsewhere in this book Dr. Eagon and his colleagues have considered the ultrastructure of *P. aeruginosa* as related to resistance. Consequently, it is proposed to take the envelope structure largely for granted and only very briefly to consider those features especially significant from the point of view of resistance. Although not strictly a structural part of the envelope, slime constitutes an important external layer when present. After a consideration of slime the involvement in resistance of the various structural layers will be dealt with using mainly the model of Costerton *et al.* (1974).

Slime

The role of slime in the drug resistance of *P. aeruginosa* has received little attention. It seems possible that a viscous slime layer could offer a penetration barrier to some drugs, perhaps by binding, especially to highly active drugs acting in small concentrations. Furthermore, slime may protect the cell against *in vivo* body defence mechanisms such as phagocytosis (Schwarzmann & Boring, 1971; Roe and Jones, 1974; Sensakovic & Bartell, 1974). An early and persistent problem was that the composition of the slime was in doubt. A clear idea of the degree of the genetically and phenotypically determined variation would help predict drug–slime interaction. The literature on this subject is contradictory, perhaps partly due to differences in extraction procedures. Warren & Grey (1954) found that hyaluronidase depolymerized a polysaccharide extracted from *P. aeruginosa*. Electron microscopy showed that hyaluronidase treatment removed extracellular material surrounding the cells (Warren & Grey, 1955). Bonde, Jensen & Thamsen (1957) also gave similar evidence for the presence of hyaluronic acid in *P. aeruginosa* slime. Concurrently Eagon & Randles (1954) found that *P. aeruginosa* strain OSU-64 (originally referred to as *P. fluorescens*, but subsequently shown to be *P. aeruginosa*) produced large amounts of high molecular weight extracellular polysaccharide composed of mannose sub-units. Eagon (1956) excluded amino sugars and also uronic acids as being components of the slime and found mannose as the sole carbohydrate constituent. Subsequently, Eagon (1962) estimated that the mannose constituted about 50% of the slime and there were appreciable amounts of DNA and RNA with small quantities of protein. Halleck, Durkin & Guschlbaüer (1960) found that slime of two strains of *Pseudomonas* species (unspecified) was highly polymerized DNA. Brown, Foster & Clamp (1966, 1969) found that slime hydrolysate contained glucuronic acid and glucosamine, suggesting about 5% hyaluronic acid. This was supported by zone electrophoresis of unhydrolysed slime as well as by the infrared spectra. They showed that slime produced by each of 8 strains of *P. aeruginosa* in a variety of culture media was qualitatively constant with minor quantitative variations. The main constituent (50–60%) was a polysaccharide composed mainly of glucose with some mannose. It was not shown if the sugar were present as a co-polymer or as a mixture of a glucan and mannan. DNA and RNA made up about 20% and 5% hyaluronic acid was present. Other, minor, components were protein, rhamnose and glucosamine. Slime was not produced in some chemically defined media with glucose as sole carbon source: it was produced with gluconate. *P. aeruginosa* slime obtained by ethanol precipitation, gel filtration and ion exchange chromotography gave on hydrolysis: rhamnose, glucose, mannose, glucosamine, galactosamine and glucuronic acid, protein and trace amounts of nucleic acids (Bartell, Orr & Chudio, 1970).

Liu, Abe & Bates (1961) and Liu & Mercer (1963) related *P. aeruginosa* toxicity to the slime, especially the DNA, without detailed analysis of the slime contents. Purified slime was found to be two to three times more toxic than lipopolysaccharide for mice (Sensakovic & Bartell, 1974). Characteristically, a capsule is absent (Wilson & Miles, 1964) but some mucoid varieties isolated from pathological conditions are encapsulated (Doggett, Harrison & Wallis,

1964, Cetin, Töreci & Anğ, 1965; Elston & Hoffman, 1967). Doggett *et al.* (1964, 1965) showed that *P. aeruginosa* strains isolated from the respiratory tract of cystic fibrosis patients differed from those isolated from control patients. The former strains were mucoid and the capsular material was greater both in quantity and in viscosity. The slime of mucoid strains contained two unidentified polysaccharides, fucose, mannose, glucose, glucosamine, galactose and galactosamine. Other workers have analysed the polysaccharide produced by mucoid strains of *P. aeruginosa* and found it consisted of uronic acids (Linker & Jones, 1964), mainly mannuronic acid, (Carlson & Matthews, 1966): these latter workers found that mucoid strains of *P. aeruginosa* also occurred in the respiratory tract of patients not suffering from cystic fibrosis. Klyhn & Gorrill (1967) found that slime produced by numerous clinical isolates of *P. aeruginosa* from various sources contained glucose, mannose, fucose, galactose, ribose and rhamnose as well as glucosamine and galactosamine. More recently, Evans & Linker (1973) studied the slime polysaccharide produced by *P. aeruginosa* isolated from a variety of human infections. It is significant that all the polysaccharides produced by strains from these *in vivo* sources were similar to each other and to seaweed alginic acids, although with large differences in mannuronic to guluronic ratio. No carbohydrates other than polyuronides were found. Much further work is needed, but nevertheless, in cystic fibrosis, for example, it would seem that antibiotic treatment eventually selects *P. aeruginosa* mucoid strains as the main pathological problem (for references see Evans & Linker, 1973).

Brown & Scott Foster (1971) used two chemically defined media identical except that one had glucose and the other gluconate as a carbon source, in which it was possible to grow cultures producing slime (from gluconate) or no slime (from glucose). The sensitivities of these two batches of *P. aeruginosa* were tested to EDTA and to polymyxin using log phase, early stationary and 6-day old cultures. Slime was found to have an initial blocking effect, greater for polymyxin than for EDTA. Once sufficient agent was present to overcome this effect, slime appeared not to contribute further to sensitivity. Cells, 6-days old, both glucose- and gluconate-grown, were more sensitive to changes in concentration of both agents than were log phase cells. It would thus seem unlikely that slime plays a major role in resistance *in vitro* to these particular agents. Its role in providing either a diffusion barrier or a drug–slime interacting barrier with other drugs is not yet clear.

Outer Membrane

Introduction

Several general lines of evidence have been indicated as especially significant in terms of the mechanism of resistance of *P. aeruginosa* (Brown, 1971, 1972). It would now seem highly likely that these lines of evidence converge on the special nature of the outer membrane of *P. aeruginosa*. This evidence will now be outlined briefly before proceeding in more detail when considering the outer membrane structure. Sensitivity to EDTA (Wilkinson, 1967) and to polymyxin (Gilardi, 1968) is characteristic of several Gram-negative species, but especially of *P. aeruginosa*. These agents, and also some non-ionic surfactants (Brown & Winsley, 1971) in concentrations which are relatively non-toxic, enhance the penetration and activity of a wide variety of antibacterial agents against Gram-negative bacteria, especially *P. aeruginosa*. These enhancing effects, as discussed below, are probably the consequence of an action on the structure of the outer membrane. Furthermore, the extraordinary sensitivity of Gram-negative bacteria, especially *P. aeruginosa* to cold shock (Gorrill & McNiel, 1960) as well as to rapid changes in pH, temperature or tonicity (Brown & Winsley, 1969) is also probably related to the structure of the outer membrane. The effects of cold shock on the physical state of the cytoplasmic membrane lipid (Farrell & Rose, 1968) probably apply also to the outer membrane lipid. However, these effects may be compounded as a result of the special structure of the outer membrane of *P. aeruginosa*. In addition it now seems likely that changes in the outer membrane are involved in the release of periplasmic enzymes after cold shock and other treatment (Costerton *et al.*, 1974). There is a species-specific antagonism by cations of antimicrobial action against *P. aeruginosa* for aminoglycoside antibiotics (Zimelis & Jackson, 1973) and polymyxin (Newton, 1953, 1954; Davis, Iannetta & Wedgewood, 1971). Once again a special feature of the wall of *P. aeruginosa* would seem to be involved, as discussed below.

It is now apparent that the Gram-negative outer membrane structure and composition are profoundly influenced by the environment, particularly conditions of specific nutrient growth limitation (McDonald & Adams, 1971; Ellwood & Tempest, 1972; Holme, 1972; Robinson & Tempest, 1973). Magnesium limitation of *P. aeruginosa* resulted in loss of sensitivity to EDTA and to polymyxin (Brown & Melling, 1969a,b), enhanced sensitivity to silver (Brown & Anderson, 1968) and was associated with structural changes in the outer membrane (Gilleland, Stinnett & Eagon, 1974).

Numerous workers have reported drug sensitivity changes associated with genetically induced changes in a variety of Gram-negative species, especially with respect to the lipopolysaccharide (LPS) (Tamaki & Matsuhashi, 1973; Gustafsson, Nordström & Normark, 1973; Sanderson, MacAlister, Costerton & Cheng, 1973). Polymyxin-trained variants of *P. aeruginosa* were also found to have changes in wall composition, probably associated with changes in the outer membrane (Brown & Watkins, 1970). This ready variation in outer membrane composition resulting from environmental or genetic (see also Chapter 1) change would seem to confer considerable survival advantages in terms of resistance.

The model of the outer membrane (Figure 1) proposed by Costerton (1974) involves a protruding 'picket-fence' pattern on both surfaces consisting of LPS oligosaccharides carrying the 'O' antigen at their distal tips. The basic continuum consists of proteins and phospholipids with the same molecular architecture as a typical membrane (Forge & Costerton, 1973). These components are exposed between the LPS oligosaccharides to a greater or lesser

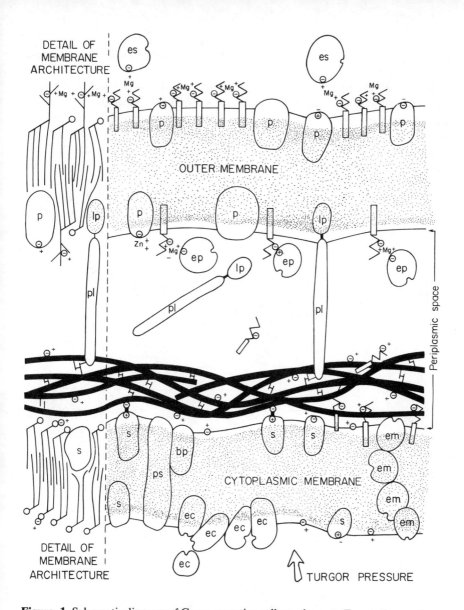

Figure 1. Schematic diagram of Gram-negative cell envelope. +, Free cation; −, free anion; ⊕ bound cation; ⊖ bound anion; ⚡ adhesion point produced by ionic bonding; ▒ hydrophobic zone; ⊃—⊂ covalent bond; ⊷═⊸ cross-linking polypeptide in the peptidoglycan; ▬▬▬ polysaccharide portion of peptidoglycan; ⌇ enzymatically active protein; ⌐º phospholipid; ⌐ lipopolysaccharide; ▭▬⊗ lipopolysaccharide (schematic); bp, binding protein; ec, enzymes associated with the cytoplasmic membrane whose function is directed to the cytoplasm; em, enzymes associated with the cytoplasmic membrane which synthesize macromolecular components of the cell wall; ep, enzymes localized in the periplasmic zone; es, enzymes localized at the cell surface; lp, lipid portion of Braun's lipoprotein; p, structural and enzymatic proteins of the outer membrane; pl, protein portion of Braun's lipoprotein; ps, permease; s, structural protein of cytoplasmic membrane. Reproduced with permission from J. W. Costerton, J. M. Ingram & K.-J. Cheng, *Bact. Revs.*, **38**, 87–110 (1974) Figure 1

extent, possibly acting as specific receptor sites. This layer forms a hydrophobic barrier in the outer cell wall which is structurally strengthened by the interaction of the protruding oligosaccharides and by the presence of structural proteins. It has been suggested that the major force holding the wall together is a hydrophobic interaction between the various protein components (Schnaitman, 1971b). Lipoprotein anchors the inner aspect of this layer to the peptidoglycan by hydrophobic interaction with the outer membrane and covalent links with the peptidoglycan. The outer membrane of *P. aeruginosa* (Figure 2) probably conforms in general to this basic pattern but with some special characteristics (see below and Meadow, 1974).

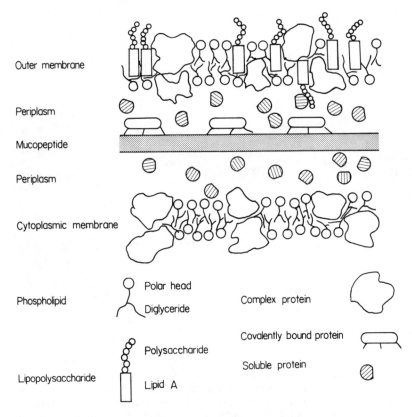

Figure 2. Diagram to show the chemical composition of the wall and membrane layers of *P. aeruginosa*. Reproduced from P. Meadow in *The Biochemistry and Genetics of Pseudomonas* (Ed. P. H. Clarke & M. H. Richmond) John Wiley, London, 1974

External Layer of Outer Membrane

Apart from any slime or appendage such as flagella, the most external envelope structure in contact with the environment will be the distal ends of the oligosaccharide parts of the LPS. Thus any drug would have to penetrate an ordered and cross-linked 'mat' of polysaccharide chains. The hydrophobic lipid A part of the LPS anchors these chains by being associated with the hydrophobic zones of the outer membrane. A rough strain of *Salmonella typhimurium* with relatively short chains of sugars distal to the lipid A gave relatively easy penetration by antibiotics and lysozyme (Sanderson *et al.*, 1973). Furthermore, periplasmic enzymes were released more readily during growth (Lindsay, Shelagh, Wheeler, Sanderson & Costerton, 1973). Schlecht & Westphal (1968, 1970) obtained similar results. In addition to the polysaccharide 'mat' this model envisages patches or specific 'sites'. These could consist of specialized LPS (phage receptors, Lindberg & Hellerquist, 1971), glycoprotein (colicin receptors, Sabet & Schnaitman, 1973) and phospholipid (see below and Glauert & Thornley, 1969) with the polar heads at the surface. The polar heads in the case of *P. aeruginosa* will characteristically be mainly of phosphatidylethanolamine (Meadow, 1974).

The overall physical shape and structure of LPS has been reviewed by Shands (1971). In an aqueous environment LPS may exist as a bilayer of polysaccharide and lipid with the non-polar lipids occupying the interior of the bilayer. LPS has been broken into small fragments by sodium dodecyl sulphate (Beer, Staehelin, Douglas & Braude, 1965), sodium deoxycholate (Ribi *et al.*, 1966) and Tween 80 (Shands, 1971). It seems that hydrophobic forces are the major ones joining the two halves of the LPS polymer and that these forces are contributed by the non-polar lipids of the inner part of the bilayer. Hydrophobic interactions also contribute to the linear polymerization of LPS. Metal cation binding also probably contributes to the linking of LPS sub-units (Olins & Warner, 1967). The mechanism is presumably by cross-linking the polar region of the amphipath by combination with negatively charged phosphate or carboxyl groups. In the outer membrane the LPS lipid A is associated with the inner hydrophobic zone. In this connection the observations of Mitchell (1970) are probably worth repeating: ' . . . the factors contributing to the stability of structure and composition of membranes in living cells may be presumed to be fundamentally similar to those factors of close packing, electric charge neutralization and segregation of hydrophobic and hydrophilic groups that have been shown to be dominant in determining the tertiary folding and sub-unit assembly of smaller scale biochemical complexes such as proteins and nucleic acids. For this reason, the functional inclusion of a given component in a lipid membrane may be less dependant upon its atomic composition—for example, whether it is classed as a protein (polypeptide) or lipid—than upon its configuration and its polar or non-polar secondary bonding characteristics.'

Lack of antibiotic uptake has been associated with resistance. Few & Schulman (1953) found a correlation between uptake and polymyxin E sensitivity for whole cells and walls of several species. Similar results were obtained with walls prepared from polymyxin-sensitive and a polymyxin-resistant strain of *P. aeruginosa* (Newton, 1954, 1956). Earlier in this chapter reference was made to the finding that the wall could be either an adsorbing or non-adsorbing barrier (Hamilton, 1968, 1970). In a manner similar to phage or colicin reception, specific outer membrane components have high affinity for specific drugs. It would seem highly likely that these components are involved in the 'sites' which take up the drug. Their absence or depletion may, in effect, constitute a penetration barrier. Qualitative changes in the outer membrane components could cause altered lipid/drug interaction in the case of LPS (e.g. polymyxin B, Bader & Teuber, 1973; ampicillin, Monner, Jonsson & Boman, 1971; numerous agents including detergents, Ennis & Bloomstein, 1974) or phospholipid (e.g. polymyxin E, Few, 1955; polymyxin B, Teuber, 1973 and HsuChen & Feinfold, 1973; penicillins, Padfield & Kellaway, 1973, 1974; gramicidin S and polymyxin B, Pache, Chapman & Hillaby, 1972).

The proteins of the outer membrane differ from those of the cytoplasmic membrane; they consist of three major proteins and a probable main function is to stabilize the outer membrane (*E. coli*: Schnaitman, 1970, 1971a,b; *P. aeruginosa*: Stinnett, Gilleland & Eagon, 1973 and also see Chapter 4). In passing, it is perhaps worth noting that the role of protein/drug interaction has received little attention in this respect.

On the basis of uptake data for cetyltrimethyl ammonium bromide (CTAB) by *E. Coli*, Salt & Wiseman (1970) proposed that individual cells first took up CTAB until a single close-packed monolayer built up on the surface of the wall outer membrane. This surface adsorption was reversible. With higher concentrations of CTAB the data was compatible with the idea that a second monolayer was built up at the cytoplasmic membrane. After completion of this second layer further uptake resulted in penetration of the cytoplasmic membrane concurrently with membrane disruption.

Specificity of polymyxin action on P. aeruginosa.   An understanding of the mode of action of polymyxin still requires a reading of the superb, classic papers of B. A. Newton (Newton, 1956). Despite much work in this general area in the last two decades (Brown & Watkins, 1970; Brown & Wood, 1972; HsuChen & Feingold, 1973; Teuber, 1973; Feingold, HsuChen & Sud, 1974) it is surprising to find what relatively little advance has been made from these early studies. In the present context a critical question concerns the high specificity of polymyxin for Gram-negative bacteria and especially *P. aeruginosa* (Gilardi, 1968; Brown, 1971). The main site of action is probably phospholipids of the cytoplasmic membrane. After this interaction the cell's osmotic barrier function is reduced probably as well as other membrane associated functions such as transport and synthesis. It would seem that it is not any special character of the cytoplasmic membrane of *P. aeruginosa* which confers special sensitivity (or resistance) to polymyxin. Spheroplasts and protoplasts of various bacterial species have been found to be relatively sensitive to a variety of membrane active agents including polymyxin (see previous section on sensitivity in absence of wall). Resistance occurred as a result of lack of penetration through the wall. This probably does not apply to mammalian membranes where the absence of specific target phospholipids may account for relative insensitivity to polymyxin (HsuChen & Feinfold, 1973). The special nature of the outer membrane of *P. aeruginosa*, which reacts with and allows access to polymyxin, is the probable cause of the organism's exceptional sensitivity. Of the various outer membrane components, some phospholipids and also LPS have been shown to have high affinity for polymyxin. In the earlier work it was often assumed that polymyxin/phospholipid interaction occurred exclusively at the cytoplasmic membrane. After considering the broad evidence indicating the importance of the outer membrane in general for polymyxin specificity, attention will be paid to polymyxin interactions with phospholipid and lipopolysaccharide.

The evidence that polymyxin has a significant action on the outer layers of envelope is now conclusive. Newton (1955) treated *P. aeruginosa* and *B. megaterium* with a fluorescent derivative of polymyxin. The latter organism took up the antibiotic at a site beneath the wall and 10% of the fluorescence was associated with the wall and 90% with the membrane fraction. Uptake by *P. aeruginosa* wall and membrane fractions was almost equal. It was suggested that because wall and membrane were closely associated in the Gram-negative bacterium any distinction about uptake was difficult. Nevertheless, in retrospect, it would seem possible that polymyxin associated with components of the outer membrane of *P. aeruginosa*. Warren, Gray & Yurchenco (1957) found that pre-treatment of several Gram-negative bacteria with polymyxin rendered them more sensitive to lysozyme, suggesting an effect of polymyxin on the outer envelope layers. Cerny & Teuber (1971) found that polymyxin treatment of *E. coli* released periplasmic proteins, presumably by an effect on an outer penetration (outwards) barrier. Koike & Iida (1971) found that polymyxin caused the appearance of projections from the surface of *E. coli*, visible by electron microscopy. Furthermore, the cells also lost their ability to adsorb lipopolysaccharide-specific phages but not lipoprotein-specific phages. Pretreatment of the cells with LPS-specific phage prevented the appearance of the polymyxin-induced projections. Smooth strains of Gram-negative bacteria are protected by their polysaccharide chains with 'O' antigen from complement- and antibody-induced damage. On the other hand, rough strains, with their shortened polysaccharide chains, are susceptible. However, smooth strains are also sensitive to immune sera after their protective LPS structure has been modified by polymyxin (Pruul & Reynolds, 1972) and also by Tris and/or EDTA (Reynolds & Pruul, 1971). Mathieu & Legault-Hetu (1973) found a decreased sensitivity to polymyxin B in colicin K-tolerant cells of *E. coli* K-12 in the presence of colicin K. It is interesting that some early workers found that polymyxin agglutinated only bacteria lacking the O antigen (Latterrade & Macheboeuf, 1950). In this connection Newton (1956) quoted previously unpublished results of McQuillen in which a rough strain of *P. aeruginosa* was agglutinated by polymyxin, unlike several smooth strains. He also found that the rough strain had a relatively high electrophoretic mobility ($4\cdot5$ μ/sec/v/cm compared to about $2\cdot1$ μ/sec/v/cm for smooth strains using M/300 phosphate buffer, pH $7\cdot0$). The loss of sensitivity to polymyxin and the related outer membrane changes in magnesium-depleted cultures of *P. aeruginosa* is further evidence of the effect of outer membrane composition on polymyxin sensitivity/resistance (Brown & Melling, 1969b; Gilleland, Stinnett & Eagon, 1974).

Polymyxin/phospholipid specificity. Not all published work has been in agreement. Few (1955) studied the reaction of polymyxin E with monolayers of various bacterial phospholipids and lipids. Strong complexes occurred with cephalin (he reported that his preparation contained phosphatidyl serine as well as phosphatidylethanolamine). Moderate complex formation occurred with cardiolipin, but no reaction occurred with lecithin. It was suggested that with lecithin monolayers the positively charged choline group effectively shields the ionized phosphate group. This prevents an electrostatic bonding between the monolayer phosphate groups and the amino groups of polymyxin E, which would be necessary for penetration of the monolayer to occur. More recently, Pache, Chapman & Hillaby (1972) used a variety of physical techniques to study the interaction of polymyxin B with a lecithin–water model system. They found that polymyxin did interact with both the polar and non-polar regions of the phospholipid. They concluded that an electrostatic interaction occurred between the amino groups of the antibiotic and the phosphate group of the lecithin, and that the fatty acid tail of the polymyxin penetrated into the lipid bilayer. The peptide ring seemed not to be incorporated into the lipid. Interaction occurred with various negatively charged phospholipids. Barrett-Bee, Radda & Thomas (1972) studied the effects of polymyxin on *E. coli* whole cells, using nuclear magnetic resonance and fluorescence techniques. Their evidence supported the idea that the non-polar region penetrates into a membrane while the polar groups are less immobilized. The contribution to these results of the outer and inner membranes was not distinguished. Teuber & Bader (1971) found that extraction of isolated cell envelopes from *Salmonella typhimurium* with chloroform–methanol (i.e. REL) reduced their binding capacity for radioactive polymyxin B by 70%. Subsequently Teuber (1973) used chromatography and chloroform extraction to show that polymyxin B formed stable complexes with phosphatidic acid and phosphatidylglycerol but not with phosphatidylethanolamine, phosphatidylserine or cardiolipin. A role for the polymyxin-complexing phospholipids was proposed in terms of the penetration of polymyxin to its site of action. HsuChen & Feingold (1973) studied the action of polymyxin B in releasing trapped glucose marker from lipid spherules (liposomes) in aqueous suspension. They found that this model system differentiated among phospholipids with various polar head structures: specifically between liposomes of phosphatidylethanolamine (sensitive, but compare above with Teuber, 1973) and *N*-methylated analogs (insensitive). Wolf-Watz & Normark (1974) briefly reported a comparison of some aspects of the composition of the outer membrane from an antibiotic supersensitive mutant of *E. coli* K12 (*env* A) and from its wild type. The permeable strain *env* A showed a relative decrease in phosphatidylglycerol compared to the wild type. Furthermore, spontaneous revertants of the *env* A strain were isolated which regained the wild-type barrier properties to varying extents. A linear relationship was reported between the relative content of phosphatidylglycerol in the outer membrane and the permeability properties of the cell envelope. The *env* A mutation also mediated a cell division abnormality, causing inadequate separation of dividing cells.

In the case of polymyxin sensitivity it has been proposed that wall phospholipid is specifically required for significant antimicrobial activity against *P. aeruginosa* and other Gram-negative bacteria (Brown & Watkins, 1970; Brown & Wood, 1972; Teuber, 1973). A stable polymyxin-resistant variant obtained by a mutagenic effect of drying was found to have much less wall phospholipid (and magnesium) than the wild type (Brown & Wood, 1971). Brown & Wood (1972) found a relative lack of wall phospholipid (not defined) in the polymyxin resistant *Proteus vulgaris* (4 strains) and a resistant strain of *K. aerogenes*. On the other hand, a polymyxin-sensitive *K. aerogenes* and *P. aeruginosa* had relatively high wall phospholipid contents. Presumably these results reflected gross differences between the wall outer membranes of these strains. The affinity of polymyxin for *P. vulgaris* phospholipid was not significantly different from that for *P. aeruginosa* phospholipid. Sud & Feingold (1970) found that the lipid composition of polymyxin-sensitive and -resistant strains of *P. mirabilis* were similar and it was proposed that lipid content was not important in polymyxin resistance. They postulated the presence of a wall (periplasmic factor responsible for polymyxin resistance. These workers did not distinguish between wall lipid and cytoplasmic membrane lipid and their findings are compatible with the hypothesis of Brown & Watkins (1970). However, a strong interaction between surface phospholipid and drug has been used to explain drug resistance in the case of penicillin (Padfield & Kellaway, 1973) and viomycin (MacKenzie & Jordan, 1970). In these cases strong surface interaction was proposed as the reason why the drug remained at the surface without penetration to inner sensitive sites. This is discussed later in this chapter in terms of ideal drug lipophilicity.

Polymyxin/lipopolysaccharide specificity. The general evidence above regarding polymyxin/wall interaction implicates the LPS as a possible receptor for polymyxin. Teuber & Bader (1972), Teuber (1973) and Bader & Teuber (1973) have suggested the specific involvement of the lipid A region of the LPS in the penetration of polymyxin B to its main site of action. These workers found that about 0·5 moles polymyxin were bound per mole phosphate and that electrostatic and hydrophobic bonds were probably involved (as also suggested by work reported above for polymyxin/phospholipid interaction).

Specificity of EDTA action on P. aeruginosa. Sensitivity to EDTA is characteristic of a range of Gram-negative species, but is remarkable in the case of *P. aeruginosa*. Furthermore, non-toxic concentrations render the organism permeable to a variety of agents. Treatment by EDTA makes *P. aeruginosa* osmotically fragile to an exceptional degree. Leive (1974) has remarked on this action of EDTA alone resembling that of EDTA plus lysozyme on the walls of other Gram-negative bacteria. The mode of action is described in detail in Chapter 5 (see also Chapter 4 as well as Leive, 1974). Only a brief comment is necessary here. The LPS core polysaccharide of *P. aeruginosa* is characteristically highly substituted by polyphosphate residues with metal-binding capacity. It seems likely that this polyphosphate-rich core is located at the outer surface of the outer membrane and the binding to other membrane components (e.g. proteins and phospholipids) by cation bridges is important for stability. EDTA treatment extracts these cations and releases a complex of protein and lipopolysaccharide (Chapter 4). It is of interest to note that cations are important in the structure both of phospholipids (Rand & Sengupta, 1972) and of lipopolysaccharides (see Chapter 5).

Brown & Melling (1969b) have reported on the striking similarity of the changes in sensitivity both to polymyxin and EDTA by growth in low magnesium concentrations. Either a relationship between their sites of action or else one common site was suggested. Further, unpublished, work showed similar effects on growth in low-phosphate media. The possibility of a common site in the outer membrane seems compatible with these findings. Thus, the specificity of action of both these agents might be explained by an initial action on a common *P. aeruginosa*-specific structure.

It is tempting to identify the possible polymyxin-combining polyphosphate loci of Newton referred to above at least partly with the polyphosphate-rich core of the lipid A and associated cation bridges sensitive to EDTA. The work of Bader & Teuber (1973) showing LPS lipid A affinity for polymyxin is of interest in this context. After an initial site on the outer membrane (lipid A or phospholipid), the main target for polymyxin is the cytoplasmic membrane (phospholipid). The initial site may coicide with that of the prime EDTA site.

Specificity of antagonism of antimicrobial action by cations. Zimelis & Jackson (1973) found a species-specific antagonism by cations for aminoglycoside activity against *P. aeruginosa*. Using carbenicillin-induced spheroplasts it was also shown that divalent cations exerted their antagonism only in the presence of the intact wall (see also Chapter 2). A similar specificity for *P. aeruginosa* has also been indicated for polymyxin antagonism by cations (Newton, 1953, 1954; Davis, Iannetta & Wedgwood, 1971). HsuChen & Feinfold (1972) also proposed that divalent cation antagonism of polymyxin action occurred via a wall effect and not at the cytoplasmic membrane. The classic study by Newton (1954) involved the use of a fluorescent dye technique to investigate competition between polymyxin and various cations for sites on saline-washed cells of *P. aeruginosa*. He compared the affinities of the various cations for the polymyxin-combining groups of the cells with the ability of these ions to reverse the charge on certain types of colloids after the manner of Bungenburg de Jong (1949). There was a close relationship between the cation sequence for the reversal of charge on 'phosphate colloid' and the affinities of these ions for the polymyxin-combining groups of saline-washed cells of *P. aeruginosa*.

This was indicative of a combination of polymyxin with phosphate groups near the surface. Uranyl ion (UO_2^{2+}) was exceptional in forming a relatively undissociated complex with the cells so that polymyxin did not combine with uranyl-treated cells even after long exposure to the antibiotic. Uranyl ion could be removed by washing only by polymerized phosphates (e.g. sodium hex-ametaphosphate, sodium pyrophosphate) and not by inorganic phosphate. On the basis of this work it was suggested that the polymyxin-combining loci of the cell surface may be polyphosphates. This hypothesis received indirect support from the work of Rothstein & Larrabee (1948) and Rothstein & Meier (1951). They also found that uranyl ions formed a very undissociated complex at the surface of yeast cells, probably with phosphate polymers. Newton (1954), in using his fluorescent dye technique, assumed that polymyxin altered cell permeability and allowed the dye to penetrate into the cell where it combined with cell protein. As discussed above in the section on the Gram-reaction, any retrospective interpretation should consider the possibility of dye also combining with protein at an external site such as the wall outer membrane as a result of polymyxin disruption of that layer. Nevertheless, in view of the work of HsuChen & Feingold (1972) and of Zimelis & Jackson (1973), a new hypothesis would be that polymyxin combines with polyphosphates on the outer-surface of the wall outer membrane. Subsequently, the major disruptive effects take place at the cytoplasmic membrane involving phospholipids.

Interaction with non-ionic surfactants.   Brown & Richards (1964) and Brown (1966) found that the sensitivity of *P. aeruginosa* to various drugs was enhanced by the non-ionic surface active agent polyoxyethylene sorbitan mono-oleate (polysorbate 80). This effect was more pronounced for *P. aeruginosa* than for *E. coli*. Polysorbate 80 alone (up to about 5%) had no measurable effect on growth rate or lysis. *P. aeruginosa* is especially sensitive to cold shock (Gorrill & McNeil, 1960; Farrell & Rose, 1968). This effect, probably involving the outer membrane (Costerton *et al.*, 1974), is enhanced by contact with polysorbate 80; indeed this surfactant enhanced the effects of rapid changes of temperature, pH and tonicity on cell leakage and viability of *P. aeruginosa* (Brown & Winsley, 1969). Evidence from dye penetration studies (referred to in the section on the basis for the Gram-reaction) suggested that the effects of polysorbate 80 included disrupting the outer layers of the envelope. Further work showing synergism between polymyxin and polysorbate 80 with respect to leakage, lysis and death of cells supported this suggestion (Brown & Winsley, 1971). Birdsell & Cota-Robles (1968) found that the non-ionic surfactant Triton X-100 lysed spheroplasts of *E. coli*. More recently, polysorbate 80 was found to be an effective lytic agent against spheroplasts of *P. aeruginosa* (Brown, 1974). The lytic activity was additive with respect to polymyxin. This is unlike the effect with *P. aeruginosa* whole cells referred to above, which was synergistic.

The precise mechanism of action of non-ionic agents is probably complex. Polysorbate 80 has been shown to alter lipopolysaccharide, probably by penetrating into the hydrophobic region of the molecule (Shands, 1971). Schnaitman (1971a) found that Triton X-100 selectively extracted proteins of the cytoplasmic membrane but not of the wall of *E. coli*. Schnaitman (1971b) also found that Triton X-100 (with or without EDTA) extracted phospholipid and LPS lipid A from the cell wall of *E. coli*.

In this later paper it was shown that whereas EDTA alone did not release any protein from the Triton-insoluble wall fraction, re-extraction with Triton X-100 in the presence of EDTA resulted in substantial solubilization of cell wall protein. The amount solubilized ranged from about 35 to 50% of the total wall protein and was not increased by repeated extraction attempts. These results are similar to those of other workers. The outer membrane isolated from *E. coli* was found to be resistant to Triton X-100 (De Pamphilis & Adler, 1971). However, Triton X-100 together with EDTA completely disaggregated the outer membrane of *E. coli* (De Pamphilis, 1971). Thus, divalent cations were thought to stabilize the cell wall, perhaps by forming cation bridges between the phosphate groups in the LPS core and charged groups on adjacent proteins or phospholipids.

The influence of non-ionic surfactant type on the movement of a drug across a membrane(s) has been studied by Gillan & Florence (1973). Although goldfish were used as a model system, the results may have relevance to bacteria. Not all non-ionics enhanced drug absorption. Increase in drug absorption rate appeared to be related to the configuration of the surfactant molecule rather than the hydrophile–lipophile balance or surface activity. The effectiveness of the non-ionic surfactants in enhancing drug penetration was related to the ease with which the surfactant penetrated lipid membranes.

Middle of Outer Membrane

The hydrophobic middle of the outer membrane is composed mainly of lipids which are readily extractable with chloroform–methanol mixtures. They consist mainly of the tails of phospholipids penetrating from both surfaces of the outer membrane and include free fatty acids and neutral lipids. In *E. coli* about half the cell phospholipid is in the wall (Schnaitman, 1971b). In addition the lipid A extends into the membrane, probably anchoring the LPS. As indicated earlier, the outer membrane contains protein which differs from that of the cytoplasmic membrane. The position is still being clarified (see Chapter 4). Schnaitman (1971b) suggested that the major force holding the wall together is a hydrophobic interaction between the various protein components. Protein from *E. coli* walls showed a very strong tendency towards aggregation into regular lamella structures even in the absence of native lipid and LPS and in the presence of Triton X-100.

In terms of resistance by an exclusion mechanism, the middle of the outer membrane is thus essentially a hydrophobic zone. Earlier in this chapter, in the section on lipid and resistance, it was proposed that the enormous literature on this subject is perhaps most usefully considered in terms of the envelope structures. Already considered is the high affinity of different drugs for specific lipids. It is now proposed to consider the role in exclusion of the hydrophobic membrane layer. Much of the evidence will also apply to the hydrophobic layer of the cytoplasmic membrane.

The nature of the fatty acid composition of cells has been correlated with resistance. It is clearly established that the nature of the fatty acid composition of membranes, such as chain length and degree of unsaturation, profoundly affects membrane stability and function. A relatively small increase in unsaturation can significantly lower the melting point of the lipids (Lyons & Asmundson, 1965). Dunnick & O'Leary (1970) found that although the amount of whole cell REL was the same for a variety of antibiotic-sensitive and -resistant Gram-negative bacteria, the fatty acid composition was different. Three types of fatty acid extracts from Gram-negative whole cells were studied: fatty acids collected after alkaline hydrolysis of whole cells, fatty acids of REL lipids and fatty acids of phosphatidylethanolamine fractions. In all fatty acid extracts from the antibiotic-resistant Gram-negative organisms there was a higher concentration of unsaturated acids and a lower concentration of cyclopropane acids than was found in corresponding extracts from sensitive organisms. The difference was not observed between sensitive and resistant Gram-positive bacteria. Anderes, Sandine & Elliker (1971) compared the whole cell lipid content of antibiotic-sensitive and -resistant strains of *P. aeruginosa* grown in a variety of ways. They found that increased whole cell lipid apparently was not necessary for resistance, although unsaturated fatty acids increased in both phospholipid and free fatty acid fractions of whole cells resistant to a quaternary ammonium compound and similar results occurred with a culture resistant to chloramphenicol. An interesting observation was that the growth temperature significantly affected lipid composition of *P. aeruginosa*. Although this phenomenon is well established (Farrell & Rose, 1968; Patching & Rose, 1971) it is nevertheless significant from the point of view of the potentially very varied growth temperatures of organisms in factory or hospital which might contaminate pharmaceutical preparations or infect wounds.

Sud & Feingold (1970) found that the fatty acid contents of polymyxin-sensitive and -resistant *Proteus mirabilis* were the same. Furthermore, liposomes prepared from the lipids of both organisms were sensitive to polymyxin B. Subsequently, HsuChen & Feingold (1973) and Feingold, HsuChen & Sud (1974) proposed that polymyxin-sensitive membranes require both the presence of specific 'target' phospholipids such as phosphatidylethanolamine and a threshold density of these molecules on the membrane surface. Vaczi (1973) found, in general, that in antibiotic-sensitive bacteria unsaturated fatty acids are more common than in resistant bacteria. Nevertheless, *P. aeruginosa* contained substantially more unsaturated fatty acids than the other Gram-negative resistant strains tested. Surdy & Hartsell (1963) found a correlation between lack of unsaturated fatty acids and resistance to lysozyme for *Achromobacter*. An increase in unsaturation of the fatty acids of the outer membrane leads to enhanced penetration by lysozyme as well as to facilitated release of periplasmic enzymes after osmotic shock (Rosen & Hackette, 1972). Generalizations about antibiotic-resistant bacteria, although useful in some circumstances, can be dangerous if the resistance is not defined precisely. Brown, Fenton & Watkins (1972) reported that trained polymyxin-resistant cultures of *P. aeruginosa* were cross-resistant to carbenicillin, gentamicin and several membrane-active agents. However, they showed increased sensitivity to tetracycline. These polymixin-resistant, tetracycline-sensitive *P aeruginosa* cultures had previously been shown to have an altered lipid composition, notably in the wall. Thus, whatever correlations occurred between lipid (i.e. outer or inner membrane) composition and polymyxin resistance, the inverse correlation existed for tetracyline resistance with these bacteria cultured and tested under the conditions specified. Similarly, Adair, Geftic, Gelzer & Hoffman (1971) found that benzalkonium-resistant *P. aeruginosa* became more sensitive to lysis by sodium lauryl sulphate.

Chemical antimicrobial agents penetrate through the cell envelope by either passive or facilitated diffusion. The majority of agents gain access by passive diffusion, in some cases enhancing penetration by membrane damage (Franklin, 1973). It seems likely that, for Gram-negative bacteria in general, the outer membrane does not carry out active transport (Costerton *et al.*, 1974).

The rate at which low molecular weight organic non-electrolytes diffuse across biological membranes correlates with their lipid–water partition coefficient, within limits. Tute (1971), in his introduction to a review on Hansch analysis, discusses the early work correlating high drug partition coefficient with narcotic activity. Positive correlations occurred until lipid solubility was so high that the drug was virtually insoluble in water and narcotic activity was reduced. Modern quantitative approaches to structure activity correlations are well reviewed by Hansch (1973). Detailed consideration is inappropriate in the present context. Nevertheless, the large number of structure activity correlations studied permit at least one generalization similar to that about narcotic activity made by early workers. Lien, Hansch & Anderson (1968) studied a large range of mainly membrane-active antibacterial agents for activity against Gram-positive and Gram-negative bacteria. They found that the ideal lipophilic character ($\log P_0$) for a set of congeneric drugs was much higher for Gram-positive bacteria (about 6) than for Gram-negative bacteria (about 4). This difference was attributed to the relatively lipid-rich wall of Gram-negative bacteria which retained lipophilic drugs and hindered penetration. A similar concept was proposed earlier, where high affinity between drug and external phospholipid was a possible cause of non-penetration.

Penicillins offer an interesting series for study in this context since the target enzymes are located outside the cytoplasmic membrane. Barber (1962) suggested that penicillin resistance may be due to 'intrinsic resistance' rather than penicillinase production. The work of Strominger and co-workers has indicated that the insensitivity of *E. coli* to penicillin G is due to lack of penetration to an otherwise sensitive target (Izaki, Matsuhashi & Strominger, 1966). Furthermore, ampicillin sensitivity is perhaps related to ease of penetration (Strominger, Izaki & Matsuhashi, 1967). It seems likely that a feature of the activity of carbenicillin against *P. aeruginosa* is relative access to its target. Conversely, carbenicillin resistance in *P. aeruginosa* may be related in many cases to lack of penetration (Brumfitt, Percival & Leigh, 1967; Smith & Finland, 1968; Watanakunakorn, Phair & Hamburger, 1970; Garber &

Friedman, 1970; Bobrowski & Borowski, 1971; Thomas & Broadbridge, 1972; Rosselet & Zimmerman, 1973). Curtis, Richmond & Stanisich (1973) found that a variant of R-factor RP1 (originally detected in *P. aeruginosa* strain 1822) specified penicillin resistance by a mechanism other than enzyme destruction. The hydrolytic activities of the neutral β-lactamases produced by *P. aeruginosa* NCTC 8203 and NCTC 10490 for different penicillins were related to the degree of the hydrophobic nature of these antibiotics, i.e. cephaloridine > benzylpenicillin > ampicillin (Thomas & Broadbridge, 1972). The least hydrophobic antibiotic, carbenicillin, was not hydrolysed. It may well be that the degree of the hydrophobic nature of the penicillin molecule may also profoundly affect penetration to the site of action. Biagi, Guerra, Barbaro & Gamba (1970) studied the activity of a series of cephalosporins and penicillins against *E. coli, Staph. aureus* and *Treponema pallidum*. The compounds most active against *E. coli* were more hydrophilic than those most active against *Staph. aureus*. This was also (cf. Lien *et al.*, 1968 above) attributed to the retention of the lipophilic drugs by the relatively lipid-rich wall of *E. coli. T. pallidum*, which lacks a cell wall, behaved in a similar manner to *Staph. aureus*. The introduction of a hydrophilic α side-chain has been shown to increase the Gram-negative activity of the penicillin molecule (Nayler, 1971).

It would thus seem, for Gram-negative bacteria, that high affinity by a drug either for specific external envelope molecules (e.g. LPS carbohydrate) or lipid in general, could result in lack of penetration. On the other hand, some degree of affinity for a surface layer could assist uptake and provide a concentrating effect which could enhance penetration.

Internal Layer of Outer Membrane

The layer between the hydrophobic zone and the periplasmic space resembles that of the external layer (Figures 1 and 2). Thus protein, LPS oligosaccharides and phospholipid heads probably form a similar structural barrier. The model of the Gram-negative outer membrane proposed by Leive (1974), however, omits LPS from the internal surface. There is little evidence about the role of this surface in terms of drug resistance. It would seem reasonable to assume that specific component–drug interaction would contribute to ease or difficulty of penetration depending on affinity, as discussed above.

Periplasmic Zone

The function of this zone is discussed in detail elsewhere (Costerton, Ingram & Cheng, 1974; Meadow, 1974). Its role in terms of enzyme inactivation of antibiotics has been referred to earlier in this chapter and also more fully in Chapter 1. Of interest is the presence of periplasmic lipoprotein linking the inner surface of the outer membrane to the structurally robust peptidoglycan layer. There is evidence that *P. aeruginosa* contains less bound lipoprotein than in *E. coli* (Meadow, 1974). Wilkinson (Chapter 5) points out that various EDTA-sensitive bacteria may contain less lipoprotein than EDTA-resistant strains. These observations may explain the relative fragility of *Pseudomonad* walls (see, however, Chapter 4).

If one assumes the periplasmic zone to extend between the two membranes, then the passage of drugs is essentially across an aqueous phase containing some potentional drug-binding molecules (e.g. protein and peptidoglycan). Although the lipoprotein may play a role in stabilizing the outer membrane (perhaps a typically small role for *P. aeruginosa*), there seems little evidence that the periplasmic zone significantly hinders drug penetration.

Peptidoglycan Layer

There is some evidence that this layer may constitute a penetration barrier. Burman, Nordström & Bloom (1972) found that the sensitivity of *P. aeruginosa* Ps 18S to the membrane-active agent sodium cholate was markedly enhanced by prior growth in the presence of benzylpenicillin. Similar results were obtained with *E. coli* (also with lysozyme) and *Proteus mirabilis*. These workers have suggested that this layer may act as a molecular sieve and may also act as a foundation for outer wall layers. Gustafsson, Nordström & Normark (1973) showed that growth in the presence of lysozyme and sub-lethal concentrations of penicillin increased the rate of uptake of gentian violet. It would seem likely that these results are the consequence of peptidoglycan damage exerting an indirect effect on the outer membrane. Nevertheless, these authors also suggested that peptidoglycan may itself constitute a drug penetration barrier. Because of the interdependence of the peptidoglycan layer and the outer membrane Costerton, Ingram & Cheng (1974) have emphasized the danger of drawing conclusions from studies in which specific wall layers are destroyed by digestion.

In conclusion, it would seem unlikely that the peptidoglycan layer directly constitutes a penetration barrier significantly contributing to drug resistance.

Cytoplasmic Membrane

The limited available evidence suggests that the cytoplasmic membrane of *P. aeruginosa* is characteristically similar to that in other bacteria, Gram-negative and Gram-positive, in structure, composition and function (Meadow, 1974). The protein composition varies from that of the outer membrane and there is no lipopolysaccharide. The role of specific phospholipids in drug sensitivity has been discussed earlier, as has the role of the hydrophobic zone in general. Membrane composition will vary to some extent, depending on genotype and environment: this will obviously affect permeability to drugs. There have been some reports of the cytoplasmic membrane of *P. aeruginosa* acting as a drug barrier. Cheng, Costerton, Singh & Ingram (1973) obtained such evidence for Actinomycin D. Nevertheless, in view of the general evidence reported earlier for drug sensitivity in the absence of the wall, it seems unlikely that the cytoplasmic membrane is characteristically the major drug penetration barrier for *P. aeruginosa* or other Gram-negative bacteria. This is not to say that reports of changes in cell lipid content associated with resistance do not in some cases reflect changes in the lipid composition of the cytoplasmic membrane. As indicated earlier, in the case of Gram-positive bacteria, the location of such lipid changes has rarely been studied.

CONCLUSIONS

The available evidence outlined above overwhelmingly implicates the envelope of Gram-negative bacteria as having a crucial role in resistance. The envelope contributes to resistance by target alteration, by contributing to the efficiency of drug-inactivating enzymes and by drug exclusion. The contribution of the outer membrane to these mechanisms seems crucial. The outer membrane allows an enhanced degree of specificity in the movement of compounds between the Gram-negative cell and its environment. In particular, it characteristically affords a protection against many antibiotics and preservatives and *in vivo* protects against body defence mechanisms.

Genetic and environmental influences profoundly affect the structure and composition of the envelope and hence the resistance of *P. aeruginosa* as they do for Gram-negative bacteria in general. Nevertheless, several features stand out in seeking an explanation of the pre-eminence of *P. aeruginosa* as a drug-resistant pathogen and spoilage organism. There are some resistance properties of *P. aeruginosa* which, although shared by some Gram-negative bacteria, seem *characteristically* highly specific for the organism (i.e. under pre-determined enviromental circumstances). These properties are especially the species-specific sensitivity to EDTA and to polymyxin. Significant to a lesser extent is the species-specific antagonism by some cations of certain drugs and also the sensitizing effects of non-ionic surfactants. Furthermore, the mechanism of these effects seems related to certain structural features characteristic of the envelope, especially the outer membrane of *P. aeruginosa*.

The outer membrane of *P. aeruginosa* appears to be relatively labile, possibly due to relative lack of lipoprotein acting as an anchor to the peptidoglycan. The peptidoglycan fraction also appears characteristically low. The lability of the outer membrane may be related to the exceptional sensitivity of *P. aeruginosa* to rapid changes of temperature, pH or tonicity: these effects being enhanced by non-ionic surfactants. A characteristic feature of the stability of the outer membrane is the reliance on cation bridges, probably linking the exceptionally polyphosphate-rich LPS core polysaccharide to other components such as proteins or phospholipids at the surface(s) of the outer membrane. Although similar links occur in other Gram-negative bacteria, there are significant differences as indicated by the action of EDTA (see earlier and Chapter 5). The contribution of protein to the special nature of the outer membrane of *P. aeruginosa* has yet to be established.

In addition to the affinity of polymyxin for specific phospholipids, it has an affinity for the lipid A of the LPS. Consequently, the point of attachment of the LPS to the surface(s) outer membrane, probably involving lipid A, could well be the first site of action both by EDTA and polymyxin. The work reported above, about the action of Triton X-100, alone and with EDTA, on the wall supports the idea of cation bridges between phosphate groups on the LPS core and charged groups on adjacent proteins or phospholipids. The LPS may not attach to the outer membrane solely by cation bridges (Leive, 1974). Nevertheless, the apparently linked change in sensitivity both to EDTA and to polymyxin upon magnesium (and phosphate) depletion by cultures of *P. aeruginosa* suggest a common *P. aeruginosa*-specific initial site(s) of action. Conversely, lack of sensitivity by other Gram-negative species suggests lack of such a site. A temptation to find a single, unifying hypothesis leads to the idea that the *P. aeruginosa*-specific antagonism by cations involves the same characteristic EDTA/polymyxin sensitive LPS-attachment site on the surface(s) of the outer membrane. It would be helpful to know the spectrum of envelope changes brought about by both genetic *and environmental* influences for *P. aeruginosa*. More work is needed in correlating the chemical structure of the envelope and the spectrum of drug sensitivity for such envelope variants. Such work will illuminate part of the way ahead for advances in chemotherapy. One might hope that the production of a 'drug resistant' variant, (i.e. relative to one or more drugs) due to a mechanism of exclusion, might simultaneously render the cell more 'drug sensitive' to another agent(s) of appropriate chemical structure. Despite the attraction of a unifying hypothesis, it is nevertheless prudent to consider, in conclusion, other relevant characteristics which may contribute to the difficulties of combating *P. aeruginosa* in a wide variety of *in vivo* and *in vitro* situations. The organism is widely distributed, grows over a wide temperature range with simple nutrient requirements and may be regarded as a permanent potential hazard. Disregarding any mechanisms of drug exclusion, *P. aeruginosa* secretes metabolites *in vivo* which inhibit phagocytosis, attack leucocytes, destroy tissue and reduce the inflammatory response. The special genetic features of *P. aeruginosa*, controlling the production of antibiotic-inactivating enzymes, have been described earlier in Chapter 1, and extend to the capacity to inactivate a wide variety of preservatives and disinfectants. Thus, under the selective pressure of drugs, strains arise with decreased sensitivity to the drug by mechanisms of exclusion or inactivation or both.

On the basis of available evidence, the general phenomenon of *P. aeruginosa* drug resistance is complex and involves the whole variety of characteristics outlined. These characteristics are qualitatively typical of Gram-negative bacteria in general. The very distinguishing character of Gram-negative bacteria involves relatively little dye penetration into the cell. It is difficult not to conclude that this same barrier to dyes is also responsible for lack of drug penetration. Thus, in summary, the resistance of *P. aeruginosa* is closely related to its complex Gram-negative character, especially its Gram-negative envelope with outer membrane. An outstanding characteristic feature of the

Gram-negative outer membrane is the lipopolysaccharide. The outstanding feature of the outer membrane of *P. aeruginosa* is the characteristic cation links between the exceptionally polyphosphate-rich LPS core polysaccharide and other components. There is thus a certain simplicity about the idea of *P. aeruginosa* owing the special nature of its complex Gram-negative resistance characteristics mainly to the special nature of the structure of its outer membrane involving its lipopolysaccharide.

REFERENCES

Adair, F. W., Geftic, S. G., Gelzer, J. & Hoffmann, H-P. (1971). Effect of a hostile environment on *Pseudomonas aeruginosa*. *Transactions N.Y. Acad. Sci. Series II*, **33**, 799–813.

Anderes, E. A., Sandine, W. E. & Elliker, P. R. (1971). Lipids of antibiotic-sensitive and -resistant strains of *Pseudomonas aeruginosa*. *Can. J. Microbiol.*, **17**, 1357–1365.

Anderson, J. S., Matsuhashi, M., Haskin, M. A. & Strominger, J. L. (1967). Biosynthesis of the peptidoglycan of bacterial cell walls II. Phospholipid carriers in the reaction sequences. *J. Biol. Chem.*, **242**, 3180–3190.

Asbell, M. A. & Eagon, R. G. (1966a). The role of multivalent cations in the organization and structure of bacterial cell walls. *Biochem. Biophys. Res. Commun.*, **22**, 664–671.

Asbell, M. A. & Eagon, R. G. (1966b). Role of multivalent cations in the organization structure and assembly of the cell wall of *Pseudomonas aeruginosa*. *J. Bacteriol.*, **92**, 380–387.

Bader, J. & Teuber, M. (1973). Action of polymyxin B on bacterial membranes, I. Binding to the O-Antigenic lipopolysaccharide of *Salmonella typhimurium*. *Z. Naturforsch*, **23c**, 422–430.

Barber, M. (1962). Resistance of bacteria to the penicillins, in *CIBA Foundation Study Group*, (Eds. A. V. S. de Reuck & M. P. Cameron), J. & A. Churchill, London, p. 89.

Barrett-Bee, K., Radda, G. K. & Thomas, N. A. (1972). Interactions, perturbations and relaxations of membrane-bound molecules. *Mitochondria/Biomembranes*, North-Holland, Amsterdam.

Bartell, P. F., Orr, T. E. & Chudio, B. (1970). Purification and chemical composition of the protective slime antigen of *Pseudomonas aeruginosa*. *Infect. immun.*, **2**, 543–548.

Beer, H., Staehelin, T., Douglas, H. & Braude, A. (1965). Relationship between particle size and biological activity of *E. coli*. bovin endotoxin. *J. Clin. Invest.*, **44**, 592–602.

Biagi, G. L., Guerra, M. C., Barbaro, A. M. & Gamba, M. F. (1970). Influence of lipophilic character on the antibacterial activity of cephalosporins and penicillins. *J. Med. Chem.*, **13**, 511–516.

Birdsell, D. C. & Cota-Robles, E. H. (1968). Lysis of spheroplasts of *E. coli* by a non-ionic detergent. *Biochem. Biophys. Res. Commun.*, **31**, 438–446.

Biswas, K. & Mukerjee, S. (1967). Studies on the mechanism of action of polymyxin on *Cholera vibrio*. *Proc. Soc. Expl. Biol. Med.*, **126**, 103.

Bobrowski, M. & Borowski, E. (1971). Interaction between carbenicillin and β-Lactamases from Gram-negative bacteria. *J. gen. Microbiol.*, **68**, 263–272.

Boman, H. G., Nordström, K. & Normak, S. (1974). Penicillin resistance in *Escherichia Coli* K12: Synergism between penicillinases and a barrier in the outer part of the envelope. *Annals N.Y. Acad. Sci.*, **235**, 569–586.

Bonde, G. J., Jensen, C. E. & Thamsen, J. (1957). Studies on a water soluble, fluorescing bacterial pigment which depolymerises hyaluronic acid. *Acta. pharmacol. toxicol.*, **13**, 184–193.

Brown, M. R. W. (1966). Turbidimetric method for the rapid evaluation of anti-microbial agents. Inactivation of preservatives by non-ionic agents. *J. Soc. Cosmetic Chem.*, **17**, 185–195.

Brown, M. R. W. (1971). Inhibition and destruction of *Pseudomonas aeruginosa*. In *Inhibition and Destruction of the Microbial Cell*, (Ed. W. B. Hugo), Academic Press, London, p. 357.

Brown, M. R. W. (1972). Antibiotic resistance in *Pseudomonas aeruginosa*: surface layers. *J. gen. Microbiol.*, **73**, v–vi.

Brown, M. R. W. (1974). Effect of sodium dodecylsulphate, sodium deoxycholate, polymyxin B sulphate and Tween 80 on lysis of whole cells and spheroplasts of *Pseudomonas aeruginosa. Polish Academy of Science Monograph*, **1**, 13–14.

Brown, M. R. W. & Anderson, R. A. (1968). The bactericidal effect of silver ions on *Pseudomonas aeruginosa. J. Pharm. Pharmac.*, **20**, Suppl. 1S–3S.

Brown, M. R. W., Clamp, J. R. & Foster, J. H. S. (1966). The presence of hyaluronic acid in the extracellular slime of *Pseudomonas aeruginosa. J. gen. Microbiol.*, **45**, v.

Brown, M. R. W., Fenton, E. M. & Watkins, W. M. (1972). Tetracycline-sensitive/polymyxin-resistant *Pseudomonas aeruginosa. Lancet*, **ii**, 86.

Brown, M. R. W., Foster, J. H. S. & Clamp, J. R. (1969). Composition of *Pseudomonas aeruginosa* slime. *Biochem. J.*, **112**, 521–525.

Brown, M. R. W. & Melling, J. (1969a). Loss of sensitivity to EDTA by *Pseudomonas aeruginosa* grown under conditions of Mg-limitation. *J. gen Microbiol.*, **54**, 439–444.

Brown, M. R. W. & Melling, J. (1969b). Role of divalent cations in the action of polymyxin B and EDTA on *Pseudomonas aeruginosa. J. gen. Microbiol.*, **59**, 263–274.

Brown, M. R. W. & Richards, R. M. E. (1964). Effect of polysorbate 80 on the resistance of *Pseudomonas aeruginosa* to chemical inactivation. *J. Pharm. Pharmac.*, **16**, Suppl. 51T–55T.

Brown, M. R. W. & Scott Foster, J. H. (1971). Effect of slime on the sensitivity of *Pseudomonas aeruginosa* to EDTA and polymyxin. *J. Pharm. Pharmac.*, **23**, Suppl. 236S.

Brown, M. R. W. & Winsley, B. E. (1969). Effect of polysorbate 80 on cell leakage and viability of *Pseudomonas aeruginosa* exposed to rapid changes of pH, temperature and tonicity. *J. gen. Microbiol.*, **56**, 99–107.

Brown, M. R. W. & Winsley, B. E. (1971). Synergism between polymyxin and polysorbate 80 against *Pseudomonas aeruginosa. J. gen. Microbiol.*, **68**, 367–373.

Brown, M. R. W. & Watkins, W. M. (1970). Low magnesium and phospholipid content of cell walls of *Pseudomonas aeruginosa* resistant to polymyxin. *Nature*, **227**, 1360–1361.

Brown, M. R. W. & Wood, S. M. (1971). Effects of drying on polymyxin sensitivity of *Pseudomonas aeruginosa. J. Pharm. Pharmac.*, **23**, Suppl. 235S–236S.

Brown, M. R. W. & Wood, S. M. (1972). Relation between cation and lipid content of cell walls of *Pseudomonas aeruginosa, Proteus vulgaris* and *Klebsiella aerogenes* and their sensitivity to polymyxin B and other antibacterial agents. *J. Pharm. Pharmac.*, **24**. 215–218.

Brumfitt, W., Percival, A. & Leigh, D. A. (1967). Clinical and laboratory studies with carbenicillin. *Lancet*, **i**, 1289–1293.

Bungenburg de Jong, H. G. (1949). Reversal of charge phenomena, equivalent weight and specific properties of the ionized groups. *Colloid Science*, (Ed. H. R. Kruyt), vol. II, Elsevier, London, p. 259.

Burke, V. & Barnes, M. W. (1929). The cell wall and the Gram reaction. *J. Bacteriol.*, **18**, 69–92.

Burman, L. G., Nordström, K. & Bloom, G. D. (1972). Murein and the outer penetration barrier of *Escherichia coli* K-12, *Proteus mirabilis* and *Pseudomonas aeruginosa. J. Bacteriol.*, **112**, 1364–1374.

Carlson, D. M. & Matthews, L. W. (1966). Polyuronic acids produced by *Pseudomonas aeruginosa*. *Biochemistry*, **5**, 2817–2822.

Carson, K. J. & Eagon, R. G. (1966). Lysozyme sensitivity of the cell wall of *Pseudomonas aeruginosa*: further evidence for the role of the non-peptidoglycan components in cell wall rigidity. *Can. J. Microbiol.*, **12**, 105–108.

Cerny, G. & Teuber, M. (1971). Differential release of periplasmic versus cytoplasmic enzymes from *Escherichia coli* B by polymyxin. *B. Arch. Mikrobiol.*, **78**, 166–179.

Cetin, E. T., Töreci, K. & Ang, Ö. (1965). Encapsulated *Pseudomonas aeruginosa* (*P. aeruginosa* mucosus) strains. *J. Bacteriol.*, **89**, 1432–1434.

Cheng, K. G., Costerton, J. W., Singh, A. P. & Ingram, J. M. (1973). Susceptibility of whole cells and spheroplasts of *Pseudomonas aeruginosa* to Actinomycin D. *Antimicrob. Ag. Chemother.*, **3**, 399–406.

Clarke, K., Gray, G. W. & Reaveley, D. A. (1967). The extraction of cell walls of *Pseudomonas aeruginosa* with aqueous phenol. The insoluble residue and material from the aqueous layers. *Biochem. J.*, **105**, 759–765.

Costerton, J. W. (1970). The structure and function of the cell envelope of Gram-negative bacteria. *Rev. Can. Biol.*, **29**, 299–316.

Costerton, J. W., Ingram, J. M. & Cheng, K.-J. (1974). Structure and function of the cell envelope of Gram-negative bacteria. *Bact. Revs.*, **38**, 87–110.

Cox, S. T. & Eagon, R. G. (1968). Action of EDTA, tris and lysozyme on cell walls of *Pseudomonas aeruginosa*. *Can. J. Microbiol.*, **14**, 913–922.

Curtis, N. A. C., Richmond, M. H. & Stanisich, V. (1973). R-factor mediated resistance to penicillins which does not involve a β-Lactamase. *J. gen. Microbiol.*, **79**, 163–166.

Davis, S. D., Iannetta, A. & Wedgewood, R. J. (1971). Activity of colistin against *Pseudomonas aeruginosa*: inhibition by calcium. *J. Infect. dis.*, **124**, 610–612.

De Pamphilis, M. L. (1971). Dissociation and reassembly of *Escherichia coli* outer membrane and of lipopolysaccharide and their reassembly onto flagellar basal bodies. *J. Bacteriol.*, **105**, 1184–1199.

De Pamphilis, M. L. & Adler, J. (1971). Attachment of flagellar basal bodies to the cell envelope: specific attachment to the outer lipopolysaccharide membrane and cytoplasmic membrane, *J. Bacterial.*, **105**, 396–407.

Doggett, R. G., Harrison, G. M. & Wallis, E. S. (1964). Comparison of some properties of *Pseudomonas aeruginosa* isolated from infections in persons with and without cystic fibrosis. *J. Bacteriol.*, **87**, 427–431.

Dogget, R. G., Harrison, G. M., Stillwell, R. N. & Wallis, E. S. (1965). Antibody response to *Pseudomonas aeruginosa* infections associated with cystic fibrosis of the pancreas. *S. Med. J.*, **58**, 1595.

Dunnick, J. K. & O'Leary, W. M. (1970). Correlation of bacterial lipid composition with antibiotic resistance. *J. Bacteriol.*, **101**, p. 892–900.

Eagon, R. G. (1956). Studies on polysaccharide formation by *Pseudomonas fluorescens*. *Can. J. Microbiol.*, **2**, 673–676.

Eagon, R. G. (1962). Composition of an extracellular slime produced by *Pseudomonas aeruginosa*. *Can. J. Microbiol.*, **8**, 585–586.

Eagon, R. G. & Carson, K. J. (1965). Lysis of cell walls and intact cells of *Pseudomonas aeruginosa* by EDTA and by lysozyme. *Can. J. Microbiol.*, **11**, 193–201.

Eagon, R. G. & Randles, C. I. (1954). Production of a mannose polysaccharide by *Pseudomonas fluorescens* from low molecular weight carbon sources. *Bacteriol. Proc.*, p. 100.

Ellwood, D. C. & Tempest, D. W. (1972). Effects of environment on bacterial wall content and composition. *Advances in Microbiol Physiology*, **7**, 83–117.

Elston, H. R. & Hoffman, K. C. (1967). Increasing incidence of encapsulated *Pseudomonas aeruginosa* strains. *Am. J. Clin. Path.*, **48**, 519.

Ennis, H. L. & Bloomstein, M. I. (1974). Antibiotic-sensitive mutants of *Escherichia Coli* possess altered outer membranes. *Annals N. Y. Acad. Sci.*, **235**, 593–600.

Evans, L. R. & Linker, A. (1973). Production and characterization of the slime polysaccharide of *Pseudomonas aeruginosa. J. Bacteriol.*, **116**, 915–924.

Farrell, J. & Rose, A. H. (1967). Temperature effects in micro-organisms. In *Thermobiology*, (Ed. A. H. Rose), Academic Press, London, pp. 123–146.

Farrell, J. & Rose, A. H. (1968). Cold shock in a mesophilic and a psychrophilic Pseudomonad. *J. gen. Microbiol.*, **50**, 429–439.

Feingold, D. S., Hsuchen, C. C. & Sud, I. J. (1974). Basis for the selectivity of action of the polymyxin antibiotics on cell membranes. *Annals. N. Y. Acad. Sci.*, **235**, 480–492.

Few, A. V. (1955). The interaction of polymyxin E with bacterial and other lipids. *Biochim. Biophys. Acta.*, **16**, 137–145.

Few, A. V. & Schulman, J. H. (1953). The absorption of polymyxin E by bacteria and bacterial cell walls and its bactericidal action. *J. gen. Microbiol.*, **9**, 454–466.

Forge, A. & Costerton, J. W. (1973). The effects of phospholipid depletion on the cleavage pattern of the cell wall of frozen Gram-negative bacteria. *Can. J. Microbiol.*, **19**, 1056–1057.

Franklin, T. J. (1973). Antibiotic transport in bacteria. *CRC Crit. Rev. Microbiol.*, **2**, 253–272.

Gale, E. F., Cundliffe, E., Reynolds, P. E., Richmond, M. H. & Waring, M. J. (1972). *The Molecular Basis of Antibiotic Action*, John Wiley, London.

Garber, N. & Friedman, J. (1970). β-Lactamase and the resistance of *Pseudomonas aeruginosa* to various penicillin and cephalosporins. *J. gen. Microbiol.*, **64**, 343–352.

Gilardi, G. L. (1968). Diagnostic criteria for differentiation of Pseudomonads pathogenic for man. *Appl. Microbiol.*, **16**, 1497–1502.

Gillan, J. M. N. & Florence, A. T. (1973). The influence of non-ionic surfactant type on the transport of a drug across a biological membrane. *J. Pharm. Pharmac.*, Suppl. **25**, 136P–137P.

Gilleland, H. E., Stinnett, J. D. & Eagon, R. G. (1974). Ultrastructural and chemical alteration of the cell envelope of *Pseudomonas aeruginosa* associated with resistance to EDTA resulting from growth in a Mg^{2+}-deficient medium. *J. Bacteriol.*, **117**, 302–311.

Glauert, A. M. & Thornley, M. J. (1969). The topography of the bacterial cell wall. *Ann. Rev. Microbiol.*, **23**, 159–198.

Gorrill, R. H. & McNeil, E. M. (1960). The effect of cold diluent on the viable count of *Pseudomonas pyocyanea. J. gen. Microbiol.*, **22**, 437.

Gustafsson, P., Nordström, K. & Normark, S. (1973). Outer penetration barrier of *Escherichia* coli K-12: kinetics of the uptake of gentian violet by wild type and envelope mutants. *J. Bacteriol.*, **116**, 893–900.

Halleck, F. E., Durkin, M. A. & Guschlbauer, W. (1960). DNA-ases of two *Pseudomonas* cultures and their relation to slime production. *Bact. Prot.*, p. 100.

Hamilton, W. A. (1970). The mode of action of membrane active antibacterials. *FEBS Symposium*, **20**, 71–79.

Hamilton, W. A. (1974). Recent research on the action of antibiotics on microbial membranes. *Industrial Aspects of Biochem.*, (Ed. B. Spencer), Federation of European Biochemical Societies.

Hamilton-Miller, J. M. T. (1965). Modes of resistance to benzylpenicillin and ampicillin in twelve *Klebsiella* strains. *J. gen. Microbiol.*, **41**, 175–184.

Hansch, C. (1973). Quantitative approaches to pharmacological structure–activity relationships. In *Structure–Activity Relationships*, Vol. I, (Ed. C. J. Cavallito), Pergamon Press, London.

Henning, U., Höhn, B. & Sonntag, I. (1973). Cell envelope and shape of *Escherichia coli* K12. The ghost membrane. *Eur. J. Biochem.*, **39**, 27–36.

Hill, M. J., James, J. M. & Maxted, W. R. (1963). Some physical investigations of the behaviour of bacterial surfaces. The occurrence of lipid in the streptococcal cell wall. *Biochim. Biophys. Acta*, **75**, 414–424.

Holme, T. (1972). Influence of environment on the content and composition of bacterial envelopes. *J. appl. Chem. Biotechnol.*, **22**, 391–399.

HsuChen, C-C. & Feingold, D. S. (1972). Locus of divalent cation inhibition of the bactericidal action of polymyxin B. *Antimicrob. Agents. Chemother.*, **2**, 331–335.

HsuChen, C-C. & Feingold, D. S. (1973). The mechanism of polymyxin B action and selectivity toward biologic membranes. *Biochem.*, **12**, 2105–2111.

Hugo, W. B. (1967). The mode of action of antibacterial agents. *J. appl. Bact.*, **30**, 17–50.

Hugo, W. B. & Stretton, R. J. (1966). The role of cellular lipid in the resistance of Gram-positive bacteria to penicillins. *J. gen. Microbiol.*, **42**, 133–138.

Hurwitz, J., Furth, J. J., Malamy, M. & Alexander, M. (1962). The role of deoxyribonucleic acid in ribonucleic acid synthesis. III. The inhibition of the enzymatic synthesis of ribonucleic acid and deoxyribonucleic acid by antinomycin D and proflavin. *Proc. Nat. Acad. Sci. U.S.A.*, **48**, 1222–1230.

Ivanov, Von W., Markov, K. I., Golowinsky, E. & Charisanova, T. (1964). The importance of surface lipids for some biological properties of a *Pseudomonas aeruginosa* strain. *Z. Naturforschg.*, **19b**, 604–606.

Izaki, K., Matsuhashi, M. & Strominger, J. L. (1966). Glycopeptide transpeptidase and D-alanine carboxypeptidase; penicillin-sensitive enzymatic reactions. *Proc. Nat. Acad. Sci. U.S.A.*, **55**, 656–663.

Izaki, K., Matsuhashi, M. & Strominger, J. L. (1968). Biosynthesis of the peptidoglycan of bacterial cell walls. XIII. Peptidoglycan transpeptidase and D-alanine carboxypeptidase: penicillin sensitive enzymatic reactions in strains of *Escherichia coli. J. Biol. Chem.*, **243**, 3180–3192.

Klyhn, K. M. & Gorrill, R. H. (1967). Studies on the virulence of hospital strains of *Pseudomonas aeruginosa. J. gen. Microbiol.*, **47**, 227–235.

Koike, M. & Iida, K. (1971). Effect of polymyxin on the bacteriophage receptors of the cell walls of Gram-negative bacteria. *J. Bacteriol.*, **108**, 1402–1411.

Latterrade, C. & Macheboeuf, M. (1950). Recherches biochimiques sur le mode d'action de la polymyxine. *Ann. inst. Pasteur*, **78**, 753–758.

Leive, L. (1974). The barrier function of the Gram-negative envelope. *Annals. N.Y. Acad. Sci.*, **235**, 109–129.

Lien, E. J., Hansch, C. & Anderson, S. M. (1968). Structure-activity correlations for antibacterial agents of Gram-positive and Gram-negative cells. *J. Med. Chem.*, **11**, 430–441.

Lindberg, A. A. & Hellerquist, C. G. (1971). Bacteriophage attachment sites, serological specificity and chemical composition of the lipopolysaccharides of semirough and rough mutants of *Salmonella typhimurium. J. Bacteriol.*, **105**, 57–64.

Lindsay, S. S., Shelagh, S., Wheeler, B., Sanderson, K. E. & Costerton, J. W. (1973). The release of alkaline phosphates and of lipopolysaccharide during the growth of rough and smooth strains of *Salmonella typhimurium. Can. J. Microbiol.*, **19**, 335–343.

Linker, A. & Jones, R. S. (1964). A polysaccharide resembling alginic acid from a *Pseudomonas* microorganism. *Nature (London)*, **204**, 187–188.

Liu, P. V., Abe, Y. & Bates, J. L. (1961). The roles of various fractions of *Pseudomonas aeruginosa* in its pathogenesis. *J. Infect. Dis.*, **108**, 218–228.

Liu, P. V. & Mercer, C. B. (1963). Growth, toxigenicity and virulence of *Pseudomonas aeruginosa. J. Hyg. Comb.*, **61**, 485–491.

Lyons, J. M. & Asmundson, C. M. (1965). Solidification of unsaturated/saturated fatty acid mixtures and its relationship to chilling sensitivity in plants. *J. American Oil Chemists Society*, **42**, 1056–1058.

MacAllister, T. J., Costerton, J. W. & Cheng, K. J. (1972). Effect of the removal of outer cell wall layers on the actinomycin sensitivity of a Gram-negative bacterium. *Antimicrob. Ag. Chemother.*, **I**, 447–449.

Mach, B. & Tatum, E. L. (1963). Ribonucleic acid synthesis in protoplasts of *Escherichia coli*: inhibition by actinomycin D. *Science*, **139**, 1051–1052.

MacKenzie, C. R. & Jordan, D. C. (1970). Cell wall phospholipid and viomycin resistance in *Rhizobium meliloti*. *Biochem. Biophys. Res. Comm.*, **40**, 1008–1012.

Mager, J., Kuczynski, M., Schatzberg, G. & Avi-Dor, Y. (1956). Turbidity changes in bacterial suspensions in relation to osmotic pressure. *J. gen. Microbiol.*, **14**, 69.

Mao, J. C. H. & Putterman, M. (1968). Accumulation in Gram-positive and Gram-negative bacteria as a mechanism of resistance to erythromycin. *J. Bacteriol.*, **95**, 1111–1117.

Mathieu, L. G. & Legault-Hetu, D. (1973). Decreased sensitivity to polymyxin B in colicin K tolerant cells of *Escherichia coli* K-12 in the presence of colicin K. *Can. J. Microbiol.*, **19**, 345–351.

Matsuhashi, M., Ohara, I. & Yoshiyama, Y. (1970). Inhibition of bacterial cell wall synthesis *in vitro* by enduracidin, a new polypeptide antibiotic. Progress in antimicrobial and anticancer chemotherapy (*Proc. 6th Int. Congr. Chemother.*, **1**. University of Tokyo Press, Tokyo, 226–229).

McDonald, I. J. & Adams, G. A. (1971). Influence of cultural conditions on the lipopolysaccharide composition of *Neisseria sicca*. *J. gen. Microbiol.*, **65**, 201–207.

Meadow, P. (1975). Wall and membrane structure. In *The Biochemistry and Genetics of Pseudomonas*, (Ed. P. H. Clarke & M. H. Richmond), John Wiley, London.

Mitchell, P. (1970). Membranes of cells and organells: morphology, transport and metabolism. *In 20th Symposium Society for Gen. Microbiol.*, (Ed. H. P. Charles & B. C. J. G. Knight), University Press, Cambridge.

Monner, D. A., Jonsson, S. & Boman, H. G. (1971). Ampicillin-resistant mutants of *Escherichia coli* K-12 with lipopolysaccharide alterations affecting mating ability and susceptibility to sex-specific bacteriophages. *J. Bacteriol.*, **107**, 420–432.

Montgomerie, J. Z., Kalmanson, G. M. & Guze, L. B. (1966). The effects of antibiotics on the protoplasts and bacterial forms of *Streptococcus faecalis*. *J. Lab. Clin. Med.*, **68**, 543–551.

Nayler, J. H. C. (1971). Structure-activity relationships in semi-synthetic penicillins. *Proc. R. Soc. Lond. (Biol).*, **179**, 357.

Newton, B. A. (1953). Reversal of the antibacterial activity of polymyxin by divalent cations. *Nature (Lond.)*, **172**, 160–161.

Newton, B. A. (1954). Site of action of Polymyxin on *Pseudomonas aeruginosa*: antagonism by cations. *J. gen. Microbiol.*, **10**, 491–499.

Newton, B. A. (1955). A fluorescent derivative of polymyxin: its preparation and use in studying the site of action of the antibiotic. *J. gen. Microbiol.*, **12**, 226–236.

Newton, B. A. (1956). The properties and mode of action of the polymyxins. *Bact. Revs.*, **20**, 14–27.

Norrington, F. E. & James, A. M. (1970). The cell wall lipids of cells of tetracyline-sensitive and tetracyline-resistant strains of *Streptococcus pyogenes*. *Biochim. Biophys. Acta*, **218**, 269–277.

Olins, A. L. & Warner, R. C. (1967). Physiochemical studies on a lipopolysaccharide from the cell wall of *Azotobacter vinelandii*. *J. Biol. Chem.*, **242**, 4994–5001.

Pache, W., Chapman, D. & Hillaby, R. (1972). Interaction of antibiotics with membranes: polymyxin B and gramicidin S. *Biochim. Biophys. Acta*, **255**, 358–364.

Padfield, J. M. & Kellaway, I. W. (1973). The interaction of penicillins with phospholipids. *J. Pharm. Pharmac.*, **25**, 285–292.

Padfield, J. M. & Kellaway, I. W. (1974). The influence of phospholipids on the transport of antibacterial agents across non-aqueous barriers, and the methods used to quantitate the rate processes. *J. Pharm. Pharmac.*, **26**, 552–530.

Patching, J. W. & Rose, A. H. (1971). Effect of growth temperature on cold osmotic shock in *Escherichia coli* ML 30. *J. gen. Microbiol.*, **69**, 429–432.

Pechey, D. T. & James, A. M. (1973). Surface lipid of cells of *Pseudomonas aeruginosa* and its relation to gentamicin-resistance. *Biomedicine*, **19**(4), 127–129.

Percival, A., Brumfitt, W. & de Louvois, J. (1963). The role of penicillinase in determining natural and acquired resistance of Gram-negative bacteria to penicillins. *J. gen. Microbiol.*, **32**, 77–89.

Perkins, H. R. & Rogers, H. J. (1959). The products of the partial acid hydrolysis of the mucopeptide from cell walls of *Micrococcus lysodeikticus*. *Biochem. J.*, **72**, 647–654.

Postgate, J. R. & Hunter, R. (1962). The survival of starved bacteria. *J. gen. Microbiol.*, **29**, 233.

Pruul, J. & Reynolds, B. L. (1972). Interaction of complement and polymyxin with Gram-negative bacteria. *Infect. Immunity*, **6**, 709–717.

Rand, R. P. & Sengupta, S. (1972). Cardiolipin forms hexagonal structures with divalent cations. *Biochem. Biophys. Acta*, **255**, 484–492.

Reynolds, B. L. & Pruul, H. (1971). Protective role of smooth lipopolysaccharide in the serum bactericidal reaction. *Infect. Immunity*, **4**, 764–771.

Ribi, E., Anacker, R. L., Brown, R., Haskins, W. T., Malmgren, B., Milner, K. C. & Rudbach, J. A. (1966). Reaction of endotoxin and surfactants. I. Physical and biological properties of endotoxin treated with sodium deoxycholate. *J. Bacteriol.*, **92**, 1493–1509.

Richmond, M. H. & Sykes, R. B. (1973). The β-lactamases of Gram-negative bacteria and their possible physiological role. In *Advances in Microbiol Physiology*, **9**, 31–88, Academic Press, London, (Ed. Rose, A. H. & Tempest, D. W.).

Robinson, A. & Tempest, D. W. (1973). Phenotypic variability of the envelope proteins of *Klebsiella aerogenes*. *J. gen. Microbiol.*, **78**, 361–370.

Roe, E. A. & Jones, R. J. (1974). Intracellular killing of different strains of *Pseudomonas aeruginosa* by human leucocytes. *Brit. J. exp. path.*, **55**, 336–343.

Roe, E. A., Jones, R. J., Lowbury, E. J. L. (1971). Transfer of antibiotic resistance between *Pseudomonas aeruginosa*, *Escherichia coli*, and other Gram-negative bacilli in burns. *Lancet*, **i**, 149–152.

Rogers, H. J. (1965). In *15th Symp. Soc. gen. Microbiol.*, Cambr. Univ. Press.

Rosen, B. P. & Hackette, S. L. (1972). Effects of fatty acid substitution on the release of enzymes by osmotic shock. *J. Bacteriol.*, **110**, 1181–1189.

Rosselet, A. & Zimmermann, W. (1973). Mutants of *Pseudomonas aeruginosa* with impaired β-lactamase inducibility and increased sensitivity to β-lactam antibiotics. *J. gen. Microbiol.*, **76**, 455–457.

Rothstein, A. & Larrabee, C. (1948). The cell surface of yeast at the site of inhibition of glucose metabolism by uranium. *J. Cellular Comp. Physiol.*, **32**, 247–259.

Rothstein, A. & Meier, R. (1951). The chemical nature of uranium-complexing groups of the cell surface. *J. Cellular Comp. Physiol.*, **38**, 245–270.

Sabet, S. F. & Schnaitman, C. A. (1973). Purification and properties of the colicin E_3 receptor of *Escherichia coli*. *J. Biol. Chem.*, **248**, 1797–1806.

Salt, W. G. & Wiseman, D. (1970). The relation between the uptake of cetyl-trimethylammonium bromide by *Escherichia coli* and its effects on cell growth and viability. *J. Pharm. Pharmac.*, **22**, 261–264.

Salton, M. R. J. (1963). The relationship between the nature of the cell wall and the Gram stain. *J. gen. Microbiol.*, **30**, 223–235.

Salton, M. R. J. (1964). In *The Bacterial Cell Wall*, Elsevier, Amsterdam.

Sanderson, K. E., MacAlister, T. J., Costerton, J. W. & Cheng, K. J. (1973). Permeability of lipopolysaccharide-deficient (rough) mutants of *Salmonella typhimurium* to antibiotics, lysozyme and other agents. In press. Quoted by Costerton, Ingram & Cheng (1974).

Schlect, S. & Westphal, O. (1968). Antibiotica-enpfindlichkeit bei S- und R-formen von *Salmonella minnesota*. *Naturwissenchaften*, **55**, 494.

Schlect, S. & Westphal, O. (1970). Untersuchungen zur typisierung von *Salmonella* R-formen 4. Mitteilung: Typisierung von *S. minnesota* -R- mutanten mittels antibiotica. *Bakteriol.*, **213**, 356–381.

Schnaitman, C. A. (1970). Protein composition of the cell wall and cytoplasmic membrane of *Escherichia coli*. *J. Bacteriol.*, **104**, 890–901.

Schnaitman, C. A. (1971a). Solubilization of the cytoplasmic membrane of *Escherichia coli* by Triton X-100, *J. Bacteriol.*, **108**, 545–552.

Schnaitman, C. A. (1971b). Effect of ethylendiaminetetraacetic acid, Triton X-100 and lysozyme on the morphology and chemical composition of isolated cell walls of *Escherichia coli*. *J. Bacteriol.*, **108**, 533–563.

Schwarzmann, S. & Boring, J. R. (1971). Antiphagocytic effect of slime from a mucoid strain of *Pseudomonas aeruginosa*. *Infection and Immunity*, **3**, 762–767.

Sensakovic, J. W. & Bartell, P. F. (1974). The slime of *Pseudomonas aeruginosa*: biological characterization and possible role in experimental infection. *J. Infect. Dis.*, **129**, 101–109.

Shands, J. W. (1971). The physical structure of bacterial lipopolysaccharides In *Microbial Toxins*, Vol. 4, (Ed. Weinbaum, G., Kadis, S. & Ajl, S. J.), Academic Press, London, pp. 127–144.

Siewert, G. & Strominger, J. L. (1967). An inhibitor of the dephosphorylation of lipid pyrophosphate, an intermediate in the biosynthesis of the peptidoglycan of bacterial cell walls. *Proc. Nat. Acad. Sci., U.S.A.*, **57**, 767–773.

Smith, C. B. & Finland, M. (1968). Carbenicillin: activity *in vitro* and absorption and excretion in normal young men. *Applied Microbiol.*, **16**, 1753–1760.

Smith, D. G. (1971). A simple technique for the quantitative assessment of Gram positivity. *J. appl. Bact.*, **34**, 361–368.

Smith, J. T., Hamilton-Miller, J. M. T. & Knox, R. (1969). Bacterial resistance to penicillins and cephalosporins. *J. Pharm. Pharmac.*, **21**, 337–358.

Spicer, A. B. & Spooner, D. F. (1974). The inhibition of growth of *Escherichia coli* spheroplasts by antibacterial agents. *J. gen. Microbiol.*, **80**, 37–50.

Stinnett, J. D., Gilleland, J. E. & Eagon, R. G. (1973). Proteins released from the cell envelopes of *Pseudomonas aeruginosa* on exposure to ethylenediaminetetraacetate: comparison with dimethylformamide-extractable proteins. *J. Bacteriol.*, **114**, 399–407.

Strominger, J. L., Izaki, K. & Matsuhashi, M. (1967). Peptidoglycan transpeptidase and D-alanine carboxypeptidase: penicillin sensitive enzymatic reactions. *Fed. Proc.*, **26**, 9–22.

Sud, I. J. & Feingold, D. S. (1970). Mechanism of polymyxin B resistance in *Proteus mirabilis*. *J. Bacteriol.*, **104**, 289–294.

Surdy, T. E. & Hartsell, S. E. (1963). Lipids and lysozymic lysis of *Achromobacter*. *J. Bacteriol.*, **85**, 1174–1175.

Tamaki, S. & Matsuhashi, M. (1973). Increase in sensitivity to antibiotics and lysozyme on deletion of lipopolysaccharides in *Escherichia coli* strains. *J. Bacteriol.*, **114**, 453–454.

Tamaki, S., Sato, T. & Matsuhashi, M. (1971). Role of lipopolysaccharides in antibiotic resistance and bacteriophage adsorption of *Escherichia coli* K-12. *J. Bacteriol.*, **105**, 968–975.

Taubeneck, U. (1962). Susceptibility of *Proteus mirabilis* and its stable L-forms to erythromycin and other macrolides. *Nature (Lond.)*, **196**, 195.

Teuber, M. (1969). Susceptibility to polymyxin B of penicillin G-induced *Proteus mirabilis* L forms and spheroplasts. *J. Bacteriol.*, **98**, 347–350.

Teuber, M. (1973). Formation of lipophilic complexes with phosphatidic acid and phosphatidylglycerol. *Z. Naturforsch.*, **28c**, 476–477.

Teuber, M. & Bader, J. (1971). *FEBS Letters*, **16**, 195.

Thomas, A. H. & Broadbridge, R. A. (1972). The nature of carbenicillin resistance in *Pseudomonas aeruginosa*. *J. gen. Microbiol.*, **70**, 231–241.

Tulasne, R. & Minck, R. (1952). Sensibilité comparée des formes normales et des formes L de deux souches de *Proteus* vis-à-vis de quelques antibiotiques. *Compt. Rend. Soc. Biol.*, **146**, 778–780.

Tute, M. S. (1971). Principles and practice of Hanseh analysis: a guide to structure-activity correlation for the medicinal chemist. *Advances in Drug Research*, **6**, 1–77.

Vaczi, L. (1966). The lipid composition of *Straphylococci* in relation to their antibiotic resistance. *Postepy Mikrobiologii t. V. z.*, **2**, 361–368.

Vaczi, L. (1973). The biological role of bacterial lipids. *Akademiai Kiado*, Budapest.

Warren, G. H. & Gray, J. (1954). The depolymerization of bacterial polysaccharide by hyaluronidase preparations. *J. Bacteriol.*, **67**, 167–170.

Warren, G. H. & Gray, J. (1955). Studies on the properties of a polysaccharide constituent produced by *Pseudomonas aeruginosa*. *J. Bacteriol.*, **70**, 152–157.

Warren, G. H., Gray, J. & Yurchenco, J. A. (1957). Effect of polymyxin on the lysis of *Neisseria catarrhalis* by lysozyme. *J. Bacteriol.*, **74**, 788.

Watanakunakorn, C., Phair, J. P. & Hamburger, M. (1970). Increased resistance of *Pseudomonas aeruginosa* to carbenicillin after reversion from spheroplast to rod form. *Infection & Immunity*, **1**, 427–430.

Wilkinson, S. G. (1967). The sensitivity of pseudomonads to EDTA. *J. gen. Microbiol.*, **47**, 67–76.

Wilson, G. S. & Miles, A. A. (1964). In *Principles of Bacteriology and Immunity*, Edward Arnold, London.

Wistreich, G. & Bartholomew, J. W. (1969). The binding of crystal violet by isolated bacterial cell wall material. *J. gen. Microbiol.*, **59**, 223–227.

Wolf-Watz, H. & Normark, S. (1974). Chemical and enzymatic comparison of outer membrane from a chain-forming antibiotic hypersensitive *env* A mutant of *Escherichia coli* K12 and its wild type. *Proc. Soc. Gen. Microbiol.*, **1**, 40–41.

Zimelis, M. & Jackson, G. G. (1973). Activity of aminoglycoside antibiotics against *Pseudomonas aeruginosa*: specificity and site of calcium and magnesium antagonism. *J. Infect. Diseases*, **127**, 663–669.

CHAPTER 4

Ultrastructure of *Pseudomonas aeruginosa* as Related to Resistance

R. G. EAGON, J. D. STINNETT and H. E. GILLELAND, JR.

INTRODUCTION

Pseudomonas aeruginosa is resistant to a wide spectrum of antibiotics in current usage. This resistance is due in some instances to enzymes which destroy the antimicrobial activity of the antibiotic by chemically modifying or altering its structure (Brzezinska *et al.*, 1972; Garber & Friedman, 1970; Kobayashi, Yamaguchi & Mitsuhashi, 1971a,b). This type of resistance may be mediated either by chromosomal mutation or by R-factors (Ayliffe, Lawbury & Roe, 1972; Bryan, Van Den Elzen & Tseng, 1972; Bryan *et al.*, 1973; Holloway, Krishnapilli & Stanisich, 1971; Olsen & Shipley, 1973; Saunders & Grinsted,

1972). In many instances, however, resistance of *P. aeruginosa* cannot be attributed to destruction or modification of the antibiotic. The concept of a 'permeability barrier' has been advanced as an explanation for this latter type of resistance. In fact, the high intrinsic resistance of *P. aeruginosa* to antibiotics and antimicrobial agents, concomitant with the observation that most resistant strains in natural populations are not the result either of antibiotic inactivation or of acquired resistance by antibiotic-sensitive sites, lends credence to the concept of 'protection by exclusion' (Tseng, Bryan & Van Den Elzen, 1972); Tseng & Bryan, 1973).

Taubeneck (1962) observed that macrolide antibiotics were more effective against L-forms of *Proteus mirabilis* than against intact cells. He suggested that these antibiotics were unable to penetrate the envelope of *P. mirabilis*. Similar reports followed, ascribing resistance to actinomycin D to a permeability barrier (Mach & Tatum, 1963). This concept, coupled with the growing awareness that drug resistance was not always due to drug destruction/modification, has stimulated investigation into the role played by the cell envelope of Gram-negative bacteria in resistance. The concept of a permeability barrier, moreover, includes both (a) the exclusion of the antimicrobial agent by the outer surface of the cell and (b) the inability of the bacterial cell to transport the agent across the cell membrane. This has been the subject of an excellent recent review (Franklin, 1973).

In this chapter, we propose to review the ultrastructure of *P. aeruginosa* in the light of its role in resistance. Toward this end we will limit our presentation to studies of *P. aeruginosa per se*, introducing findings in other bacterial species only as required to support basic hypotheses and as points of comparison or contrast.

As a beginning point, we define the cell envelope, as did Brown (1971), as being all structures external to the cytoplasm to include the cytoplasmic membrane, peptidoglycan (murein) layer and outer cell wall membrane.

ULTRASTRUCTURE OF THE CELL ENVELOPE

Electron Microscopy

P. aeruginosa exhibits an ultrastructure typical of Gram-negative bacteria. The thin-sectional cell envelope profile consists of an outer cell wall membrane, an electron transparent space, a single dense layer of peptidoglycan (murein), another electron transparent space and the cytoplasmic membrane. Most recently, freeze-etching has been employed to further elucidate the ultrastructure of *P. aeruginosa* (Gilleland *et al.*, 1973; Lickfeld *et al.*, 1972; Weiss & Fraser, 1973).

Cells freeze-etched without cryoprotection by glycerol exhibited as convex fracture surfaces a smooth outer cell wall layer, a middle wall layer and the convex cytoplasmic membrane (Figure 1). The smooth outer wall layer exhibited the presence of pili and flagella and was identified as the outermost

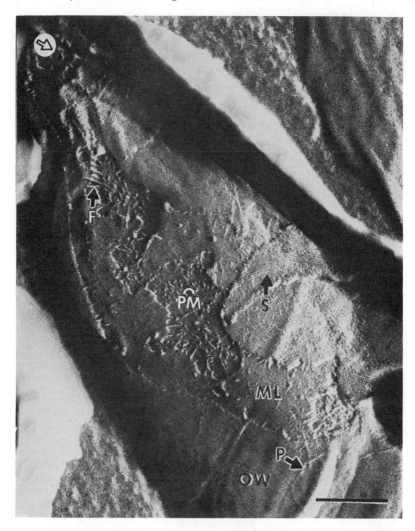

Figure 1. Freeze-etched cell without a cryoprotective agent. The smooth outer wall layer (OW), middle cell wall layer (ML), convex cytoplasmic membrane (PM), pili (P), fibrils (F) and, in the outer cell wall layer, a regular array of sub-units (S) are shown. The arrowhead in the upper left corner of this and all subsequent electron micrographs of freeze-etched preparations indicates the direction from which the metal was evaporated in the production of the replica. The horizontal bar in all figures represents 200 nm. Reproduced with permission from H. E. Gilleland *et al.*, *J. Bacteriol.*, **113**, 417–432 (1973)
Figure 2

layer of the outer membrane. A regular arrangement of sub-units in the outer cell wall layer was also observed. The middle layer was thought to be the inner track of the outer membrane. The cytoplasmic membrane was believed to split down the hydrophobic centre, as suggested for other membranes by other

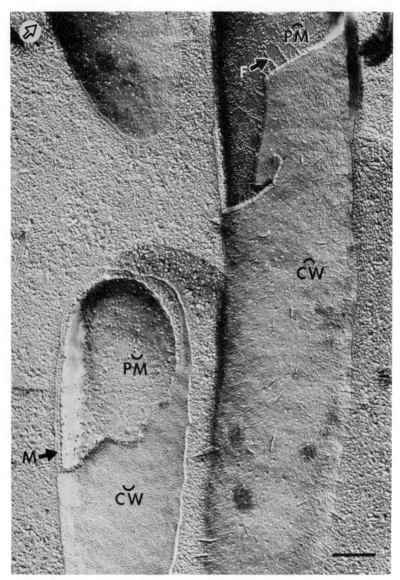

Figure 2. Freeze-etched cells after cryoprotection with glycerol. The cells shown here were washed twice in HEPES buffer prior to glycerol treatment. The four fracture surfaces encountered in glycerol-protected cells are shown: convex cell wall layer (CŴ), convex cytoplasmic membrane (PM̂), concave cell wall layer (CW̃), and concave cytoplasmic membrane (PM̃). Fibrils (F) can be seen running between the convex cell wall and the convex cytoplasmic membrane. A profile murein layer (M) can be seen between the concave cell wall and cytoplasmic membrane layers. A closely packed layer of rodlets 20–25 nm in length, composed of spherules 6 nm in diameter, make up in part the concave cell wall. Reproduced with permission from Gilleland *et al.*, *J. Bacteriol.*, **113**, 417–432 (1973) Figure 3

workers (Branton, 1966; Branton, 1969; Deamer & Branton, 1967; Nanninga, 1971; Sleytr, 1970; Van Gool & Nanninga, 1971). The resulting convex fracture, therefore, represents the inner track of the membrane. This surface was studded with particles believed to be proteins (Fox, 1972; Mühlethaler, Moor & Szarkowski, 1965).

When cells of *P. aeruginosa* were freeze-etched in the presence of 30% glycerol, the convex fractures revealed were a convex cell wall layer, which was felt to be the middle layer seen in non-cryoprotected cells, and the convex cytoplasmic membrane (Figure 2). The smooth outer cell wall layer and the flagella and pili were not seen, owing to the fracture plane now occurring within the cell wall, i.e. down the hydrophobic centre of the outer membrane. The concave fractures were the concave cytoplasmic membrane and the concave cell wall layer. The concave cytoplasmic membrane was thought to be the inside surface of the outer track of the membrane and thus complementary to the convex cytoplasmic membrane fracture. This was supported by the observation of depressions in the concave cytoplasmic membrane in a pattern which matched the pattern of particles on the convex membrane surface.

The concave cell wall layer had spherical units of approximately 6 to 7 nm in diameter, embedded in, or resting upon, an underlying smooth layer. The spherical units appeared to form rodlets composed primarily of three or four spherical units. The concave cell wall layer was thought to be the inside surface of the outer track of the outer cell wall membrane. It is of interest to point out that both the outer cell wall membrane and the cytoplasmic membrane appeared to fracture down their centres.

The peptidoglycan layer could not be unequivocally identified in freeze-etched cells of *P. aeruginosa*. The fibrils which extended from the convex cell wall layer onto the convex cytoplasmic membrane might represent the peptidoglycan as seen in the convex fracture, although they might be artifactual instead. In concave fractures the peptidoglycan layer appeared as a profile layer between the concave cytoplasmic membrane and the concave cell wall layer.

Chemistry

Clarke, Gray & Reaveley (1967) reported that cell envelopes of *P. aeruginosa* grown in a complex medium were similar to other Gram-negative bacteria. They contained lipid and lipopolysaccharide (55–65%), protein (30%) and peptidoglycan (5–15%). Heilmann (1972) showed that the peptidoglycan of *P. aeruginosa* consisted of a macromolecular bag-shaped network of covalently linked repeating units. The only components were glutamic acid (glu), 2,5-diaminopimelic acid (DAP), alanine (ala), N-acetylglucosamine and N-acetylmuramic acid. The backbone was a repeating unit of β-1,4-N-acetylglucosaminyl-β-1,4-N-acetylmuramic acid. The carboxyl groups of the muramic acid were the attachment sites of peptide side-chains with the sequence NH_2-(L-ala,D-glu)-DAP-D-ala-COOH. Approximately 1 out of 4

DAP residues was cross-linked. The lipopolysaccharide was not covalently linked to the peptidoglycan layer and cations played no role in the structure of peptidoglycan. Covalently bound lipoprotein, however, was found linked to the peptidoglycan layer by a trypsin/chymotrypsin-sensitive linkage. It was originally thought that *P. aeruginosa* lacked such peptidoglycan-bound protein (Martin, Heilman & Preusser, 1972). It was suggested that this may be the reason for the extreme ethylenediaminetetraacetate (EDTA) sensitivity of this organism (Stinnett, Gilleland & Eagon, 1973). It is now known, however, that *P. aeruginosa* is similar to *Escherichia coli* in that about 1 out of 10 DAP residues bears one of these protein molecules, bound by lysine (Braun, 1973; Heilmann, 1972). The lipoprotein apparently extends outward from the peptidoglycan layer and provides a backbone and support for the outer (LPS) membrane.

Lysozyme, which attacks the glycosidic bond between the acetyl amino sugars in the peptidoglycan layer and causes lysis of Gram-positive bacteria, is generally ineffective against Gram-negative bacteria. Although this ineffectiveness has generally been attributed to exclusion, Eagon & Carson (1965) and Carson & Eagon (1966) presented evidence that lysozyme actually attacked the peptidoglycan of *P. aeruginosa*. These authors suggested that the peptidoglycan layer was not solely responsible for cell wall rigidity. These findings were further supported by Asbell & Eagon (1966a,b) and by Cox & Eagon (1968) who reported that cations played a major role in maintaining the structural integrity of the envelope.

The lipopolysaccharide of *P. aeruginosa* has received considerable attention (Clarke, Gray & Reavley, 1965; Chester, Gray & Wilkinson, 1972; Chester, Meadow & Pitt, 1973; Fensom & Gray, 1969; Ikeda & Egami, 1973). It appears to be generally similar to the lipopolysaccharide of the Enterobacteriaceae. Major differences are the high phosphorus content (4·3%) and low sugar content (16–17%). Moreover, only about 20% of the polysaccharide moiety is released by treatment with dilute acetic acid. Also, the hydroxy acids present in the lipid A moiety differ from those of the Enterobacteriaceae (Hancock, Humphreys & Meadow, 1970).

The lipid composition of the cell envelope is typical of Gram-negative bacteria, consisting primarily of phosphatidyl ethanolamine and diphosphatidyl glycerol (Bobo & Eagon, 1968; Brown, 1971; Clarke, Gray & Reaveley, 1967). Brown (1971), moreover, suggested that, as a generalization, phosphatidyl ethanolamine is the major phospholipid in Gram-negative bacteria, while in Gram-positive bacteria it is phosphatidylglycerol.

Lipopolysaccharide has been shown to be released from *P. aeruginosa* as a complex with protein (PrLPS) on exposure to EDTA (Rogers, Gilleland & Eagon, 1969). Except for their role in endotoxin (Homma, 1968; Homma & Suzuki, 1964, 1966), the protein components of this cell wall have not been studied until recently. Using techniques developed by Schnaitman (1970a), which involve protein solubilization by the use of acidic N,N'-dimethylformamide (DMF) and sodium dodecyl sulphate (SDS)-

polyacrylamide gel electrophoresis, it was shown that the cell envelope of
P. aeruginosa, when grown in Tryptic Soy broth at 30°C, contained three major
proteins (Figure 3) (Stinnett, Gilleland & Eagon, 1973). The molecular
weights of these proteins were estimated to be 43,000 daltons (Protein A),
16,500 daltons (Protein B) and 72,000 daltons (Protein C). Comparative
staining of gels for protein with Coomassie blue and with the Periodate–Schiff
base reaction for carbohydrate gave preliminary evidence that proteins A and
B were glycoproteins.

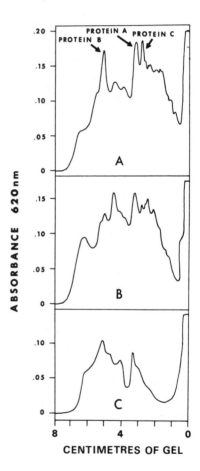

Figure 3. Densitometric tracing of electrophoresis gels to which 100 μg of protein was applied; all gels were stained with Coomassie Blue. Gel A, proteins extracted from cell envelopes with *N,N'*-dimethylformamide (DMF); gel B, proteins extracted with DMF from the 100,000 xg supernatant fraction of the material solubilized from cell envelopes by EDTA; and gel C, proteins extracted from the protein–lipopolysaccharide complex (PrLPS) by DMF. Protein A (43,000 daltons), protein B (16,500 daltons), and protein C (72,000 daltons) are identified in gel A. This Figure shows that protein A and protein B are components of the PrLPs complex (gel C). A wide variety of proteins was released from the cell envelope by EDTA (gel B). The tops of the gels are to the right. The tracing was done with a Gilford scanner at 620 nm. Reproduced with permission from J. D. Stinett, H. E. Gilleland, Jr. & R. C. Eagon, *J. Bacteriol.*, **114**, 399–407 (1973) Figure 3

Resolution of envelope preparations into cytoplasmic- and outer-
membranes by discontinuous sucrose density gradient centrifugation and
subsequent analysis by SDS-polyacrylamide gel electrophoresis showed that
proteins A and B were the major protein components of the outer membrane
(Figure 4) (Stinnett & Eagon, 1973). As will be discussed later, proteins A and
B are part of the PrLPS complex found in the outer membrane (Stinnett,
Gilleland & Eagon, 1973).

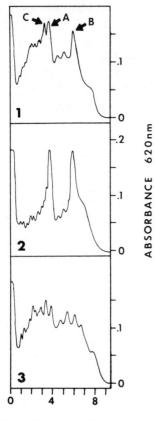

Figure 4. Densitometric tracing of electrophoresis gels to which 100 μg of protein was applied; all gels were stained with Coomassie Blue. Gel 1, crude cell envelope membranes; gel 2 outer (cell wall) membrane; gel 3, cytoplasmic membrane. The tops of the gels are to the left, the tracing was done with a Gilford scanner at 620 nm. Reproduced by permission of the National Research Council of Canada from the *Canadian Journal of Microbiology*, Vol. **19**, pp. 1469–1471 (1973)

The exact role of protein in the cell envelope is not known. Many of the proteins, especially those associated with the cytoplasmic membrane, may be the classical membrane-bound enzymes, transport proteins, etc. The outer membrane of Gram-negative bacteria, however, is essentially devoid of the high levels of enzymatic activity that is characteristic of the cytoplasmic membrane (Bell *et al.*, 1971; White *et al.*, 1971). This implies that the outer membrane either has undiscovered enzymatic activities, or that at least some of the protein serves only in a structural role. As will be shown later, there is highly suggestive circumstantial evidence that proteins A and B, in conjunction with lipopolysaccharide, serve to stabilize the cell envelope of *P. aeruginosa* and that they are necessary to maintain the structural integrity of the cell envelope.

Suzuki & Goto (1972) conducted studies on surface monolayers of protein and lipopolysaccharide from *P. aeruginosa*. By determining the surface properties of such monolayers, they found that the protein film was stiffened and stabilized by the addition of lipopolysaccharide. Lipopolysaccharide alone would not form a monolayer. Unfortunately, this was a protein–lipopolysaccharide system that did not include phospholipid. Monolayers composed of phospholipid–protein–lipopolysaccharide would probably be more representative of the native outer membrane. Additionally, it has been shown that the protein of the outer membrane is complexed with lipopolysaccharide (Stinnett, Gilleland & Eagon, 1973; Stinnett & Eagon, 1973). Thus, it would seem more logical to use a PrLPS complex in the presence of phospholipid than purified protein and purified lipopolysaccharide.

The protein composition of the cell envelope appears to vary with growth conditions (Gilleland, Stinnett & Eagon, 1974). Changes in cell envelope proteins of other bacteria as a result of growth in different media have also been noted by other workers (Bennett, Lopes & Rothfield, 1973). The significance of these changes, however, is not understood.

In summary, the chemical composition of the cell envelopes of *P. aeruginosa* is quite typical of Gram-negative bacteria. The peptidoglycan is essentially the same as that of *E. coli*, possessing bound lipoprotein which apparently serves as an anchor for the outer membrane. When grown in complex media, the cell envelopes contain three major proteins, two of which reside in the outer membrane and are associated with lipopolysaccharide. The presence of protein and lipopolysaccharide in the outer membrane is thought to stabilize the membrane and may affect the permeability of that membrane.

ANTIMICROBIAL EFFECTS OF EDTA ON THE OUTER MEMBRANE: A MODEL SYSTEM

The lysis of *P. aeruginosa* by EDTA will be discussed in full elsewhere in this volume (Chapter 5). Nevertheless, we wish to present a brief description of the lytic effects of EDTA in order to develop a model system for studying the effects of antimicrobial agents against this organism.

Ultrastructural Effects as Determined by Electron Microscopy

The effect of treatment with EDTA on the ultrastructure of cells of *P. aeruginosa* was studied using the freeze-etch technique (Gilleland *et al.*, 1973). When cells of *P. aeruginosa* in a hypertonic sucrose medium were treated with EDTA-tris(hydroxymethyl)aminomethane (Tris)-hydrochloride, osmotically fragile rods, which have been termed osmoplasts (Asbell & Eagon, 1966a,b), resulted. Freeze-etching of osmoplasts revealed that the concave cell wall layer had been ultrastructurally altered (Figure 5). Approximately one-half of the spherical units which were embedded in the underlying smooth layer were extracted by EDTA–Tris treatment. This ultrastructural observation correlated well with the chemical finding that one-half of the lipopolysaccharide within the cell envelope was extracted by EDTA (Thota, 1972). The extracted lipopolysaccharide has been shown to be in the form of a complex with protein, i.e. PrLPS (Rogers, Gilleland & Eagon, 1969; Roberts, Gray & Wilkinson, 1970). The PrLPS complex extracted from cell envelopes of

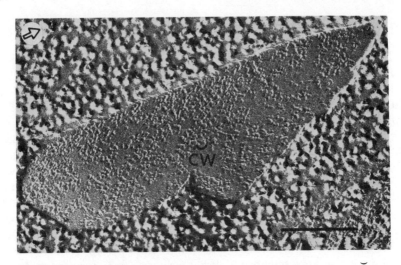

Figure 5. Freeze-etch of osmoplasts. The concave cell wall layer (C̆W) is shown to have lost many of the spherical units (PrLPS). Reproduced with permission from Gilleland *et al.*, *J. Bacteriol.*, **113**, 417–432 (1973)
Figure 8

P. aeruginosa had previously been shown to possess an ultrastructural appearance of short rodlets 20–25 nm long by 7 nm in width which, in turn, appeared to be comprised of spherical sub-units approximately 7 nm in diameter (Rogers, Gilleland & Eagon, 1969). These dimensions agreed well with those of the spherical units seen in the concave cell wall layer. When the supernatant fluid from an osmoplast preparation was examined using the negative staining technique, spherical units and rodlets composed of spherical units were again seen (Figure 6). These findings indicated that the spherical units in the concave cell wall layer represented an EDTA-sensitive site within the cell envelope.

Asbell & Eagon (1966a,b) showed that osmoplasts could be restored to osmotic stability by the addition of excess Mg^{2+}. They termed such cells 'restored' cells. When restored cells were freeze-etched, the concave cell wall layer again had an altered ultrastructure (Gilleland *et al.*, 1973). This layer, in restored cells, had a disorganized, crowded appearance with the spherical units so closely packed that the underlying smooth layer could not easily be seen (Figure 7). It appeared as though the units had reaggregated into the cell wall to restore the osmotic stability of the cells, but were not in the same configuration or orientation as in untreated cells. The observation that restored cells respired normally but were not viable supports this interpretation. Moreover, restored cells were found to be 'hypersensitive' to the effects of EDTA–Tris (Eagon, Gilleland & Stinnett, unpublished observations).

The effect of EDTA on isolated cell envelopes of *P. aeruginosa* was investigated using negative staining techniques (Stinnett, Gilleland & Eagon, 1973). The cell envelopes had a smooth, close-knit appearance prior to EDTA

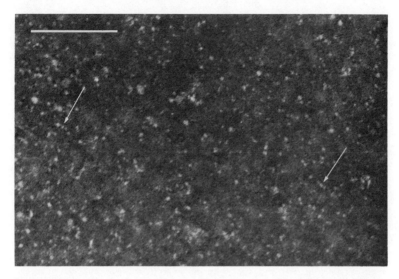

Figure 6. Negatively stained (phosphotungstic acid) preparation of the supernatant fraction from an osmoplast suspension. Sperical units and rodlets (arrows) are shown. Some of the rodlets can be seen to be composed of three spheres in a chain-like fashion. Reproduced with permission from Gilleland *et al.*, *J. Bacteriol.*, **113**, 417–432 (1973) Figure 9

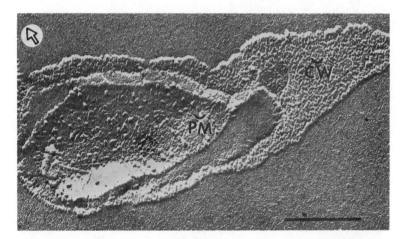

Figure 7. Freeze-etch of restored cells. This cell shows the concave cytoplasmic membrane (PM) and the concave cell wall (CW). The concave cell wall can be seen to be closely packed with spherical units. Reproduced with permission from Gilleland *et al.*, *J. Bacteriol.*, **113**, 417–432 (1973) Figure 10

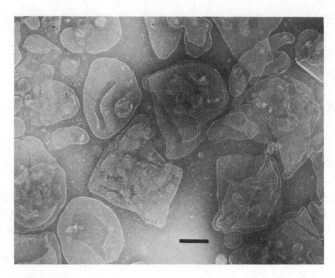

Figure 8. Electron micrograph of a negatively stained (phosphotungstic acid) preparation of cell envelopes. Note the smooth close-knit appearance of the cell envelopes. Reproduced with permission from J. D. Stinnett, H. E. Gilleland & R. C. Eagon, *J. Bacteriol.*, **114**, 399–407 (1973) Figure 1

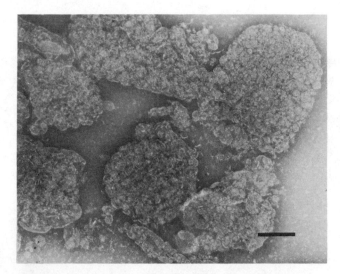

Figure 9. Electron micrograph of a negatively stained (phosphotungstic acid) preparation of cell envelopes after EDTA treatment. Note the gaps in the envelope structure and the loss of the smooth, close-knit appearance. Reproduced with permission from J. D. Stinnett, H. E. Gilleland & R. C. Fagon, *J. Bacteriol.*, **114**, 399–407 (1973) Figure 5

treatment (Figure 8). Following such treatment, the cell envelopes retained their cell-like morphology but the smooth, close-knit appearance was lost with gaps appearing which were apparently due to the loss of cell envelope material (Figure 9). Electron microscopic examination of the material solubilized by EDTA from the cell envelopes revealed the presence of rodlets approximately 7 nm by 20 to 25 nm. These rodlets were comparable to those released from osmoplasts (ref. Figure 6) and they corresponded to the purified PrLPS fraction of the supernatant fluid. The results obtained from treatment of isolated cell envelopes with EDTA–Tris were entirely compatible, therefore, with the understanding of the effect of EDTA–Tris on the cell envelope as gained through freeze-etch analysis of whole cells.

Chemical Effects

Eagon & Carson (1965) showed that EDTA-extracts of whole cells of *P. aeruginosa* in hypertonic sucrose contained CA^{2+}, Mg^{2+} and Zn^{2+}. Asbell & Eagon (1966a,b), Cox & Eagon (1968) and Eagon (1969) made similar observations on both intact cells and isolated cell envelopes. These authors suggested that EDTA lysed *P. aeruginosa* by extracting divalent cations which were involved in intra- and intermolecular cross-linkages via phosphate groups contained in phospholipid and lipopolysaccharide components of the cell envelope.

The material extracted from cell envelopes by EDTA contained phosphorus, carbohydrate (lipopolysaccharide) and protein (Gray & Wilkinson, 1965a; Cox & Eagon, 1968). Subsequent studies have shown that the protein and lipopolysaccharide is extracted as a complex (Rogers, Gilleland & Eagon, 1969; Roberts, Gray & Wilkinson, 1970). As described previously, this complex has been visualized by electron microscopy. Analysis of the proteins released from isolated cell envelopes by EDTA (ref. Figure 3) has shown that a wide variety of proteins were extracted by this treatment (Stinnett, Gilleland & Eagon, 1973). Obviously, all of these proteins may not be subject to extraction by EDTA in whole cells. That is, proteins which are bound to the cytoplasm side of the cytoplasmic membrane would normally be inaccessible to EDTA but the proteins could be extracted when isolated cell envelopes were used as the substrate. Of those proteins released by EDTA, two have been shown to be associated with the PrLPS complex (ref. Figure 3) (Stinnett, Gilleland & Eagon, 1973). These are proteins A and B, which have already been described.

It seems likely that protein A (43,000 daltons) is the same as the endotoxin protein (42,000 daltons) previously described by Homma and coworkers (1964, 1966, 1968). This observation has received support from other workers (Roberts, Gray & Wilkinson, 1970) who found that the amino acid composition of the PrLPS complex was very similar to that of Homma's endotoxin protein. The presence of proteins A and B in the PrLPS complex is probably not surprising since they were shown to be localized in the outer membrane (ref. Figure 4) (Stinnett & Eagon, 1973).

The osmoplast/restoration experiments, described in the preceding section of this chapter, lend strong circumstantial evidence to the role of protein and lipopolysaccharide in maintaining the structural integrity of the envelope. Supernatant fluids from osmoplast preparations contained approximately 100 μg of protein per millilitre; following restoration of these cells to osmotic stability, the protein concentration dropped to about 10 μg per millilitre (Gilleland *et al.* 1973). Furthermore, the protein present in the supernatant fluid was necessary for restoration, since osmoplasts centrifuged and resuspended in hypertonic sucrose could not be restored to osmotic stability by the addition of cations.

Discussion

At this point it seems fairly certain that EDTA exerts its lytic effect on *P. aeruginosa* by extracting divalent cations (primarily Mg^{2+} and Ca^{2+}) which anchor a complex of protein and lipopolysaccharide in the outer membrane. This process has been described in some detail, in terms of both visual and chemical events. More importantly, this has demonstrated how judicial application of electron microscopic and chemical techniques *together* can provide a better description of the effects of antimicrobial agents on bacteria.

ACQUISITION OF RESISTANCE TO EDTA BY GROWTH ON Mg^{2+} DEFICIENT MEDIA: A MODEL SYSTEM

Ultrastructural Changes as Determined by Electron Microscopy

Brown & Melling (1969a,b) reported that cells of *P. aeruginosa* became resistant to the lytic action of EDTA when grown in a Mg^{2+}-limited basal medium. We hoped that this shift from EDTA sensitivity to EDTA resistance would involve an observable ultrastructural alteration in the concave cell wall layer of the envelope which we had identified as an EDTA-sensitive site. Employing two different basal media (Gilleland, Stinnett & Eagon, 1974), *P. aeruginosa* was grown in Mg^{2+}-sufficient media containing a concentration of 0·5 mM Mg^{2+} and in Mg^{2+}-deficient media containing a concentration of 0·005 mM Mg^{2+}. The cells grown in Mg^{2+}-sufficient media retained their sensitivity to EDTA and, upon freeze-etching, untreated cells exhibited an ultrastructure identical to that of untreated cells grown in Tryptic Soy broth (ref. Figure 2). When osmoplasts were prepared from cells grown in Mg^{2+}-sufficient medium, spherical units were observed to have been extracted from the concave cell wall layer identically to that of cells grown in Tryptic Soy broth (ref. Figures 5 and 6). Cells grown in the Mg^{2+}-deficient media were, on the other hand, resistant to lysis by EDTA (Brown & Melling, 1969a,b; Gilleland, Stinnett & Eagon, 1974). These cells exhibited an altered ultrastructure upon freeze-etching, with the concave cell wall layer having a disorganized, crowded appearance which appeared to contain more spherical units (Figure 10). When

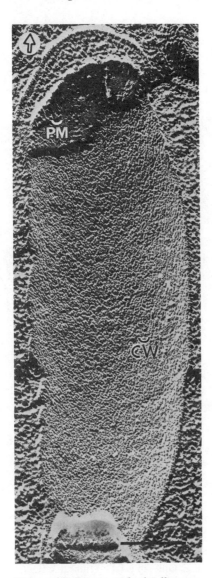

Figure 10. Freeze-etched cell grown in Mg^{2+}-deficient medium. The concave cell wall fracture (CW̆) appears disorganized and more crowded with spherical units. The underlying smooth layer cannot be seen clearly. Reproduced with permission from H. E. Gilleland, J. D. Stinnett & R. C. Eagon, *J. Bacteriol.*, **117**, 302–311 (1974) Figure 6

treated with EDTA, these cells did not form osmoplasts and the concave cell wall layer remained unchanged.

It is of interest to point out that the cytoplasmic membrane also appeared affected by growth in the Mg^{2+}-deficient media. In Tryptic Soy broth-grown cells (ref. Figure 2) and in cells grown in Mg^{2+}-sufficient media (Figure 11), the

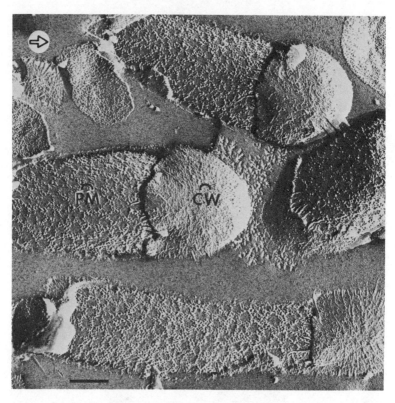

Figure 11. Freeze-etched cells grown in Mg^{2+}-sufficient medium. Convex cell wall (CW) and convex cytoplasmic membrane (PM) are shown. The convex cytoplasmic membrane reveals a netlike array of particles resting upon, or embedded in, a smooth underlying layer. Reproduced with permission from H. E. Gilleland, J. D. Stinnett & R. C. Eagon, *J. Bacteriol.*, **117**, 302–311 (1974) Figure 5

convex cytoplasmic membrane exhibited a netlike array of particles under the conditions of freeze-etching employed. On the other hand, the EDTA-resistant cells grown in the Mg^{2+}-deficient media exhibited an alteration of this netlike pattern (Figure 12) under identical freeze-etch conditions. This suggested that there must be some difference between the membrances since they responded differently under the same conditions of freeze-etching.

The netlike pattern of particles in the convex cytoplasmic membrane is now believed to be due to aggregation of the particles induced by the use of a

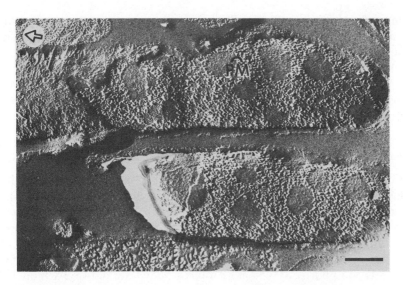

Figure 12. Freeze-etched cells grown in Mg^{2+}-deficient medium. The convex cytoplasmic membrane (PM) appears disorganized with the disruption of the netlike array of particles and the appearance of large smooth areas of exposed underlying layer. Reproduced with permission from H. E. Gilleland, J. D. Stinnett & R. C. Eagon, *J. Bacteriol.*, **117**, 302–311 (1974) Figure 8

temperature of 4 °C for incubation of the cells in the glycerol mixture prior to harvesting and freezing the cells. James & Branton (1973), using *Acholeplasma laidlawii*, showed that temperatures at or near the phase transition temperature of lipids in the cytoplasmic membrane caused aggregation of the particles but, at temperatures well above the transition temperature the convex cytoplasmic membrane exhibited a random distribution of particles. Similarly, Speth & Wunderlich (1973) showed that the convex plasma membrane surface of *Tetrahymena* exhibited a random distribution of particles at 28 °C, but at 5 °C the particles had aggregated into a netlike pattern.

The cytoplasmic membrane of *P. aeruginosa* has now been shown to respond similarly to the effects of temperature (H. E. Gilleland, Jr., unpublished observations). Thus, when *P. aeruginosa* was freeze-etched after being incubated with glycerol at 30 °C and followed by centrifugation at ambient temperature, the convex cytoplasmic membrane exhibited a random distribution of particles. When the same procedures were performed at 4 °C, the netlike pattern of particles resulted. If the cells were fixed by glutaraldehyde (final concentration 2%) for 1 hour prior to incubation in glycerol at 4 °C and centrifugation at 4 °C, random distribution of particles was observed. Nevertheless, the different aggregational patterns of particles observed in cytoplasmic membranes of freeze-etched preparations of cells grown in Mg^{2+}-sufficient and Mg^{2+}-deficient media do suggest a difference between the membranes, especially in the lipids. This is true since the aggregating of particles is considered to be a function of the transition temperature of the lipids in the cytoplasmic membrane.

The distribution of spherical units in the outer cell wall membrane, however, was not affected by temperature (H. E. Gilleland, Jr., unpublished observations). Thus, the altered ultrastructural appearance of the outer membrane of cells grown in Mg^{2+}-deficient media was a response to conditions of growth.

Chemical Changes

Cell envelopes were prepared from cells of *P. aeruginosa* grown in Mg^{2+}-sufficient and Mg^{2+}-deficient media, then analysed for protein, total phosphorus, total carbohydrate and 2-keto-3-deoxy-octonate (KDO) (Gilleland, Stinnett & Eagon, 1974). Although there was no difference in the total protein content of the two envelopes, there were significant changes in the other components. Envelopes of cells grown in Mg^{2+}-deficient medium contained 18% less phosphorus, 16·4% more total carbohydrate and 13·3% more KDO. These analyses compared favourably with the reports of Wilkinson (1968; 1970) who found lower phosphorus and higher carbohydrate content in cell envelopes of *Pseudomonas* species resistant to EDTA. A correlation between the phosphorus content of the envelope and sensitivity to EDTA is not surprising when the probable cation-binding role of phosphate groups in lipopolysaccharide is considered (Wilkinson, 1970).

The absence of a quantitative change in protein content of the cell envelopes seemed inconsistent with the ultrastructural observation that the concave cell wall layer of EDTA-resistant cells was apparently crowded with spherical units, i.e. PrLPS (Gilleland, Stinnett & Eagon, 1974). Several explanations for this apparent discrepancy may be offered. One proposal is that the 'crowding' seen in the concave cell wall layer was actually due to a configurational or orientational change in the PrLPS rather than an actual increase in the number of protein molecules. Another alternative may be that the composition of these spherical units, which we assume are analogous to the PrLPS complex in Tryptic Soy broth-grown cells (Stinnett, Gilleland & Eagon, 1973; Gilleland *et al.*, 1973), may have changed and they are no longer composed of 60% protein and 30% lipopolysaccharide, but now have a greater proportion of lipopolysaccharide. Unfortunately, firm evidence cannot be offered for any of these explanations at this time.

Even though there was no overall quantitative change in protein content, considerable qualitative differences were found (Gilleland, Stinnett & Eagon, 1974). SDS-Polyacrylamide gel electrophoresis (Figure 13) revealed that cell envelopes from cells grown in Mg^{2+}-sufficient medium contained four distinct proteins, including proteins A, B and C which were previously described (Stinnett, Gilleland & Eagon, 1973). In addition, a new band (protein E) having a molecular weight of approximately 100,000 daltons was found. Cell envelopes prepared from cells grown in Mg^{2+}-deficient medium had almost no

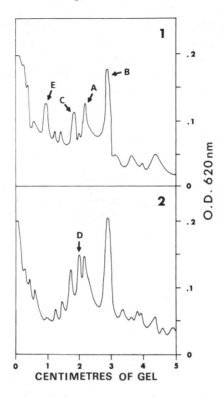

Figure 13. Densitometric tracing of electrophoresis gels to which 50 μg of protein was applied. Both gels were stained with Coomassie blue. Panel 1: Proteins extracted from envelopes grown in Mg^{2+}-sufficient medium. Panel 2: proteins from envelopes of cells grown in Mg^{2+}-deficient medium. The tops of the gels are to the left. The tracing was done with a Gilford scanner at 620 nm. Protein A (43,000 daltons), protein B (16,500 daltons), protein C (72,000 daltons), and protein E (100,000 daltons) are identified in panel 1. This Figure shows that envelopes from cells grown in Mg^{2+}-deficient medium (panel 2) differ from those of cells grown in Mg^{2+}-sufficient medium (panel 1) by having almost no protein E and having a greater proportion of protein D (50,000 daltons). Reproduced with permission from H. E. Gilleland, J. D. Stinnett & R. C. Eagon, *J. Bacteriol.*, **117**, 307–311 (1974) Figure 9

protein E but a new band (protein D), having an approximate molecular weight of 50,000 daltons, appeared in greater proportion. Since protein D is one-half the molecular weight of protein E, perhaps protein D, when produced by cells grown in Mg^{2+}-deficient medium, cannot be dimerized to protein E. Such a dimerization, however, would involve a covalent linkage since samples were reduced with mercaptoethanol prior to electrophoresis in SDS and urea.

Proteins A, B and C have been previously identified as major proteins in the cell envelope from Tryptic Soy broth-grown cells (Stinnett, Gilleland & Eagon, 1973). In addition, proteins A and B were shown to be associated with lipopolysaccharide. Proteins D and E, however, were not observed as major proteins in cell envelopes of Tryptic Soy broth-grown cells. Thus, the proteins of cell envelopes from cells grown in the chemically defined Mg^{2+}-sufficient media and in Tryptic Soy broth differed qualitatively. Changes in cell envelopes proteins of other bacteria as a result of growth in different media have also been noted by other workers (Bennett, Lopes & Rothfield, 1973).

Discussion

To our knowledge there has been no other instance where the freeze-etching technique has been employed to study the ultrastructure of cells made resistant to an agent to which the cells were normally sensitive. One could speculate that ultrastructural changes might be detected in cells in which resistance involved a significant change in the chemical properties of the cell envelope. Such a possibility is the exclusion of antibiotics by resistant cells through increased impermeability of the cell envelope owing to a change in lipid, lipopolysaccharide or protein content. It would certainly be interesting to investigate such cells toward this end. In particular, it would be worthwhile comparing an EDTA-resistant mutant of *P. aeruginosa*, which otherwise grew and behaved normally, with the EDTA-sensitive parent to determine if the concave cell wall layer was ultrastructurally altered. Likewise, it would be of interest to compare the concave cell wall ultrastructure of an EDTA-resistant species of *Pseudomonas* with that of the highly EDTA-sensitive *P. aeruginosa*.

While the interpretation of these data is incomplete at this time, a useful model has been presented. Crucial problems remaining are the lack of quantitative difference in total protein content between the two cell envelopes and the inavailability of more chemical data, especially with respect to lipids. In addition, it would be useful to know if the protein content of the PrLPS complex has changed and if the density of the outer membrane been altered under Mg^{2+}-limitation. The latter would be expected from the electron microscopic evidence. Such comparative studies will be useful and will finally serve to define the role of the outer membrane, particularly with respect to the protein and lipopolysaccharide components, in conferring the so-called 'intrinsic drug resistance' upon *P. aeruginosa*.

ULTRASTRUCTURAL FACTORS IMPLICATED IN RESISTANCE TO OTHER ANTIMICROBIAL FACTORS

There is relatively little information in the literature concerning physical and chemical ultrastructural factors which contribute to either the acquired or intrinsic resistance of *P. aeruginosa* to antimicrobial agents. Sufficient information is available, however, to permit one to conclude that ultrastructural factors, particularly those associated with the cell envelope, are involved in resistance. Moreover, ultrastructural factors associated with resistance would appear to offer a fertile field of study.

Polymyxins

The mechanism of sensitivity and of resistance of *P. aeruginosa* to polymyxin has received considerable attention. The antimicrobial action of polymyxin against Gram-negative bacteria can be explained in terms of a disorganization of the cell membrane with resultant disruption of the osmotic equilibrium of the cell and leakage of the cell contents (Newton, 1956; Muschel, Ahl & Fisher, 1969). It has been proposed that polymyxin combines with phospholipids in the cell envelope (Newton, 1956; Few, 1955) but evidence has also been reported that polymyxin acts on lipopolysaccharide as well (Koike & Iida, 1971). Polymyxin, therefore, is considered to bind to the cell envelope. Moreover, the cell envelope of resistant cells of *P. aeruginosa* was shown to have a low affinity for polymyxin (Newton, 1956; Few & Schulmann, 1953).

Sensitive strains of *P. aeruginosa* became resistant to polymyxin and to EDTA when grown in Mg^{2+}-limited media (Brown & Melling, 1969a,b). Phosphate-limited cultures also showed changes in sensitivity similar to those associated with Mg^{2+}-limitation (Brown 1972). Polymyxin-resistant mutants of *P. aeruginosa* had a low cell wall content of magnesium, phospholipid and phosphorus (Brown & Watkins, 1970). Similarly, low cell wall contents of phospholipid and cations also occurred with other polymyxin-resistant Gram-negative species (Brown & Wood, 1972).

Brown and Melling (1969b) pointed out that there is a striking similarity in the changes in sensitivity to polymyxin and to EDTA produced in *P. aeruginosa* by growth in Mg^{2+}-limited media. EDTA and polymyxin, however, cannot have a common site of action (but see Chapter 3, pages 90–98). EDTA is an anionic agent which functions to chelate divalent cations while polymyxin is a cationic cyclic polypeptide. Moreover, the action of polymyxin is antagonized by divalent cations. Newton (1956) reported that the antagonism was due to competition between polymyxin and the cations for binding sites on the cells.

Chen & Feingold (1972) suggested that divalent cations antagonized the bactericidal effect of polymyxin B indirectly through interaction with the cell wall rather than at the primary cell membrane locus of action. Thus, the interaction of divalent cations with the cell wall prevented the access of polymyxin B to the cell membrane by mechanisms that remain unclear. Nevertheless, this evidence appears to substantiate Hamilton's (1968) hypothesis that resistance to membrane-active agents is due to the agent not penetrating through the cell wall.

A change in lipid composition appears to be a common finding in resistant strains of *P. aeruginosa*. Anderes, Sandine & Elliker (1971) reported that cells resistant to a quaternary ammonium compound (QAC) contained 77% more total lipid than sensitive cells. When grown in a medium lacking QAC, the cells retained their resistance and had 27% more total lipid than sensitive cells. Similarly, Thomas & Broadbridge (1972) found that the cell wall from cells of *P. aeruginosa* which had been habituated to the presence of carbenicillin possessed a higher lipid content than walls of the parent-sensitive strain. Brown & Watkins (1970) showed that the cell walls of a strain of *P. aeruginosa* resistant to polymyxin contained 70% more readily extractable lipid than the cell walls of sensitive cells, although the resistant cells walls contained only one-fourth the phospholipid and one-tenth the Mg^{2+} of the sensitive cell walls. These changes in lipid composition of the cell envelope could conceivably cause the outer cell wall membrane to become more impermeable to the chemical agent so that it is blocked from the active site of its action on the cytoplasmic membrane as proposed by Hamilton (1968). It would be most interesting to see, therefore, if a polymyxin-resistant strain of *P. aeruginosa* showing normal growth in a Mg^{2+}-sufficient medium possessed an ultrastructurally altered outer cell wall membrane similarly to cells of a sensitive strain which was grown in Mg^{2+}-deficient media as reported by Gilleland, Stinnett & Eagon (1974).

Quaternary Ammonium Compounds

The quaternary ammonium compounds are a group of chemical agents to which *P. aeruginosa* has demonstrated the ability to develop strains which are resistant to their bactericidal activity. Adair and co-workers (1969, 1971a) reported on a mutant of *P. aeruginosa* which developed a tolerance for benzalkonium chloride (BC). Ultrastructural analysis by thin-sectioning of cells of a sensitive strain and of a resistant strain grown in the presence of BC was performed (Adair, Geftic & Gelzer, 1971b; Hoffman *et al.*, 1973). The sensitive strain presented an ultrastructure typical of Gram-negative bacteria. The cell envelope consisted of an inner cytoplasmic membrane and an outer cell wall membrane. These layers were separated by an electron-dense periplasmic area owing to the particular fixation procedure they employed (i.e. other staining techniques generally depict the periplasmic space as being electron transparent). The cytoplasm appeared typical, with an electron-transparent area containing filamentous material representing the nuclear material. The surrounding cytoplasm contained ribosomal particles. No cytoplasmic membranous structures were observed.

The ultrastructure of the resistant cells grown in the presence of BC, however, was drastically altered from that of sensitive cells. The cytoplasm contained centrally located, round, electron-transparent areas which were not bounded by a membrane. Surrounding these areas was a diffuse substance that differed in appearance from the ribosomal or nuclear material. The nuclear material was fragmented into pockets near the periphery of the cell instead of being centrally located within the cytoplasm. The cell envelope was altered so that the membraneous layers seen in the cell envelope of sensitive cells could not be clearly resolved in the resistant cells grown in BC. Furthermore, the cell surface of BC-grown cells appeared to have a covering substance which had not been found on the surface of the sensitive cells.

These studies showed, therefore, that ultrastructural changes resulted from growth in BC. Unfortunately for our purpose in this chapter, these studies did not answer the question whether there were detectable ultrastructural differences between sensitive cells and resistant cells not grown in the presence of BC. The ultrastructural alterations described above for resistant cells grown in the presence of BC most likely resulted from the presence of BC. When sensitive cells were treated with 1 mg of BC per millilitre for 1 hour before fixation and embedding, the cells showed similar alterations beginning to occur (Hoffman *et al.*, 1973). The cytoplasmic membrane no longer exhibited the trilaminar profile and centrally located, round, electron-transparent areas containing trilaminar membrane segments appeared. The latter might have been the remnants of the cytoplasmic membrane. Furthermore, the BC-resistant cells grew poorly in the presence of BC. They experienced a lag phase of 30 hr, then a generation time of 6·5 hr, and an incubation time of 72 hr was required before the late logarithmic growth phase was reached. If BC-resistant cells were grown overnight in the absence of BC, however, they exhibited a normal cytoplasmic appearance even though they remained resistant to BC (Adair, Geftic & Gelzer, 1971b). These authors, however, did not specify if the cell envelope profile exhibited a normal appearance or was altered under these conditions.

Exclusion of Antibiotics by Cell Envelope Factors

P. aeruginosa acquires resistance to a variety of antibiotics by producing enzymes which catalyse chemical modifications of the antibiotics (Chapter 1). Some examples are β-lactamase, carbenicillinase, streptomycin phosphorylase and an enzyme which brings about *N*-acetylation of the deoxystreptamine moiety of gentamicin. In many cases, on the other hand, resistance appears not to be due to chemical modification of the antibiotics. The latter type of resistance has been attributed to diminished uptake and not inactivation of the antibiotics (Barrett & Asscher, 1972; Curtis, Richmond & Stanisich, 1973;

Garber & Friedman, 1970; Thomas & Broadbridge, 1972; Tseng & Bryan, 1973; Tseng, Bryan & Van Den Elzen, 1972).

It appears evident that the diminished uptake of antibiotics by resistant strains of *P. aeruginosa* is due to ultrastructural alterations of the cell envelope, particularly the cell wall. Barrett & Asscher (1972) reported that carbenicillin-resistant mutants were resistant to EDTA. These authors speculated that carbenicillin resistance was due to a change in cell wall composition, particularly a change in type, or an increase in amount of lipopolysaccharide. Such a change presumably functioned to exclude carbenicillin from its site of action.

Thomas & Broadbridge (1972) presented evidence that the cell wall of a strain of *P. aeruginosa* resistant to carbenicillin had higher lipid, phosphorus, calcium, magnesium and sodium content than the sensitive strain. These workers concluded that the cell wall of the resistant strain had reduced permeability to the antibiotic.

Zimelis & Jackson (1973) observed that calcium and magnesium antagonized the action of aminoglycoside antibiotics. These cations did not inactivate the antibiotics *per se* and they were inhibitory only if the cell wall was intact. They concluded that the interaction of calcium and magnesium with *P. aeruginosa*, resulting in resistance to aminoglycoside antibiotics, was at a locus exterior to the cell membrane, probably in the cell wall.

Mitsuhashi (1972) reported that resistant strains of *P. aeruginosa* lost their resistance to six aminoglycoside antibiotics after cold storage for twenty days. These results suggest that cold storage rendered the cell envelope permeable to these antibiotics.

Kay & Gronlund (1969) reported that the membrane of *P. aeruginosa* is made permeable to solutes at low temperature. This observation was confirmed by Midgley & Dawes (1973) who showed that washing cells of *P. aeruginosa* in ice-cold buffer resulted in the loss of over 90% of the intracellularly accumulated solute. Similarly, cold-shock loss of accumulated substrate pools in *E. coli* has been reported to approach totality (Leder, 1972). Thus, low temperature affects the membrane of mesophilic bacteria by causing the membrane to become permeable to solutes as a result of a phase transition change in membrane lipids.

These observations suggest an experimental approach to determine if certain types of antibiotic resistance of *P. aeruginosa* are due to exclusion of the antibiotics by the cell envelope. Cold-shock of *P. aeruginosa* when suspended in a solution of antibiotic will result in the intracellular accumulation of the antibiotic. Thus, if exclusion is the mechanism of resistance, then the subsequent growth of cells cold-shocked in the presence of antibiotic should be inhibited.

Penicillins

Eagon & Carson (1965) presented evidence which strongly suggested that the peptidoglycan (murein) layer was not solely responsible for the rigidity and shape of the cell envelope of *P. aeruginosa*. These authors observed that the reduction in absorbance owing to lysis of cells of *P. aeruginosa* suspended in an EDTA and lysozyme solution was greater than in a solution containing only EDTA. Lysozyme in the absence of EDTA was ineffectual in causing lysis. However, when cells were first incubated with lysozyme, then washed free of lysozyme, and then incubated with EDTA, the rate and extent of lysis were equal to that observed by incubation in the presence of both agents. This suggested that lysozyme acted against the peptidoglycan component of *P. aeruginosa* in the absence of EDTA.

Eagon & Carson (1965) then prepared a fluorescent derivative of lysozyme by labelling lysozyme with rhodamine. Cells incubated with rhodamine-labelled lysozyme showed fluorescence, indicating binding of lysozyme by the cell envelope. Fluorescence was lost upon washing the cells with water. These experimental data indicated (a) that lysozyme had indeed been removed by washing the cells and (b) that the increased rate and extent of lysis of cells pre-incubated with lysozyme upon suspension in EDTA were the result of lysozyme having broken sensitive linkages in the peptidoglycan component. Finally, Carson & Eagon (1966) presented electron microscopic evidence that the lysozyme-sensitive peptidoglycan layer of *P. aeruginosa* was accessible to lysozyme without prior incubation with EDTA.

Ashbell & Eagon (1966a,b) noted that incubation of *P. aeruginosa* with EDTA and lysozyme in a hypertonic environment resulted in the formation of osmotically fragile rods rather than spheroplasts. This confirmed an earlier and similar observation by Voss (1964). More recently, Henning, Höhn & Sonntag (1973) reported rod-shaped 'ghosts' isolated from *E. coli* cells which were devoid of peptidoglycan but which were surrounded by a unit membrane. The latter was identified as the outer (cell wall) membrane. Schnaitman (personal communication) has also concluded that the outer membrane may be involved in determining cell shape of *E. coli*.

These data offer an alternative explanation for the low level and/or intrinsic resistance to penicillins of strains of *P. aeruginosa* lacking β-lactamases. It is likely that the penicillins are not excluded by the cell envelope by these resistant strains. Instead, they may actually permeate the cell envelope and react with penicillin-sensitive sites with the resultant synthesis of a defective peptidoglycan layer. This may not be lethal in view of the fact that the data cited above suggest that *P. aeruginosa* might remain viable osmotically stable even with a defective peptidoglycan layer. This hypothesis could easily be experimentally tested and someone should do so.

Outer Membrane Proteins

The study of the outer (cell wall) membrane proteins of Gram-negative bacteria is an exciting new area. Outer membrane proteins have received little attention until recently. Instead, lipopolysaccharides have received an inordinate amount of attention.

Stinnett, Gilleland & Eagon (1973) reported that the cell envelope of *P. aeruginosa*, when grown in Tryptic Soy broth, contained three major proteins. Two of these major proteins were part of the protein-lipopolysaccharide complex of the outer membrane which was released upon exposure to EDTA (Stinnett, Gilleland & Eagon, 1973; Stinnett & Eagon, 1973). These two major proteins, furthermore, were shown to be glycoproteins. Moreover, the protein composition of the cell envelope appeared to vary with conditions of growth (Gilleland, Stinnett & Eagon, 1974).

The exact role of proteins in the outer membrane is not known. There is at present highly suggestive evidence that these proteins, in conjunction with lipopolysaccharide, serve to stabilize the cell envelope of *P. aeruginosa* and that they are necessary to maintain the structural integrity of the cell envelope. Other authors working with *E. coli* have arrived at similar conclusions (Henning, Höhn & Sonntag, 1973; C. A. Schnaitman, personal communication).

Most of the studies on bacterial outer membrane proteins have been carried out with *E. coli*. Much of this research has been pioneered by Schnaitman (1973a,b and personal communication). It has been demonstrated that the major polypeptide composition of *E. coli* is not constant. Instead, the polypeptide composition differs in different strains and it differs as a consequence of cultural conditions. The major outer membrane proteins of *E. coli*, however, may vary considerably without affecting the integrity of the outer membrane.

The outer membrane proteins are thought to represent integral proteins of the bacterial outer membrane. They may constitute as much as 70% of the total outer membrane of *E. coli*. Comparative studies on other species indicate that they are universal components of the outer membranes of Gram-negative bacteria (Schnaitman, 1970a,b; Stinnett & Eagon, 1974).

It has been noted that there is a direct relationship between the content of outer membrane protein and lipopolysaccharide (Ames, Spudich & Nikaido, 1974; Koplow & Goldfine, 1974; Rogers, Gilleland & Eagon, 1969; Stinnett, Gilleland & Eagon, 1973; Wu & Heath, 1973). The exact role played by these proteins remains unclear. The observation that *P. aeruginosa* is lysed on exposure to EDTA and that a protein–lipopolysaccharide complex is released (Rogers, Gilleland & Eagon, 1969; Gilleland *et al.*, 1973) suggests a structural role for the outer membrane proteins.

The outer membrane proteins could be the final products of genetic 'information' specifying cellular shape (Henning, Höhn & Sonntag, 1973) or specifying amount and type of lipopolysaccharide. On the other hand, these proteins might need lipopolysaccharide in order to be 'anchored' to it in the outer membrane (Ames, Spudich & Nikaido, 1974). None of these alternative explanations, however, fully accounts for the variability and interchangeability of the proteins of the major protein complex of the outer membrane of Gram-negative bacteria. It is highly probable, however, that the low level and/or intrinsic resistance of *P. aeruginosa* to antibiotics will be shown to be related to the protein content of the outer membrane.

CLINICAL IMPLICATIONS: A RATIONAL APPROACH TO CHEMOTHERAPY AND PROTECTION

Chemotherapeutic Agents

The sensitive site of attack by EDTA on *P. aeruginosa* now appears to be a protein–lipopolysaccharide complex either located on or embedded in the inside surface of the outer layer of the outer (cell wall) membrane (Gilleland *et al.*, 1973; Rogers, Gilleland & Eagon, 1969). Electron microscopy revealed that the protein–lipopolysaccharide complex occurs in the form of spherical units about 7 nm in diameter. The spherical units appeared to form rodlets composed of three or four spherical units. For reasons still not clearly understood, removal of about one-half of these spherical units (with accompanying loosely bound phospholipid) on exposure to EDTA results in osmotically fragile cells which undergo lysis. A rational approach to chemotherapy, then, would appear to be the development of antimicrobial agents specifically targeted to attack this protein–lipopolysaccharide complex in the outer membrane. EDTA would appear to be such an agent.

Cell surfaces of Gram-negative bacteria are damaged by exposure to EDTA (Eagon & Carson, 1965; Roberts, Gray & Wilkinson, 1970). Tris buffer enhances the effects of EDTA (Goldschmidt & Wyss, 1967; Neu, 1969; Voss, 1967). Exposure of Gram-negative bacteria to EDTA–Tris results in increased permeability to extracellular solutes (Hamilton-Miller, 1966; Leive, 1968a,b); sensitization of cells to lysozyme, to bactericides and to antibiotics (Brown & Richards, 1965; Haslam, Best & Durham, 1970; Monkhouse & Groves, 1967; Rawal & Owen, 1971; Repaske, 1956; Reybrouck & van de Voorde, 1969; Russel, 1967; Smith, 1970; Weiser, Assher & Wimpenny, 1968; Vymola *et al.*, 1968); release of periplasmic enzymes and cell membrane-associated proteins (Heppel, 1971); release of lipopolysaccharide, protein, phospholipid and divalent cations from the cell wall (Gilleland *et al.*, 1973; Leive, Shovlin & Mergenhagen, 1968; Roberts, Gray & Wilkinson, 1970; Rogers, Gilleland & Eagon, 1969; Stride, 1962).

EDTA-Tris is particularly active against *P. aeruginosa* and death is caused by rapid cellular lysis (Eagon & Carson, 1965; Gray & Wilkinson, 1965a). Most other Gram-negative bacterial species are also killed by exposure to EDTA–Tris provided that lysozyme is also present. A combination of EDTA, Tris and lysozyme, therefore, has potential use in chemotherapy to control infections caused by *P. aeruginosa*, particularly when the infected site can be treated by lavage or irrigation. Two groups of workers have already shown the effectiveness of this treatment. Goldschmidt, Kuhn, Perry & Johnson (1972) reported that EDTA–Tris–lysozyme lavage was effective in eradicating *Pseudomonas* and coliform bladder infections associated with indwelling catheters or genito-urinary instrumentation in human patients. Similarly, Wooley, Schall, Eagon and Scott (1974) showed that a solution of EDTA–Tris–lysozyme was effective in the treatments of experimentally induced *P. aeruginosa* cystitis in dogs. Most recently, Blue, Wooley & Eagon (unpublished observations) showed the efficacy of EDTA–Tris–lysozyme lavage in the treatment of experimentally induced *P. aeruginosa* otitis externa in dogs. In none of the cases was there any indication of detrimental effects on the bladder or ear tissue by this treatment.

EDTA–Tris would also be useful in therapy to inhibit metal-requiring toxins. For example, corneal ulcers are caused by a proteolytic enzyme produced by *P. aeruginosa* (Fisher & Allen, 1958). This protease requires calcium for activity (E. Fisher, Jr., personal communication). Thus, EDTA–Tris lavage might be useful not only to eradicate *P. aeruginosa* but to inhibit the proteolytic activity of the protease as well. Similarly, EDTA and ethylenetriaminepentaacetate have been demonstrated to have the ability to protect mice against lethal doses of *Clostridium perfringens* α-toxin (Lynch & Moskowitz, 1968). This toxin also requires calcium or other divalent cations for activity. The results discussed above demonstrate the usefulness of treatment of *P. aeruginosa* infections by lavage with a solution of EDTA–Tris–lysozyme. It is probable that this treatment would be effective without lysozyme being incorporated into the lavage solution. EDTA, moreover, has also been used in medicine for the treatment of (a) metal poisoning, (b) radioactive metal contamination, (c) hypercalcaemia, (d) atherosclerosis, (e) corneal calcification and (f) digitalis poisoning (Catsch, 1964; Cutting, 1972; Soffer *et al.*, 1964). Tris has been used in medicine (a) to treat salicylate intoxication and barbiturate poisoning, (b) to correct for hypercapnia or metabolic acidosis, (c) to produce diuresis and (d) to increase urine and plasma pH (Cutting, 1972). Thus, ample precedents have been set for the use of these agents in medicine.

Active chelating agents of the EDTA class, however, show considerable toxicity when used via systemic administration (Catsch, 1964; Cutting, 1972; Soffer *et al.*, 1964). The principal toxicity results from withdrawal of calcium from tissues and blood with resultant danger of hypocalcaemia and deposit of calcium in the kidneys. Thus, treatment with EDTA–Tris–lysozyme solution would appear to be limited to infections that could be treated by lavage or irrigation of the infected site.

The data discussed here, however, strongly suggest that EDTA–Tris(–lysozyme) therapy would be particularly useful in the treatment of infections caused by strains of *P. aeruginosa* resistant to gentamicin or to other antibiotics. Similarly, this therapy might also prove useful for the treatment of infections caused by other antibiotic-resistant Gram-negative bacteria and this therapy might be used to enhance the effectiveness of antibiotics against *Pseudomonas* and other Gram-negative bacteria. What is clear, however, is that a search is indicated for other antimicrobial agents that attack the same sensitive site as EDTA in the outer membrane of *P. aeruginosa*, but without the toxic side-effects of EDTA.

Protective Antibodies

Another rational approach to the control of infections by *P. aeruginosa* would appear to be through the production of antibodies specific for the outer membrane proteins. As antigen, one would use proteins associated with the protein–lipopolysaccharide complex which is liberated on exposure to EDTA and which appears to play an important role in the structural integrity of the cell envelope. These proteins can be isolated from the outer membrane in highly pure form. Antibodies thus produced would be expected to combine specifically with the EDTA-sensitive site in the outer membrane. The antibodies, in conjunction with complement, might very well lead to the production of osmotically unstable cells which would be killed through lysis.

Spheroplasts are formed from other Gram-negative bacteria by the action of the antibody complement system and lysozyme (Crombie & Muschel, 1965). Owing, however, to the unique sensitivity of *P. aeruginosa* to disruption of the protein–lipopolysaccharide complex in the outer membrane, lysozyme probably would not be required in conjunction with the antibody complement system for the formation of osmotically fragile cells.

The outer membrane proteins of *P. aeruginosa*, provided that they are not toxic, could be used as a vaccine for human patients. Alternatively, they could be used for the production of specific antiserum in animals. The antiserum would be used to confer passive immunity in those human patients who are pre-disposed to infection by *P. aeruginosa*, such as severely burned patients.

This approach to the control of *P. aeruginosa* infections takes advantage, therefore, of the unique ultrastructural properties of this microorganism.

REFERENCES

Adair, F. W., Geftic, S. G. & Gelzer, J. (1969). Resistance of *Pseudomonas* to quaternary ammonium compounds, I. Growth in benzalkonium chloride solution. *Appl. Microbiol.*, **18**, 299–302.

Adair, F. W., Geftic, S. G. & Gelzer, J. (1971a). Resistance of *Pseudomonas* to quaternary ammonium compounds, II. Cross-resistance characteristics of a mutant of *Pseudomonas aeruginosa*. *Appl. Microbiol.*, **21**, 1058–1063.

Adair, F. W., Geftic, S. G. & Gelzer, J. (1971b). Effect of a hostile environment on *Pseudomonas aeruginosa*. *Trans. N.Y. Acad. Sci.*, **33**, 799–813.

Ames, G. F.-L., Spudich, E. N. & Nikaido, H. (1974). Protein composition of the outer membrane of *Salmonella typhimurium*: effect of lipopolysaccharide mutants. *J. Bacteriol.*, **117**, 406–416.

Anderes, E. A., Sandine, W. E. & Elliker, P. R. (1971). Lipids of antibiotic-sensitive and -resistant strains of *Pseudomonas aeruginosa*. *Can J. Microbiol.*, **17**, 1357–1365.

Asbell, M. A. & Eagon, R. G. (1966a). The role of multivalent cations in the organization and structure of bacterial cell walls. *Biochem. Biophys. Res. Commun.*, **22**, 664–671.

Asbell, M. A. & Eagon, R. G. (1966b). Role of multivalent cations in the organization, structure, and assembly of the cell wall of *Pseudomonas aeruginosa*. *J. Bacteriol.*, **92**, 380–387.

Ayliffe, G. A. J., Lowbury, E. J. L. & Roe, E. (1972). Transferable carbenicillin resistance in *Pseudomonas aeruginosa*. *Nature New Biology*, **235**, 141.

Barrett, E. & Asscher, A. W. (1972). Action of EDTA on carbenicillin-resistant strains of *Ps. aeruginosa*. *J. Med. Microbiol.*, **5**, 355–360.

Bell, R. M., Mavis, R. D., Osborn, M. J. & Vagelos, P. R. (1971). Enzymes of phospholipid metabolism: localization in the cytoplasmic and outer membrane of the cell envelope of *Escherichia coli* and *Salmonella typhimurium. Biochim. Biophys. Acta,* **249**, 628–635.

Bennett, R. L., Lopes, J. & Rothfield, L. (1973). Identification of inducible proteins in the outer membrane of gram negative bacteria. *Abstr. Annu. Meet. Amer. Soc. Microbiol.*, p. 155.

Bobo, R. A. & Eagon, R. G. (1968). Lipids of cell walls of *Pseudomonas aeruginosa* and *Brucella abortus. Can. J. Microbiol.*, **14**, 503–513.

Branton, D. (1966). Fracture faces of frozen membranes. *Proc. Nat. Acad. Sci. U.S.A.* **55**, 1048–1056.

Branton, D. (1969). Membrane structure. *Ann. Rev. Plant Physiol.*, **20**, 209–238.

Braun, V. (1973). Molecular organization of the rigid layer and the cell wall of *Escherichia coli. J. Infect. Dis.*, **128**, S1–S8.

Brown, M. R. W. (1971). Inhibition and Destruction of *Pseudomonas aeruginosa*. In *Inhibition and Destruction of the Microbial Cell* (Ed. W. B. Hugo), Academic Press, New York, pp. 307–367.

Brown, M. R. W. (1972). Antibiotic resistance in *Pseudonomas aeruginosa*: surface layers. *J. Gen. Microbiol.*, **73**, v–vi.

Brown, M. R. W. & Melling, J. (1969a). Loss of sensitivity to EDTA by *Pseudomonas aeruginosa* grown under conditions of Mg-limitation. *J. Gen. Microbiol.*, **54**, 439–444.

Brown, M. R. W. & Melling, J. (1969b). Role of divalent cations in the action of polymyxin B and EDTA on *Pseudomonas aeruginosa. J. Gen. Microbiol.*, **59**, 263–274.

Brown, M. R. W. & Richards, R. M. E. (1965). Effect of ethylenediamine tetraacetate on the resistance of *Pseudomonas aeruginosa* to antibacterial agents. *Nature,* **207**, 1391–1393.

Brown, M. R. W. & Watkins, W. M. (1970). Low magnesium and phospholipid content of cell walls of *Pseudomonas aeruginosa* resistant to polymyxin. *Nature,* **227**, 1360–1361.

Brown, M. R. W. & Wood, S. M. (1972). Relation between cation and lipid content of cell walls of *Pseudomonas aeruginosa, Proteus vulgaris* and *Klebsiella aerogenes* and their sensitivity to polymyxin B and other antibacterial agents. *J. Pharm. Pharmac.* **24**, 215–218.

Bryan, L. E., Semaka, S. D., Van Den Elzen, H. M., Kinnear, J. E. & Whitehouse, R. L. S. (1973). Characteristics of R931 and other *Pseudomonas aeruginosa* R-factors. *Antimicrob. Agents Chemother.*, **3**, 625–637.

Bryan, L. E., Van Den Elzen, H. M. & Tseng, J. T. (1972). Transferable drug resistance in *Pseudomonas aeruginosa. Antimicrob. Agents Chemother.*, **1**, 22–29.

Brzezinska, M., Benveniste, R., Davies, J., Dánick, P. J. L. & Weinstein, J. (1972). Gentamicin resistance in strains of *Pseudomonas aeruginosa* mediated by enzymatic *N*-acetylation of the deoxy streptamine moiety. *Biochemistry*, **11**, 761–766.

Carson, K. J. & Eagon, R. G. (1966). Lysozyme sensitivity of the cell wall of *Pseudomonas aeruginosa*: further evidence for the role of the non-peptidoglycan components in cell wall rigidity. *Can. J. Microbiol.*, **12**, 105–108.

Catsch, A. (1964). *Radioactive Metal Mobilization in Medicine.* Charles C. Thomas, Springfield, Ill. 170 pp.

Chen, C.-C. H. & Feingold, D. S. (1972). Locus of divalent cation inhibition of the bactericidal action of polymyxin B. *Antimicrob. Agents Chemother.*, **2**, 331–335.

Chester, I. R., Gray, G. W. & Wilkinson, S. G. (1972). Further studies of the chemical composition of the lipopolysaccharide of *Pseudomonas aeruginosa. Biochem. J.*, **126**, 395–407.

Chester, I. R., Meadow, P. M. & Pitt, T. L. (1973). The relationship between the O-antigenic lipopolysaccharides and serological specificity in strains of *Pseudomonas aeruginosa* of different O-serotypes. *J. Gen. Microbiol.*, **78**, 305–318.

Clarke, K., Gray, G. W. & Reaveley, D. A. (1965). 'Lipid A' component from the cell-walls of *Pseudomonas aeruginosa*. *Nature*, **208**, 586–587.

Clarke, K., Gray, G. W. & Reaveley, D. A. (1967). The cell walls of *Pseudomonas aeruginosa*. General Composition. *Biochem. J.*, **105**, 749–754.

Cox, S. T., Jr. & Eagon, R. G. (1968). Action of ethylenediaminetetraacetic acid, tris(hydroxymethyl)aminomethane, and lysozyme on cell walls of *Pseudomonas aeruginosa*. *Can. J. Microbiol.*, **14**, 913–922.

Crombie, L. B. & Muschel, L. H. (1965). Quantitative studies on spheroplast formation by the antibody complement system and lysozyme on Gram-negative bacteria. *Federation Proc.*, **24**, 447.

Curtis, N. A. C., Richmond, M. H. & Stanisich, V. (1973). R-Factor mediated resistance to penicillin which does not involve a β-lactamase. *J. Gen. Microbiol.*, **79**, 163–166.

Cutting, W. C. (1972). *Handbook of Pharmacology*, 5th Edition. Meredith Corp., New York, N.Y. 659 pp.

Deamer, D. W. & Branton, D. (1967). Fracture planes in an ice-bilayer model membrane system. *Science*, **158**, 655–657.

Eagon, R. G. (1969). Cell wall-associated substances from *Pseudomonas aeruginosa*. *Can. J. Microbiol.*, **15**, 235–236.

Eagon, R. G. & Carson, K. J. (1965). Lysis of cell walls and intact cells of *Pseudomonas aeruginosa* by ethylenediamine tetraacetic acid and by lysozyme. *Can. J. Microbiol.*, **11**, 193–201.

Fensom, A. H. & Gray, G. W. (1969). The chemical composition of the lipopolysaccharide of *Pseudomonas aeruginosa*. *Biochem. J.*, **114**, 185–196.

Few, A. V., (1955). The interaction of polymyxin E with bacterial and other lipids. *Biochim. Biophys. Acta*, **16**, 137–145.

Few, A. V. & Schulman, J. H. (1953). The absorption of polymyxin E by bacteria and bacterial cell walls and its bactericidal action, *J. Gen. Microbiol.*, **9**, 454–466.

Fisher, E. Jr. & Allen, J. H. (1958). Corneal ulcers produced by cell-free extracts of *Pseudomonas aeruginosa*. *Amer. J. Ophthalmol.*, **46**, 21–27.

Fox, C. F. (1972). The structure of cell membranes. *Sci. Amer.*, **226**, 30–38.

Franklin, T. J. (1973). Antibiotic transport in bacteria. *CRC Crit. Rev. Microbiol.*, **2**, 253–272.

Garber, N. & Friedman, J. (1970). β-lactamase and the resistance of *Pseudomonas aeruginosa* to various penicillins and cephalosporins. *J. Gen. Microbiol.*, **64**, 343–352.

Gilleland, H. E., Jr., Stinnett, J. D., Roth, I. L. & Eagon, R. G. (1973). Freeze-etch study of *Pseudomonas aeruginosa*: Localization within the cell wall of an ethylenediaminetetraacetate–extractable component. *J. Bacteriol.*, **113**, 417–432.

Gilleland, H. E., Jr., Stinnett, J. D. & Eagon, R. G. (1974). Ultrastructural and chemical alteration of the cell envelope of *Pseudomonas aeruginosa*, associated with resistance to ethylenediaminetetraacetate resulting from growth in a Mg^{2+}-deficient medium. *J. Bacteriol.*, **117**, 302–311.

Goldschmidt, M. C., Kuhn, C. R., Perry, K. & Johnson, D. E. (1972). EDTA and lysozyme lavage in the treatment of *Pseudomonas* and bladder infections. *J. Urol.*, **107**, 969–972.

Goldschmidt, M. C. & Wyss, O. (1967). The role of tris in EDTA toxicity and lysozyme lysis. *J. Gen. Microbiol.*, **47**, 421–431.

Gray, G. W. & Wilkinson, S. G. (1965a). The action of ethylenediaminetetraacetic acid on *Pseudomonas aeruginosa*. *J. Appl. Bacteriol.*, **28**, 153–165.

Gray, G. W. & Wilkinson, S. G. (1965b). The effect of ethylenediaminetetra-acetic acid on the cell walls of some gram-negative bacteria. *J. Gen. Microbiol.*, **39**, 385–399.

Hamilton, W. A. (1968). The mechanism of the bacteriostatic action of tetrachlorosalicylanilide: a membrane-active antibacterial compound. *J. Gen. Microbiol*, **50**, 441–458.

140   *Resistance of Pseudomonas aeruginosa*

Hamilton-Miller, J. M. T. (1966). Damaging effects of ethylenediaminetetraacetate and penicillins on permeability barriers in Gram-negative bacteria. *Biochem. J.*, **100**, 675–682.

Hancock, I. C., Humphreys, G. O. & Meadow, P. M. (1970). Characterization of the hydroxy acids of *Pseudomonas aeruginosa* 8602. *Biochim. Biophys. Acta*, **202**, 389–391.

Haslam, D. R., Best, G. K. & Durham, N. N. (1970). Quantitation of the action of ethylenediaminetetraacetic acid and tris(hydroxymethyl)-aminomethane on a Gram-negative bacterium by vancomycin adsorption. *J. Bacteriol.*, **103**, 523–524.

Heilmann, H.-D. (1972). On the peptidoglycan of the cell walls of *Pseudomonas aeruginosa*. *Eur. J. Biochem.*, **31**, 456–463.

Henning, U., Höhn, B. & Sonntag, I. (1973). Cell envelope and shape of *Escherichia coli* K12. The ghost membrane. *Eur. J. Biochem.*, **39**, 27–36.

Heppel, L. A. (1971). The concept of periplasmic enzymes, In *Structure and Function of Biological Membranes*, (Ed. L. I. Rothfield), Academic Press, New York, N.Y., pp. 224–247.

Hoffman, H.-P., Geftic, S. G., Gelzer, J., Heymann, H. & Adair, W. F. (1973). Ultrastructural alterations associated with the growth of resistant *Pseudomonas aeruginosa* in the presence of benzalkonium chloride. *J. Bacteriol.*, **113**, 409–416.

Holloway, B. W., Krishnapilli, V. & Stanisich, V. (1971). *Pseudomonas* genetics. *Ann. Rev. Genetics*, **5**, 425–446.

Homma, J. Y. (1968). The protein moiety of the endotoxin of *Pseudomonas aeruginosa*. *Zeit. Allg. Mikrobiol.*, **8**, 227–248.

Homma, J. Y. & Suzuki, (1964). 'Cell-wall Protein A' of *Pseudomonas aeruginosa* and its relationship to 'original endotoxin protein'. *J. Bacteriol.*, **87**, 630–640.

Homma, J. Y. & Suzuki, N. (1966). The protein moiety of the endotoxin of *Pseudomonas aeruginosa*. *Ann. N.Y. Acad. Sci.*, **133**, 508–526.

Ikeda, K. & Egami, F. (1973). Lipopolysaccharide of *Pseudomonas aeruginosa* with special reference to Pyocin R receptor activity. *J. Gen. Appl. Microbiol.*, **19**, 115–128.

James, R. & Branton, D. (1973). Lipid- and temperature-dependent structural changes in *Acholeplasma laidlawii* cell membranes. *Biochim. Biophys. Acta*, **323**, 378–390.

Kay, W. W. & Gronlund, A. F. (1969). Carbohydrate metabolism in *Pseudomonas aeruginosa*: a procedure for accumulating phosphorylated intermediates. *Can. J. Microbiol.* **15**, 739–741.

Kobayashi, F., Yamaguchi, M. & Mitsuhashi, S. (1971a). Phosphorylated inactivation of aminoglycosidic antibiotics by *Pseudomonas aeruginosa*. *Japan J. Microbiol.*, **15**, 265–272.

Kobayashi, F., Yamaguchi, M. & Mitsuhashi, S. (1971b). Inactivation of dihydrostreptomycin by *Pseudomonas aeruginosa*. *Japan. J. Microbiol.*, **15**, 381–382.

Koike, M. & Iida, K. (1971). Effect of polymyxin on the bacteriophage receptors of the cell walls of gram-negative bacteria. *J. Bacteriol.*, **108**, 1402–1411.

Koplow, J. & Goldfine, H. (1974). Alterations in the outer membrane of the cell envelope of heptose-deficient mutants of *Escherichia coli*. *J. Bacteriol.*, **117**, 527–543.

Leder, I. G. (1972). Interrelated effects of cold shock and osmotic pressure on the permeability of the *Escherichia coli* membrane to permease accumulated substrates. *J. Bacteriol.*, **111**, 211–219.

Leive, L. (1968a). A nonspecific increase in permeability in *Escherichia coli* produced by EDTA. *Proc. Nat. Acad. Sci. U.S.A.*, **53**, 745–750.

Leive, L. (1968b). Studies on the permeability change produced in coliform bacteria by ethylenediaminetetraacetate. *J. Biol. Chem.*, **243**, 2373–2380.

Leive, L., Shovlin, V. K. & Mergenhagen, S. E. (1968). Physical, chemical, and immunological properties of lipopolysaccharide released from *Escherichia coli* by ethylenediaminetetraacetate. *J. Biol. Chem.*, **243**,6384–6391.

Lickfeld, K. G., Achterrath, M., Hentrich, F., Kolehmainen-Seveus, L. & Persson, A. (1972). Die Feinstrukturen von *Pseudomonas aeruginosa* in ihrer Deutung durch die Gefrierätztechnik, Ultramikrotomie und Kryoultramikrotomie. *J. Ultrastruct. Res.,* **38**, 27–45.

Lynch, K. L., & Moskowitz, N. (1968). Effects of chelates in chemotherapy of experimental gas-gangrene toxemia. *J. Bacteriol.,* **96**, 1925–1930.

Mach, B. & Tatum, E. L. (1963). Ribonucleic acid synthesis in protoplasts of *Escherichia coli*: inhibition by actinomycin D. *Science,* **139**, 1051.

Martin, H. H., Heilmann, H. D. & Preusser, H. J. (1972). State of the rigid-layer in cell walls of some Gram-negative bacteria. *Arch. Mikrobiol,* **83**, 332–346.

Midgley, M. & Dawes, E. A. (1973). The regulation of transport of glucose and methyl α-glucoside in *Pseudomonas aeruginosa*. *Biochem. J.,* **132**, 141–154.

Mitsuhashi, S. (1972). Lability of resistance to aminoglycoside antibiotics in *Pseudomonas aeruginosa*. *Chemotherapy (Tokyo),* **20**, 695–698.

Monkhouse, D. C. & Groves, G. A. (1967). The effect of EDTA on the resistance of *Pseudomonas aeruginosa* to benzalkonium chloride. *Australian J. Pharm.,* **48**, 570–575.

Mühlethaler, K., Moor, H. & Szarkowski, H. W. (1965). The ultrastructure of the chloroplast lamellae. *Planta,* **67**, 305–323.

Muschel, L. M., Ahl, L. A. & Fisher, M. W. (1969). Sensitivity of *Pseudomonas aeruginosa* to normal serum and to polymyxin. *Bacteriol.,* **98**, 453–457.

Nanninga, N. (1971). Uniqueness and location of the fracture plane in the plasma membrane of *Bacillus subtilis*. *J. Cell. Biol.,* **49**, 564–570.

Neu, H. C. (1969). The role of amine buffers in EDTA toxicity and their effect on osmotic shock. *J. Gen. Microbiol,* **57**, 215–220.

Newton, B. A. (1956). The properties and mode of action of the polymyxins. *Bacteriol. Rev.,* **20**, 14–27.

Olsen, R. H. & Shipley, P. (1973). Host range and properties of *Pseudomonas aeruginosa* R-factor R1822. *J. Bacteriol.,* **113**, 772–780.

Rawal, B. D. & Owen, W. R. (1971). Combined action of sulfamethoxazole, trimethoprim, and ethylenediaminetetraacetic acid on *Pseudomonas aeruginosa*. *Appl. Microbiol.,* **21**, 367–368.

Repaske, R. (1956). Lysis of gram-negative bacteria by lysozyme. *Biochim. Biophys. Acta,* **22**, 189–191.

Reybrouck, G. & van de Voorde, H. (1969). Effect of ethylenediaminetetraacetate on the germicidal action of disinfectants against *Pseudomonas aeruginosa*. *Acta Clinica Belgia,* **24**, 32–41.

Roberts, N. A., Gray, G. W. & Wilkinson, S. G. (1970). The bactericidal action of ethylenediaminetetra-acetic acid on *Pseudomonas aeruginosa*. *Microbios,* **2**, 189–208.

Rogers, S. W., Gilleland, Jr., H. E. & Eagon, R. G. (1969). Characterization of protein–lipopolysaccharide complex released from cell walls of *Pseudomonas aeruginosa* by ethylenediaminetetraacetic acid. *Can. J. Microbiol.,* **15**, 743–748.

Russel, A. D. (1967). Effect of magnesium ions and ethylenediaminetetraacetic acid on the activity of vancomycin against *Escherichia coli* and *Staphylococcus aureus*. *J. Appl. Bacteriol.,* **30**, 395–401.

Saunders, J. R. & Grinsted, J. (1972). Properties of RP4 an R-factor which originated in *Pseudomonas aeruginosa* S8. *J. Bacteriol.,* **112**, 690–696.

Schnaitman, C. A. (1970a). Examination of the protein composition of the cell envelope of *Escherichia coli* by pdyacrylamide gel electrophoresis. *J. Bacteriol.,* **104**, 882–889.

Schnaitman, C. (1970b). Comparisons of the envelope protein compositions of several Gram-negative bacteria. *J. Bacteriol.,* **104**, 1404–1405.

Schnaitman, C. A. (1973a). Other membrane proteins of *Escherichia coli*. I. Effect of preparative conditions on the migration of protein in polyarylamide gels. *Arch. Biochem. Biophys.*, **157**, 541–552.

Schnaitman, C. A. (1973b). Outer membrane proteins of *Escherichia coli*. II. Heterogeneity of major outer membrane polypeptides. *Arch. Biochem. Biophys.*, **157**, 553–560.

Sleytr, U. B. (1970). Fracture faces in intact cells and protoplasts of *Bacillus stearothermophilus*. A study of conventional freeze-etching and freeze-etching of corresponding fracture moieties. *Protoplasma*, **71**, 295–312.

Smith, G. (1970). Ethylene diamine tetra-acetic acid and the bactericidal efficiency of some phenolic disinfectants against *Pseudomonas aeruginosa*. *J. Med. Lab. Technol.*, **27**, 203–206.

Soffer, A., Chenoweth, N., Eichhorn, G. L., Rosoff, B., Rubin, M. & Spencer, H. (1964). *Chelation Therapy*. Charles C. Thomas, Springfield, Ill. 163 pp.

Speth, V. & Wunderlich, F. (1973). Membranes of Tetrahymena, II. Direct visualization of reversible transitions in biomembrane structure induced by temperature. *Biochim. Biophys. Acta*, **291**, 621–628.

Stinnett, J. D. & Eagon, R. G. (1973). Outer (cell wall) membrane proteins of *Pseudomonas aeruginosa*. *Can. J. Microbiol.*, **19**, 1469–1471.

Stinnett, J. D., Gilleland, Jr., H. E. & Eagon, R. G. (1973). Proteins released from cell envelopes of Pseudomonas aeruginosa on exposure to ethylenediaminetetraacetate: Comparison with dimethylformamide-extractable proteins. *J. Bacteriol.*, **114**, 399–407.

Stride, R. D. (1962). Recent developments in otitis externa. *British Med. J.* **1**, 607–609.

Suzuki, A. & Goto, S. (1972). Surface films of proteins and a protein-lipopolysaccharide complex extracted from *Pseudomonas aeruginosa*. *Biochim. Biophys. Acta*, **255**, 734–743.

Taubenek, U. (1962). Susceptibility of *Proteus mirabilis* and its stable L-forms to erythromycin and other macrolides. *Nature*, **196**, 195.

Thomas, A. H. & Broadbridge, R. A. (1972). The nature of carbenicillin resistance in *Pseudomonas aeruginosa*. *J. Gen. Microbiol.*, **70**, 231–241.

Thota, H. (1972). Comparison of extractable and non-extractable lipopolysaccharide of cell envelopes of *Pseudomonas aeruginosa* exposed to EDTA and to aqueous phenol. Ph.D. Thesis, University of Georgia.

Tseng, J. T. & Bryan, L. E. (1973). Mechanisms of R factor R931 and chromosomal tetracycline resistance in *Pseudomonas aeruginosa*. *Antimicrob. Agents Chemother.*, **3**, 638–644.

Tseng, J. T., Bryan, L. E. & Van Den Elzen, H. M. (1972). Mechanism and spectrum of streptomicin resistance in a natural population of *Pseudomonas aeruginosa*. *Antimicrob. Agents Chemother.*, **2**, 136–141.

Van Gool, A. P. & Nanninga, N. (1971). Fracture faces in the cell envelope of *Escherichia coli*. *J. Bacteriol.*, **108**, 474–481.

Voss, J. G. (1964). Lysozyme lysis of Gram-negative bacteria without production of spheroplasts. *J. Gen. Microbiol.*, **35**, 313–317.

Voss, J. G. (1967). Effects of organic cations on the Gram-negative cell wall and their bactericidal activity with ethylenediaminetetra-acetate and surface active agents. *J. Gen. Microbiol.*, **48**, 391–400.

Vymola, F., Nezval, J., Ryc, M., Taborsky, I., Pillich, J. & Pacova, Z. (1968). Prevention of the emergence of drug resistance in *Pseudomonas aeruginosa* by EDTA. *Sci. Med.*, **41**, 411–422.

Weiser, R., Asscher, A. W. & Wimpenny, J. (1968). *In vitro* reversal of antibiotic resistance by ethylenediaminetetraacetic acid. *Nature*, **219**, 1365–1366.

Weiss, R. L. & Fraser, D. (1973). Surface structure of intact cells and spheroplasts of *Pseudomonas aeruginosa*. *J. Bacteriol.*, **113**, 963–968.

White, D. A., Albright, F. R., Lennarz, W. L. & Schnaitman, C. A. (1971). Distribution of phospholipid-synthesizing enzymes in the wall and membrane subfractions of the envelope of *Escherichia coli. Biochim. Biophys. Acta,* **249**, 636–642.

Wilkinson, S. G. (1968). Studies on the cell walls of *Pseudomonas* species resistant to ethylenediaminetetra-acetic acid. *J. Gen. Microbiol.,* **54**, 195–213.

Wilkinson, S. G. (1970). Cell walls of *Pseudomonas* species sensitive to ethylenediaminetetraacetic acid. *J. Bacteriol.,* **104**, 1035–1044.

Wooley, R. E., Schall, W. D., Eagon, R. G. & Scott, T. A. (1974). The efficacy of EDTA-Tris-lysozyme lavage in the treatment of experimentally induced *Pseudomonas aeruginosa* cystitis in the dog. *Amer. J. Vet. Res.,* **35**, 27–29.

Wu, M. C. & Heath, E. C. (1973). Properties of a lipopolysaccharide–protein complex of *E. coli* cell envelope. *Federation Proc.,* **32**, 481.

Zimelis, V. M. & Jackson, G. G. (1973). Activity of aminoglycoside antibiotics against *Pseudomonas aeruginosa*: specificity and site of calcium and magnesium antagonism. *J. Infect. Dis.,* **127**, 663–669.

CHAPTER 5

Sensitivity to Ethylenediaminetetraacetic Acid

S. G. WILKINSON

INTRODUCTION

In a volume otherwise concerned with bacterial *resistance* and factors which contribute to it, the presence of a chapter on a specific example of *sensitivity* may be both unexpected and welcome. Perhaps even more remarkable is the fact that an organism so generally refractory as *Pseudomonas aeruginosa* should exhibit a type or degree of sensitivity found in few organisms outside the genus *Pseudomonas*. Thus, the antibacterial activity of ethylenediaminetetraacetic acid (EDTA) against *P. aeruginosa* is specific as well as potent. Although the main purpose of this chapter is to examine the nature and mode of action by EDTA, its prophylactic and therapeutic value (actual or potential) will also be discussed briefly.

For long it was believed that EDTA could not penetrate bacterial cells, because of the non-lipophilic character of the compound and its salts and chelates, and consequently had no antibacterial activity (Albert, 1960). The use of EDTA as a 'metal buffer' in culture media partly reflects this belief. The few early reports of the inhibition of bacterial growth by EDTA could reasonably be attributed to the sequestration of essential metal ions, rather than to direct action by EDTA on the bacteria. Similarly, the potentiation by

EDTA of recognized bactericides such as quaternary ammonium compounds (Bersworth & Singer, 1950) could largely be explained by the chelation of antagonistic metal ions. But even before the antibacterial properties of EDTA were fully appreciated, there were signs (e.g. Hatch & Cooper, 1948; Repaske, 1956, 1958; MacGregor & Elliker, 1958; Zemjanis & Hoyt, 1960; Stothart & Beecroft, 1961; Post, Krishnamurty & Flanagan, 1963; Elliott, Straka & Garibaldi, 1964) that pseudomonads were unusually sensitive to metal-binding compounds. As discussed below, there is now abundant evidence that *P. aeruginosa* and related species have high *intrinsic* sensitivity to EDTA. The antibacterial effects of EDTA and their importance in microbiology have previously been reviewed by Nezval & Ritzerfeld (1969a) and Russell (1971).

BACTERICIDAL ACTIVITY OF EDTA

Reports from many laboratories have confirmed that EDTA, used under appropriate conditions, possesses lytic, bactericidal activity against strains of *P. aeruginosa* (e.g. MacGregor & Elliker, 1958; Gray & Wilkinson, 1965a; Eagon & Carson, 1965; Wilkinson, 1967; Goldschmidt & Wyss, 1967; Brown & Melling, 1969a; Neu, 1969). Results from typical experiments are given in Table 1. Even at room temperature, the action of EDTA is rapid and almost irreversible: under conditions of high activity it is virtually complete within 2 min (Gray & Wilkinson, 1965a). The more gradual action under less toxic conditions (Gray & Wilkinson, 1965a; Brown & Melling, 1969a) probably involves secondary autolysis of damaged cells. Attempts to revive EDTA-treated cells (protected from lysis by 0·55 M sucrose) by treatment with cations known to be extracted by EDTA have met with slight success (Asbell & Eagon, 1966a,b). The few additional survivors were probably cells which had suffered only limited damage by EDTA. Likewise, the dilution fluid and recovery medium used in the determination of viable counts have relatively little influence on survival (Gray & Wilkinson, 1965a; Asbell & Eagon, 1966a,b), while EDTA-treated cells which do not produce colonies also fail to grow in nutrient broth (Gray & Wilkinson, 1965a).

Although high kills can be achieved with low concentrations of EDTA, the test suspensions of *P. aeruginosa* are not usually sterilized. In tests using

Table 1. Bactericidal effect of EDTA on *P. aeruginosa*. Examples of conditions under which viable counts were reduced by at least 99·99%

Strain	Conditions	Reference
N	0·85 mM EDTA, pH 7·4	MacGregor & Elliker (1958)
NCTC 1999	0·1 mM EDTA, pH 9·2, 10 min, 20 °C	Gray & Wilkinson (1965a)
OSU 64	0·9 mM EDTA, pH 8, 10 min, 30 °C	Eagon & Carson (1965)

0·1 mM EDTA at pH 9·2 and 20 °C, viable counts did not change significantly over the period 2 to 30 min, and the use of more concentrated EDTA did not lead to zero counts (Gray & Wilkinson, 1965a). Also, for thin suspensions of a given population, the fraction of organisms which survived EDTA-treatment was roughly independent of the number of cells used (other conditions being constant). These observations suggest that the survivors were the more resistant members of the population, although this was not confirmed by retreatment with EDTA. The cells used in the above tests were from batch cultures, in which a considerable spread of resistance might be expected: comparable tests of cells from continuous or synchronized cultures in defined media do not seem to have been made, but would be of much interest. It is likely that incomplete bactericidal action by EDTA (or similarly active compounds), followed by the growth of surviving organisms, largely explains the limited inhibition of growing cultures of 'sensitive' pseudomonads (Zemjanis & Hoyt, 1960; Post *et al.*, 1963; Elliott *et al.*, 1964), although growth can apparently be checked by EDTA without lysis (Brown & Richards, 1965). The fact of growth in the presence of EDTA seems to imply that the developing populations have enhanced EDTA-resistance. However, this needs to be verified by determining the concentration of residual (non-chelate) EDTA in the growing culture and by carrying out further tests on the new cells. Cells of *Escherichia coli* which survive EDTA-treatment do not seem to be genetically resistant (Voss, 1967; Leive, 1968). Although minimal inhibitory concentration (MIC) values for *P. aeruginosa* may vary widely with strain and growth medium, values up to about 30 mM for EDTA at pH about 7 have been obtained (Weiser, Asscher & Wimpenny, 1968; Adair, Geftic & Getzer, 1971. See, however, comments in Chapter 2).

Although high sensitivity to EDTA seems to be characteristic of mainstream pseudomonads, it is not confined to these organisms. Similar sensitivity has been reported for some other species from the order Pseudomonadales (Table 2), although not for all (e.g. *Desulphovibrio vulgaris*; Findley & Akagi, 1968).

Table 2. Species highly sensitive to EDTA

Species	Reference
Pseudomonas species	{ Shively & Hartsell (1964a) { Wilkinson (1967)
Spirillum itersonii	Garrard (1971)
Vibrio cholerae	⌠ Murti & Gupta (1960) ⎪ Adhikari & Chatterjee (1969) ⎨ Adhikari, Raychaudhuri & ⌡ Chatterjee (1969)
Vibrio eltor	{ Adhikari & Chatterjee (1969) { Adhikari *et al.* (1969)
Vibrio foetus	Zemjanis & Hoyt (1960)
Vibrio succinogenes	Wolin (1966)

Toxic action by EDTA has also been reported for other Gram-negative bacteria, including *Azotobacter vinelandii* (Socolofsky & Wyss, 1961; Goldschmidt & Wyss, 1966) and various enterobacteria (e.g. Gray & Wilkinson, 1965a; Goldschmidt, Goldschmidt & Wyss, 1967; Neu, Ashman & Price, 1967; Buller & Dobbs, 1971). However, the effect of EDTA is generally less marked and more critically dependent on the conditions of treatment, especially on the use of buffer containing 2-amino-2-(hydroxymethyl)propane-1,3-diol (tris), than in the case of *P. aeruginosa*. Also, the toxic effect on other organisms often seems to be a secondary one (Neu *et al.*, 1967): other effects associated with EDTA action (see later) can be produced without impairment to cell viability more readily than with *P. aeruginosa* (Leive & Kollin, 1967; Leive, 1968).

LYTIC ACTIVITY OF EDTA

The bactericidal action of EDTA against *P. aeruginosa* involves gross lysis of the cells, as judged by the decreased turbidity of cell suspensions and the release of intracellular solutes. In most reported studies (e.g. Repaske, 1956, 1958; Eagon & Carson, 1965), turbidity changes were rapid (comparable in rate but not in extent with viability changes): under conditions of slower lysis, the correlation is less secure (Brown & Melling, 1969a). Imperfect correlation between turbidity and viability measurements has been noted in other studies of the action of EDTA on bacteria. Thus, loss of viability can occur without comparable change in turbidity (e.g. Rodwell, 1965; Goldschmidt & Wyss, 1966; Neu *et al.*, 1967), while turbidity changes for *P. aeruginosa*, apparently including some caused by EDTA, need not imply loss of viability (e.g. Bernheim, 1963, 1969, 1972; Matula & MacLeod, 1969). Despite these limitations, the turbidimetric method has been very useful in studies of the lytic action of EDTA. In a typical experiment (Eagon & Carson, 1965), a loss of viability exceeding 99% corresponded to about 50% decrease in turbidity of the cell suspension. Almost total clearing occurred on subsequent or simultaneous treatment of the cells with lysozyme.

More direct evidence for the lysis of cells by EDTA is the loss of intracellular solutes during treatment. The leakage products are rich in phosphorus, pentose and materials with absorption maxima near 260 nm (Gray & Wilkinson, 1965a). Leakage appears to be less rapid than loss of viability, indicating that it is not the primary cause of death. In tests of thick suspensions of *P. aeruginosa* treated with 3·4 mM EDTA at pH 7·1 and 20 °C, leakage was rapid during the first hour and was largely complete within 3 hr (Gray & Wilkinson, 1965a). The above conditions (relatively low pH value and high cell: EDTA ratio) do not favour high bactericidal action by EDTA, and it is likely that rapid leakage due to lysis of some cells merges with slower processes involving partially damaged cells and autolytic reactions. Nevertheless, when determinations were made after 1 hr in similar tests using chelating agents at pH 7·1 or 9·2, a reasonably satisfactory correlation between leakage and loss of viability was obtained (Roberts, Gray & Wilkinson, 1970).

The release by EDTA of solutes absorbing at 260 nm is substantially greater than that produced by treatment of the cells with cold trichloroacetic acid (Gray & Wilkinson, 1965a). Thus, EDTA action involves more than loss of the nucleotide pool: the rapid (within 10 min) loss of this pool from *E. coli* and other enterobacteria during treatment with EDTA in tris buffer (pH 8·0) at 0 °C is not a significantly toxic process (Neu *et al.*, 1967). Fractionation of EDTA extracts from *P. aeruginosa* confirmed that most of the material absorbing at 260 nm was of high molecular weight (Roberts *et al.*, 1970). The presence in the extracts of polynucleotides (mainly RNA) is probably a direct consequence of lysis, although breakdown of RNA and decreasing viability can occur during prolonged exposure of *E. coli* to EDTA (Neu *et al.*, 1967; Leive & Kollin, 1967). Intracellular macromolecules are also released during the bactericidal, lytic action of EDTA on *Vibrio* species (Wolin, 1966; Adhikari *et al.*, 1969).

The solutes extracted from *P. aeruginosa* by EDTA at pH 9·2 include relatively little acid-precipitable protein (Roberts *et al.*, 1970), but although experimental evidence is lacking, the presence of periplasmic enzymes and various transport factors might be expected. At least one periplasmic enzyme (alkaline phosphatase) can be released from *P. aeruginosa* simply by washing with 0·2 M $MgCl_2$ at pH 8·4: other washing procedures are partially effective (Cheng, Ingram & Costerton, 1970a,b). However, the standard procedures for the release of periplasmic enzymes involve either the conversion of cells into spheroplasts using EDTA, tris buffer and lysozyme in concentrated sucrose solution, or the related treatment in which the action of EDTA in tris buffer is compounded by 'osmotic shock' (e.g. Malamy & Horecker, 1964; Neu & Heppel, 1965; Heppel, 1971). Treatment with EDTA and tris buffer alone is generally ineffective (Neu & Heppel, 1965), although exponential-phase cells of some enterobacteria grown at low Mg concentration are unusually sensitive to EDTA and release periplasmic enzymes without osmotic shock (Neu & Chou, 1967). Also, alkaline phosphatase, ribonuclease and soluble cytochrome *c* are readily released from the EDTA-sensitive organism *Spirillum itersonii* (Garrard, 1971), while even components of the cytoplasmic membrane can be extracted from EDTA-resistant *Haemophilus parainfluenzae* (Tucker & White, 1970). It therefore seems likely that the drastic action of EDTA on *P. aeruginosa* includes similar effects.

If treatment of *P. aeruginosa* with EDTA is done using hypertonic solutions of sucrose or NaCl (about 0·5 M), lysis is prevented or much reduced (Gray & Wilkinson, 1965a; Asbell & Eagon, 1966a,b; Wilkinson, 1967). Nevertheless, the treated cells are osmotically fragile and lyse when suspended in water. These fragile cells, termed 'osmoplasts' (Asbell & Eagon, 1966a), retain the bacillary form of the parent organisms, even when lysozyme is included in the preparative treatment (Voss, 1964; Asbell & Eagon, 1966a,b). Osmoplasts can be restored to an osmotically stable state by the addition of multivalent cations. The protective effect of these cations is relatively unspecific, but maximum recovery of viable cells was obtained by using a mixture of Ca^{2+},

Mg^{2+} and Zn^{2+} in the same ratio as found in the cell wall (Asbell & Eagon, 1966a,b). Other studies (Grossowicz & Ariel, 1963; Bernheim, 1972) suggest that di- and polyamines might also afford protection to cells damaged by EDTA. Despite their low viability, cation-restored cells of *P. aeruginosa* are motile and respire almost normally: if phosphate buffer is used during the EDTA treatment, the ability to form an induced permease to citrate is retained (Asbell & Eagon, 1966b). However, if EDTA is used in tris buffer, the ability to form induced permeases is lost and permease activity is absent from pre-induced restored cells (Eagon & Asbell, 1966; Kleber & Sorger, 1970). These results seem to confirm the earlier suggestion that transport factors can be released during lysis of *P. aeruginosa* by EDTA.

SENSITIZING EFFECTS OF EDTA

Whilst toxicity, the most extreme manifestation of the antibacterial properties of EDTA, is restricted to a few species, the non-lethal effects of this reagent are widespread. Reference to some of these effects, e.g. the release of periplasmic enzymes by osmotic shock, has already been made. Such effects seem to be based on the ability of EDTA to cause a relatively unspecific change in the permeability characteristics of cells, and can result in sensitization to a wide variety of other antibacterial agents. This property of EDTA has mainly been studied with *E. coli*, but sub-lethal concentrations of EDTA affect *P. aeruginosa* similarly.

The standard conditions developed by Leive (1965b; 1968) for increasing the permeability of *E. coli* are treatment of buffer-washed cells (about 5×10^9/ml) for 2 min at 37 °C with 0·2 mM EDTA in 0·12 M tris buffer (pH 8·0). *P. aeruginosa* is lysed under these conditions, but other coliform bacteria behave like *E. coli* (Leive, 1968). By avoiding prolonged exposure to EDTA and treatment with tris buffer at 0–4 °C, the permeable cells remain viable, retain their nucleotide pools and active transport functions, and grow at an almost normal rate (Leive & Kollin, 1967; Leive, 1968). Repair of the permeability barrier during growth requires energy metabolism and is complete in less than one generation time.

The enhanced permeability of EDTA-treated cells can be demonstrated in various ways. For example, the penetration of cells by enzyme substrates for which the organism lacks the necessary permeases is possible after EDTA treatment (Leive, 1965b). Similarly, treated cells can be attacked by degradative enzymes, e.g. lysozyme (Repaske, 1956, 1958) and phospholipases (Slein & Logan, 1967), to which they are normally resistant. For academic microbiology, the sensitization of Gram-negative bacteria to lysozyme is one of the most important consequences of EDTA-induced permeability. The combination of EDTA with lysozyme has been used widely for the preparation of osmotically fragile spheroplasts and for the study of bacterial surface structures. 'Membrane' preparations useful for the study of enzyme distributions can be obtained from many bacteria including *P. aeruginosa* (e.g. Campbell, Hogg &

Strasdine, 1962; Norton, Bulmer & Sokatch, 1963; Nagata, Mizuno & Maruo, 1966). Although egg-white lysozyme is the enzyme normally used, milk lysozymes are also potentiated by EDTA (Vakil, Chandan, Parry & Shahani, 1969): interestingly, the milk enzymes show significant activity against *P. aeruginosa* even without EDTA.

From the clinical point of view, sensitization to antibacterial agents is the most important result of treating Gram-negative organisms with EDTA. Compounds of which the action against *P. aeruginosa* is reported to be potentiated by EDTA are listed in Table 3. Various other compounds for

Table 3. Sensitization of *P. aeruginosa* to antibacterial agents by EDTA

Agent	Reference
Phenolic compounds	Stothart & Beecroft (1961)
	Gray & Wilkinson (1965a)
	Reybrouck & van de Voorde (1969)
	Smith (1970)
Quaternary ammonium compounds	MacGregor & Elliker (1958)
	Nezval (1964)
	Brown & Richards (1965)
	Reybrouck & van de Voorde (1969)
	Adair *et al.* (1971)
Chlorhexidine	Brown & Richards (1965)
Chloramine	Reybrouck & van de Voorde (1969)
Nalidixic acid	Nezval & Halačka (1967)
Sulphamethoxazole and trimethoprim	Rawal & Owen (1971)
2-Hydroxy-3-(dimethylhexadecyl-ammonio)-propane-1-sulphonate	Voss (1967)
Polymyxin	Brown & Richards (1965)
Neomycin	Nezval, Smékal, Skotáková & Rýc (1965)
Rifampicin	Nezval & Ritzerfeld (1969b)
Chloramphenicol	Weiser, Asscher & Wimpenny (1968)
	Weiser, Wimpenny & Asscher (1969)
	Nezval & Ritzerfeld (1970)
Tetracycline	Weiser *et al.* (1968, 1969)
Benzylpenicillin	Weiser *et al.* (1968, 1969)
Ampicillin	Weiser *et al.* (1968, 1969)
	Výmola, Nezval, Rýc, Táborský, Pillich & Páčová (1968)
Novobiocin	Cleeland, Beskid & Grunberg (1970)
Coumermycin A₁	Cleeland *et al.* (1970)

which similar observations have been made are described in the patent literature. On the other hand, the effectiveness of gentamicin and carbenicillin against *P. aeruginosa* is apparently not improved by EDTA (Nezval & Ritzerfeld, 1970). In view of the chemotherapeutic importance of these antibiotics and the potentiation reported for related agents (Table 3), confirmation of these results seems desirable. In fact, synergism between EDTA and gentamicin has recently been reported for 7 out of 10 naturally occurring strains of *P. aeruginosa* (Pechey & James, 1974).

Because of the exceptional sensitivity of *P. aeruginosa* to EDTA, potentiating effects for this organism can be particularly large, e.g. 250-fold improvement of a phenolic germicide (Stothart & Beecroft, 1961). Although bactericidal action by EDTA itself can contribute to such effects (e.g. Gray & Wilkinson, 1965a), it is not a prerequisite (e.g. Brown & Richards, 1965; Reybrouck & van de Voorde, 1969). The compounds listed in Table 3 represent widely differing modes of antibacterial action, and bacterial resistance to them can take several forms (Franklin & Snow, 1971; Benveniste & Davies, 1973). Thus, the nature of EDTA-potentiation is unlikely to be identical in all cases. Nevertheless, disruption of a permeability barrier by EDTA is probably a common cause of sensitization (Franklin, 1973). Increased permeability of Gram-negative organisms after EDTA treatment has been demonstrated or inferred for various antibiotics and bactericides, e.g. actinomycin D (Leive, 1965a), benzylpenicillin (Hamilton-Miller, 1965, 1966), puromycin (Sellin, Srinivasan & Borek, 1966), PA 114 A (Ennis, 1967), vancomycin (Russell, 1967; Haslam, Best & Durham, 1970), rifampicin (Reid & Speyer, 1970), viomycin (Yu & Jordan, 1971), erythromycin (Spicer & Spooner, 1974) and some other agents listed in Table 3. Antibacterial agents have been categorized by Muschel & Gustafson (1968) according to whether or not their effectiveness is limited by a permeability barrier disrupted by EDTA. Lack of EDTA-potentiation against *Salmonella typhi* was found for chloramphenicol, chlortetracycline and various aminoglycoside antibiotics (Muschel & Gustafson, 1968). Since potentiation of these or related antibiotics can occur with other organisms (e.g. Weiser *et al.*, 1968), it is apparent that the existence or importance of permeability barriers will vary with organism and strain as well as with antibiotic. The result obtained in a test for potentiation may also depend on the method used (Russell, 1971; see also Chapter 2, page 60). Whilst the effects of EDTA on the actions of ampicillin, chloramphenicol, tetracycline and the sulphamethoxazole–trimethoprim combination against *E. coli* and other enterobacteria seem to be additive (Neu & Winshell, 1970; Then, 1972), the corresponding effects for *P. aeruginosa* can be described as synergistic (Weiser *et al.*, 1969; Rawal & Owen, 1971). The role of the permeability barrier in the resistance of *P. aeruginosa* is discussed more fully in Chapters 3 and 4 of this volume.

FACTORS AFFECTING ANTIBACTERIAL ACTIVITY

The failure to recognize sooner the toxicity of EDTA for *P. aeruginosa* may be attributed partly to the incompleteness of the bactericidal action, and partly to the dependence of bactericidal activity on experimental conditions. Many factors seem to be involved, but the systematic studies needed to separate conclusively, establish and rationalize individual effects have not yet been made. The complexities of the biological system and our limited knowledge of the physicochemical properties of bacterial surface structures constitute major obstacles to such studies.

Chelating Ability

In the discussion so far, it has been implied that the antibacterial actions of EDTA can be attributed to its metal-binding properties. Although alternative hypotheses will be considered later, some of the evidence in favour of a mode of action based on the chelation of essential metal ions will be presented at this point. Part of this evidence comes from comparisons of the effects of different metal-binding agents (Gray & Wilkinson, 1965a; Roberts *et al.*, 1970; Haque & Russell, 1974; Spicer & Spooner, 1974). In addition to EDTA, other aminopolycarboxylic acids (Table 4) with good metal-binding properties are

Table 4. Aminopolycarboxylic acids active against *P. aeruginosa*

Ethylenediaminetetraacetic acid (EDTA)
trans-Cyclohexane-1,2-diaminetetraacetic acid (CDTA)
Diethylenetriaminepentaacetic acid (DTPA)
N-(2-Hydroxyethyl)ethylenediaminetriacetic acid (HEDTA)
[(Ethylenedioxy)diethylenedinitrilo]tetraacetic acid (EGTA)
Nitrilotriacetic acid (NTA)

toxic for *P. aeruginosa*, and their bactericidal activities can be correlated with their affinities for Mg^{2+} in particular (Roberts *et al.*, 1970). The results obtained with EGTA, which has rather greater affinity for Ca^{2+} at pH 9·2 than does EDTA, are of special interest. The fact that EGTA had the lower bactericidal activity at that pH value indicates that chelation of Ca^{2+} was not the major toxic process for the particular cells under test. Less avid aminopolycarboxylic acids (e.g. iminodiacetic acid and *trans*-cyclohexane-1,4-diaminetetraacetic acid) and other relatively weak or less hydrophilic metal-binding agents (e.g. 2,2'-bipyridyl, 1,10-phenanthroline, pyridine-2,6-dicarboxylic acid and 8-hydroxyquinoline) are inactive against *P. aeruginosa* (Gray & Wilkinson, 1965a; Eagon & Carson, 1965; Goldschmidt & Wyss, 1967; Roberts *et al.*, 1970). On the other hand, sodium hexametaphosphate has an activity similar to that of EDTA (Gray & Wilkinson, 1965a; Roberts *et al.*, 1970), indicating that structural features of the reagent other than those which contribute to chelating ability are unimportant.

Comparable evidence in support of a chelating mode of action can be derived from other studies. Repaske (1958) found that other (weaker) chelating agents could not replace EDTA in the sensitization of Gram-negative bacteria to lysozyme, but that treatment of the cells with a strong cation-exchange resin (H^+ form) had an effect similar to that of EDTA. A quantitative release of alkaline phosphatase was obtained when a chelating resin (Chelex 100) was used in osmotic shock treatment of *E. coli*, but other metal-binding reagents (apart from ATP) were less effective than EDTA (Neu & Heppel, 1965). Of the chelating agents tested, only EDTA increased the permeability of *Klebsiella aerogenes* to benzylpenicillin (Hamilton-Miller, 1965).

The dependence of antibacterial activity on chelation is also indicated by studies using various chelates of EDTA. Thus, chelates neither sensitized *E. coli* to actinomycin D (Leive, 1968) nor *P. aeruginosa* to other antibiotics (Brown & Richards, 1965; Nezval *et al.*, 1965; Weiser *et al.*, 1968). Although the magnesium chelate slightly affected the permeability barrier of *K. aerogenes* (Hamilton-Miller, 1966), this could have been due to the substitution of magnesium for calcium, which is more strongly chelated and which seemed to be extracted by EDTA itself. Like EDTA, the calcium chelate increased the rate of swelling of *P. aeruginosa* previously exposed to salt solutions, but different sites of action were indicated (Bernheim, 1972). It is not clear whether the effect of EDTA on the swelling of cells is closely related to its lytic, bactericidal effect. Finally, the stabilizing or restorative effects of multivalent metal cations on EDTA-treated cells (e.g. Repaske, 1958; Asbell & Eagon, 1966a,b; Hamilton-Miller, 1966; Findley & Akagi, 1968) also support a chelating mode of action by EDTA. The requirement of high chelating ability further indicates that the action of EDTA involves competition for metal ions firmly bound by the bacterial cells.

State of the Test Organisms

Sensitivity to EDTA has been found for *P. aeruginosa* grown under widely differing conditions. Nevertheless, the response of the organism to treatment with EDTA varies both with the age of the culture and with the growth medium used (Repaske, 1958; see also Chapter 2 of this volume). In tests using EDTA and lysozyme, Repaske noted that the percentage of the total lysis which could be obtained by the action of EDTA alone fell from 74% for 7-hr cultures (early logarithmic growth) to 36% for 48-hr cultures (total lysis was apparently similar for both young and old cultures). Similar observations on the relative fragility of logarithmic-phase cells have been made in other studies of effects involving the action of EDTA (e.g. Slein & Logan, 1967; Neu & Chou, 1967). Variations in sensitivity to EDTA with growth medium can presumably be partly attributed to differences in the growth phase of the test cultures, and possibly to slime formation in some cases (Brown & Foster, 1971). However, most studies of the effect of EDTA on *P. aeruginosa* have used complex media, and more significant factors affecting sensitivity have been revealed by the use of defined media. Unreported studies made in 1963 by R. A. Cowen (personal communication) showed that N-limited, stationary-phase, batch cultures of *P. aeruginosa* NCTC 1999 grown with an initial Mg concentration of 4 μg/ml were resistant to EDTA, whereas corresponding cultures grown at higher Mg concentration (40 μg/ml) had normal sensitivity. Similar results were obtained using Ca and, to a lesser extent, Zn. Independent studies by Brown & Melling (1969a,b) with *P. aeruginosa* NCTC 6750 also showed that increasing Mg limitation progressively decreased the sensitivity to EDTA. It should be noted that the range of Mg concentrations (0·05–4·0 µg/ml) used by Brown and Melling was substantially lower than that used by Cowen, and growth of the cultures was terminated by depletion of the C source. Extensive, rapid lysis was not observed even with the most sensitive cells (grown with Mg concentration 1 µg/ml and treated with about 3 μM EDTA (pH 7·2) at 37·5°C). Cells grown under conditions of severe Mg limitation were not made EDTA-sensitive simply by exposure to Mg^{2+}, but sensitivity was gradually recovered during growth at higher Mg concentration (Brown & Melling, 1969b). These authors also showed that Ca and Zn, in decreasing order of effectiveness, added to Mg-limited media gave cultures increased sensitivity to EDTA. The results of these and subsequent studies by Brown and his colleagues are described more fully in Chapter 2, and a possible explanation for the effect of Mg limitation is considered later in the present chapter.

The sensitivity to EDTA of test cells is also affected by treatments which precede exposure to EDTA. Repaske (1958) found that the lysis by EDTA and lysozyme of cells which had been stored for several hours was less than that of freshly harvested and washed cells. Sensitivity could be restored simply by aerating the cell suspension. The application and nature of washing procedures can also moderate EDTA sensitivity. Surprisingly, the bactericidal effect of 3·4 mM EDTA in borate buffer (pH 7·1) on unwashed cells of *P. aeruginosa* was greater than that on water-washed cells; buffer-washed cells were even less sensitive (Gray & Wilkinson, 1965a). Variation in the toxic effect with the washing procedure was also noted by Goldschmidt & Wyss (1967). However, such effects are not always apparent. Whereas washing *S. typhi* with NaCl solution instead of water considerably decreased the extent of lysis by EDTA and lysozyme (Raza Nasir & Ghatak, 1970), washing *E. coli* with either 0·85% NaCl or 10 mM tris buffer (pH 7·4) gave cells of equal sensitivity (Neu, 1969). The EDTA-induced permeability change and the effectiveness of osmotic shock on *E. coli* are also relatively insensitive to the nature of the preliminary washing procedure (Neu & Chou, 1967; Leive, 1968). As a second-order effect, the washing procedure is possibly decisive only in situations where the major factors which determine the response of the cell to EDTA are poised.

With the limited data available, the effects of washing cannot be properly characterized or interpreted. Nevertheless, possibly significant changes in the surface properties of the cells can be suggested. Gram-negative bacteria, including *P. aeruginosa* (Bernheim, 1963; Matula & MacLeod, 1969), when suspended in water shrink rapidly on the addition of salts, then slowly swell. These effects, as reflected in turbidity changes, seem to be primarily osmotic in nature and involve the cytoplasmic membrane (Knowles, 1971; Alemohammad & Knowles, 1974), although the situation for *P. aeruginosa* is less clear than that for *E. coli* (Matula & MacLeod, 1969). However, studies with whole cells and isolated walls have shown that the volume of the wall is also affected by salts, probably as a result of electrostatic interactions. The salt-induced contraction of the walls of Gram-positive bacteria and their expansion at high pH values could be rationalized by considering the walls as amphoteric polyelectrolytes (Marquis, 1968; Ou & Marquis, 1970). Similar considerations can probably be applied to the wall of *P. aeruginosa* (Shively & Hartsell, 1964b; Matula & MacLeod, 1969). Superimposed on and possibly contributing to the above effects are changes in the ionic balance of the cell wall and cytoplasmic membrane as a result of cation-uptake or cation-exchange during washing. The effects of such changes on *P. aeruginosa* may be particularly significant (e.g. Cheng *et al.*, 1970a). Differences between the surfaces of cells washed in different ways may be large and persistent enough to affect their response to EDTA treatment. The vulnerability of water-washed *P. aeruginosa* (Brown, 1968) may be related to the distended state of such cells, and the desensitizing effect of 0·2 M borate buffer (Gray & Wilkinson, 1965a) may be attributable to salt-induced contraction of the wall, possibly assisted by complexing of the buffer with carbohydrate components of the wall.

Conditions of EDTA-treatment

The sensitivity of an organism, as measured by the effect produced by a particular concentration of EDTA in a given time, depends critically on the choice of other test conditions. Most obviously, the effect can vary with the cell: EDTA ratio, if the process of chelation significantly reduces the concentration of free EDTA (Garrard, 1971). The rate and extent of leakage from *P. aeruginosa* (thick suspension) can be increased by raising the concentration of EDTA or, more significantly, by lowering the density of the cell suspension (Gray & Wilkinson, 1965a; S. G. Wilkinson, unpublished results). Other test conditions such as the pH and the ionic strength of the medium can affect not only the cell surface and thereby the response to EDTA as discussed previously, but also the chelating ability of EDTA. The optimum pH values for the chelation of Ca^{2+} and Mg^{2+} are 7·5 and 10, respectively (Ringbom, 1954), and the stabilities of the chelates are adversely affected by increasing ionic strength. Although similar considerations may also apply to the relevant metal-binding sites in bacteria, the competitive position of EDTA would be better at high pH if (poly)phosphate residues and Mg^{2+} are involved (Roberts *et al.*, 1970). The greater bactericidal action against *P. aeruginosa* of EDTA in 0·05 M borate buffer (pH 9·2) compared with 0·2 M borate buffer (pH 7·1) is consistent with the combined effects of pH value and ionic strength (Gray & Wilkinson, 1965a; Roberts *et al.*, 1970). Similar effects of pH on the toxicity of EDTA in tris buffer for *V. succinogenes* and *A. vinelandii* cysts have been reported (Wolin, 1966; Goldschmidt & Wyss, 1966). The EDTA-induced permeability changes for other Gram-negative bacteria also seem to have mildly alkaline pH optima (Hamilton-Miller, 1965; Neu *et al.*, 1967; Leive, 1968), and this probably contributes to the enhanced lysis of these organisms by EDTA and lysozyme at alkaline pH values (e.g. Repaske, 1958; Shively &

Hartsell, 1964b; Raza Nasir & Ghatak, 1970). Some failures to elicit the expected response to EDTA from sensitive organisms (e.g. Patel & Shah, 1965; Reybrouck & van de Voorde, 1969) may be attributed to the use of unbuffered solutions of the disodium salt of EDTA, which are weakly acidic. The greater lysis of *P. aeruginosa* by EDTA in phosphate buffer (pH 7·0) compared with distilled water (Shively & Hartsell, 1964a) may have the same explanation. The expected adverse effect of increased ionic strength alone on the activity of EDTA against *P. aeruginosa* has been demonstrated (Goldschmidt & Wyss, 1967). The inclusion of 0·15 M NaCl in an EDTA–tris buffer reagent increased the survival of buffer-washed cells from 13% to 23% and partially inhibited lysis by EDTA–lysozyme. Similar observations were made by Shively & Hartsell (1964b): the lysis of *P. fragi* by EDTA–lysozyme in dilute phosphate buffer (pH 7·0) was prevented by 0·17 M NaCl, and the lysis of other pseudomonads, including *P. aeruginosa*, was decreased by 0·34 M NaCl. However, Goldschmidt & Wyss (1967) also found that EDTA had a greater effect on water-washed *P. aeruginosa* in the presence of 0·15 M NaCl (but no buffer) than in its absence. This result cannot be explained on the basis of the effects discussed.

The lysis of sensitive bacteria (Table 2) by EDTA requires a hypotonic medium. Osmotic stabilization is most commonly provided by sucrose (about 0·5 M), but non-penetrating salts can also be used. Thus, the inhibition of EDTA-induced lysis of *P. aeruginosa* by 0·15 M NaCl (Goldschmidt & Wyss, 1967) could be an osmotic effect of the salt, since other results described above showed that the antibacterial activity of EDTA was not fully repressed. Solutions of NaCl (0·15 M) and sucrose (0·3 M) were equally effective in preventing lysis of *V. cholerae* and *V. eltor* (Adhikari *et al.*, 1969) and *V. succinogenes* (Wolin, 1966). However, the absence of lysis of the latter organism after treatment with EDTA in 0·15 M NaCl at pH 9·0, then washing and resuspension of the cells in a hypotonic medium, showed that the action of EDTA had been prevented or greatly attenuated. On the other hand, hypertonic solutions containing NaCl (0·5 M) as used to prevent lysis of EDTA-treated *P. aeruginosa* in other studies (Gray & Wilkinson, 1965a; Asbell & Eagon, 1966b) do not inhibit the action of EDTA in osmotic shock treatment of enterobacteria (Neu & Chou, 1967). Unlike osmoplasts of *P. aeruginosa* prepared using EDTA in 0·5 M sucrose, those prepared in 0·5M NaCl could not be restored and stabilized against lysis by multivalent cations (Asbell & Eagon, 1966b). The situation is confused even further by the report that *P. aeruginosa* is freely penetrated by NaCl, and that the salt-induced rapid increase in turbidity was not followed by a slow decrease when 0·5 M NaCl was used (Matula & MacLeod, 1969). From this limited discussion and the work of Bernheim (1963, 1969, 1972) it is apparent that further studies are necessary to clarify the complex interplay of salt effects on *P. aeruginosa* and the action of EDTA.

Following the observations of Repaske (1958), the potentiating effects of tris buffer on the antibacterial actions of EDTA have been very widely reported.

Repaske noted that the lysis of Gram-negative bacteria by EDTA–lysozyme was far more rapid in tris buffer than in others tried, and that the rate of lysis increased with buffer concentration up to a species-dependent optimum value. Tris buffers are also most effective in osmotic shock treatments (Neu & Chou, 1967), in the extraction of nucleotide pools (Neu *et al.*, 1967), and possibly in the alteration of permeability characteristics generally (Leive, 1968; Neu, 1969). Although weakly alkaline solutions of EDTA are toxic for *P. aeruginosa* even in the absence of buffer, the activity of EDTA is greater in the presence of tris buffer than phosphate (Asbell & Eagon, 1966b), borate (S. G. Wilkinson, unpublished results), or other amine-type buffers (Goldschmidt & Wyss, 1967; Neu, 1969). With other Gram-negative bacteria, the co-operative effect of tris buffer can be essential to action by EDTA. Tris has weak metal-binding properties (e.g. Hanlon, Watt & Westhead, 1966; Allen, Baker & Gillard, 1967), and it has been suggested that it potentiates the action of EDTA by forming mixed chelates of increased stability (Goldschmidt & Wyss, 1966, 1967). Possibly more significant is the fact that tris possesses separate and distinctive antibacterial activity. Thus, cold tris buffer causes the release of nucleotide pools from enterobacteria without producing the permeability changes characteristic of EDTA action (Neu *et al.*, 1967; Leive & Kollin, 1967; Leive, 1968). Most of the periplasmic alkaline phosphatase was released from *Sp. itersonii* by tris buffer, if the cells were pre-treated with EDTA then thoroughly washed with water: the reverse sequence of treatments was ineffective (Garrard, 1971). These and similar observations indicate that tris has a specific effect on bacterial surface structures. Voss (1967) suggested that tris was active as an organic cation, and showed that other organic cations had similar effects and also removed somatic antigens from *E. coli* and *S. typhi*. Tris buffer has also been shown to solubilize material from isolated walls of *P. aeruginosa* (Cox & Eagon, 1968), and this effect is likely to underlie the potentiation of EDTA action.

Finally, the effect of temperature has been included in several studies of factors which influence the antibacterial activities of EDTA. The release of intracellular solutes from *P. aeruginosa* by EDTA in borate buffer (pH 7·1) was less at 0–2 °C than at 20 °C (Gray & Wilkinson, 1965a). However, the extent of the decrease (31% or 66%, depending on the method of calculation) could not be decided because of leakage from cells treated with cold buffer only, presumably as a result of 'cold shock' (Gorrill & McNeil, 1960; Farrell & Rose, 1968; MacKelvie, Gronlund & Campbell, 1968). Evidence that the bactericidal activity of EDTA against *P. aeruginosa* is less at 2 °C than at 37 °C has been reported briefly (Haslam, Best & Durham, 1969). The adsorption of vancomycin to the cell wall of a species of *Flavobacterium* after treatment with EDTA was also less at low temperature (Haslam *et al.*, 1970). On the other hand, the EDTA-induced permeability change in *E. coli* is complete within 15 sec at either 4 °C or 37 °C (Leive, 1968). Similar results for the EDTA-induced release of periplasmic proteins from *Sp. itersonii* were obtained by Garrard (1971), although unfortunately a comparison of the viabilities of cells treated with EDTA at either 4 °C or 24 °C was apparently not made. The overall impression from these studies is that the non-toxic permeability changes induced by EDTA are rapid and largely independent of temperature, but that autolysis may be involved in the lethal or lytic effects on some organisms.

EFFECTS OF EDTA ON CELL ENVELOPES

The accumulated evidence of the antibacterial effects of EDTA points clearly to action at the cell surface, and in particular to action on the wall element of the cell envelope. For example, the release of periplasmic enzymes and the sensitization of bacteria to agents active against the cytoplasmic membrane indicate that some structure at or near the periphery of the cell is affected by EDTA. The ability of EDTA to sensitize Gram-negative bacteria to lysozyme also shows that it acts on a component of the wall which overlies and protects the peptidoglycan substrate of the enzyme. Thus, the various permeability changes induced by EDTA can be attributed to an effect on an outlying component of the cell wall which has the properties of a permeability barrier: it is now generally accepted that the characteristic 'outer membrane' of the Gram-negative cell envelope (Glauert & Thornley, 1969) has such properties. The osmotic stabilization by sucrose of osmoplasts indicates that the lysis of hypersensitive organisms such as *P. aeruginosa* does not involve further action by EDTA on the cytoplasmic membrane. Both electron microscopic studies and chemical analyses show that the cell envelope of *P. aeruginosa* has the architecture characteristic of Gram-negative bacteria. The composition and structure of the envelope have been reviewed by Meadow (1975), and aspects relevant to EDTA-sensitivity are discussed later in this chapter.

Extraction of Metal Cations

As wall cations seemed the obvious target for action by EDTA, EDTA-extracts from *P. aeruginosa* (protected against lysis by 0·55 M sucrose) were analysed for divalent cations (Eagon & Carson, 1965). The cations detected were Ca^{2+}, Mg^{2+} and Zn^{2+} in the approximate ratio (of gram-ions) 6:1·5:1. Subsequent analyses (Eagon, Simmons & Carson, 1965; Cox & Eagon, 1968; Eagon, 1969) of cell walls isolated from the strain (OSU 64) used showed that Mg^{2+} was the most abundant and Ca^{2+} the next most abundant ion present (ratio of gram-ions in the range 2·2:1 to 3·4:1). About 80% of the Mg^{2+} and about 40% of the Ca^{2+} were solubilized by treatment with EDTA in tris buffer: tris alone was ineffective but considerably enhanced the extraction of cations by EDTA. Similar results for the cation contents of the wall and the effect of EDTA have been obtained for *P. aeruginosa* NCTC 1999 (Payne, 1965). Payne also found that the isolated walls could bind Mg^{2+} but not Ca^{2+}, and that the amount bound was increased by EDTA-treatment of the walls. The extraction of wall cations by EDTA has also been demonstrated for *Rhizobium trifolii* (Humphrey & Vincent, 1962) and *Salmonella enteritidis* (Chipley, 1972;

Chipley & Edwards, 1972). Nevertheless, it is perhaps significant that cell walls contain small amounts of cations which resist extraction by EDTA, and that Mg-starved stationary-phase cells of *E. coli* retained almost all their Mg on treatment with EDTA (Lusk, Williams & Kennedy, 1968). The extraction of accessible Zn^{2+} from the wall of *S. enteritidis* was complete within a few minutes at either 4 °C or 37 °C, but the amount of Zn^{2+} removed at the higher temperature was significantly the greater (Chipley & Edwards, 1972).

Although the results obtained with *P. aeruginosa* seem to support the previous inference that Mg^{2+} is the essential cation chelated by EDTA, causing death of the bacteria, the evidence is not conclusive. Thus, the major cation in the wall and in the EDTA-extract is not necessarily the vital one. Also, the walls of *P. aeruginosa* grown under conditions in which Ca compensated for Mg inadequacy (Brown & Melling, 1969b) probably had a different cation balance and gave a different EDTA extract.

Extraction of Organic Components

The lytic effect of EDTA on whole cells of *P. aeruginosa* is paralleled by a similar turbidimetric effect on isolated cell walls (Gray & Wilkinson, 1965a; Eagon & Carson, 1965). The effect is complete within a few minutes at room temperature and is greater at pH 9·2 than 7·1. A comparison of *P. aeruginosa* with other organisms similarly showed that the effect of EDTA on the cell wall could be correlated with its bactericidal effect on the bacteria (Gray & Wilkinson, 1965a). These observations suggested that EDTA could disaggregate organic components of the wall, in addition to extracting metal ions. Analysis of EDTA extracts and infrared spectroscopy of insoluble wall residues confirmed that EDTA selectively solubilized material from the walls of sensitive organisms (Gray & Wilkinson, 1965b). The material extracted was rich in phosphorus and carbohydrate, and the suggestion that it included lipopolysaccharide has been confirmed by subsequent studies. These studies have concerned the materials extracted by EDTA in borate buffer (pH 9·2) from walls or whole cells of *P. aeruginosa* NCTC 1999 (Payne, 1965; Roberts *et al.*, 1970) and by EDTA in tris buffer (pH 8) from walls of *P. aeruginosa* OSU 64 (Cox & Eagon, 1968; Rogers, Gilleland & Eagon, 1969; Stinnett, Gilleland & Eagon, 1973). Basically similar results have been obtained by both groups of workers. In addition to lipopolysaccharide, the EDTA extracts contain protein and lipid, but not peptidoglycan. Recent studies of purified peptidoglycan from strain OSU 64 have confirmed that it is not affected by EDTA (Heilmann, 1972).

The protein, lipid and lipopolysaccharide components of the EDTA extracts from *P. aeruginosa* are apparently loosely associated in a complex or series of complexes, the composition and heterogeneity of which may depend on their origin (whole cells or isolated walls) and on the methods used to isolate and examine them. The product extracted from cell walls by Eagon and his colleagues was initially purified simply by dialysis, and consisted mainly of protein and lipopolysaccharide (weight ratio probably about 3:1) with smaller amounts of non-polar lipids (Cox & Eagon, 1968; Rogers *et al.*, 1969). The complex seemed homogeneous by polyacrylamide-gel electrophoresis and by chromatography on Sephadex G-200, but heterogeneity was revealed by ultracentrifugation and density-gradient centrifugation. The chromatographic and sedimentation data showed that the particle weights for the complex were very high, and the dimensions of particles seen in electron micrographs indicated values over 10^6 daltons. The particles consisted mainly of spherical units (diameter 6–8 nm) and rodlets (about 7 nm × 20 nm) apparently composed of spherical units, together with a few vesicles (Rogers *et al.*, 1969). Similar morphological variation has been observed for protein–lipopolysaccharide complexes from other Gram-negative bacteria (e.g. Knox, Cullen & Work, 1967; Marsh & Walker, 1968; DePamphilis, 1971) and for such endotoxins extracted from *P. aeruginosa* by various techniques, including treatment with EDTA and lysozyme (Dyke & Berk, 1973b). Recent studies have shown that the EDTA extract from *P. aeruginosa* can be 'purified' further by ultracentrifugation and by ultrafiltration or chromatography on Sepharose 4B (Rubio & Lopez, 1971, 1972; Stinnett *et al.*, 1973), by removal of some protein. Rodlets are still present in the final product (Figure 1). Proteins remaining in the complex were extracted with *NN*-dimethylformamide and

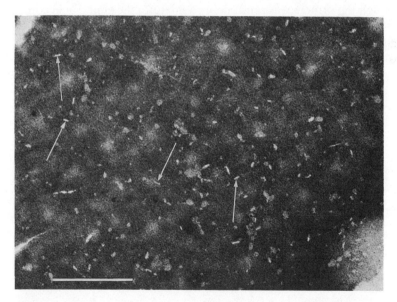

Figure 1. Electron micrograph of negatively stained (phosphotungstic acid) protein–lipopolysaccharide complex extracted by EDTA from the cell envelope of *P. aeruginosa*. Some rodlets (arrowed) are seen to be composed of spherical units. The marker bar represents 200 nm. Reproduced with permission from Stinnett *et al.*, *J. Bacteriol.*, **114**, 399–407 (1973) Figure 7

examined by gel electrophoresis (Stinnett *et al.*, 1973). Two of the major proteins, having molecular weights of 16,500 and 43,000, were possibly glycoproteins, and the latter (also found to be the major envelope protein by Schnaitman, 1970b) could correspond to the endotoxin protein studied by Homma and Suzuki (1966). It has been confirmed that the proteins associated with the EDTA extract are derived from the outer membrane of the cell envelope (Stinnett & Eagon, 1973). It should be noted, however, that the method used to solubilize the proteins has recently been shown (Inouye & Yee, 1973) to give an artificially simple electrophoretic picture of the envelope proteins of *E. coli*, with a three-component peak for proteins of molecular weight about 48,000.

In the related studies with *P. aeruginosa* NCTC 1999, EDTA extracts were prepared from whole cells, partly to avoid the loss of wall components during the isolation of cell envelopes (Roberts, Gray & Wilkinson, 1967; Cox & Eagon, 1968). The high-molecular-weight complex was separated from leakage products by gel filtration and chromatography on DEAE–cellulose (Roberts *et al.*, 1970). The absence of binding between EDTA and the complex was consistent with the results of other studies (Dvorak, 1968; Garrard, 1971), which showed that EDTA was not adsorbed by bacteria. The complex had the approximate composition: protein, 60%; lipopolysaccharide, 30%, loosely bound lipids, 10%. Other analytical data are given in Table 5. Although the protein was presumably a mixture, the amino acid composition was very similar to that of the endotoxin protein analysed by Homma & Suzuki (1966). The complex differed from that studied by Eagon and his colleagues in the presence of phospholipids (mainly phosphatidylethanolamine) in addition to free fatty acids. Although the possible presence in the complex of unnatural

Table 5. Composition of the complex extracted by EDTA from
P. aeruginosa

Component	% by weight
Protein	64
Loosely bound lipid	9
Total fatty acid	9·7
Carbohydrate[a]	5·6
2-Keto-3-deoxyoctonic acid	1·2
Glucosamine	1·0
Total amino sugar[a]	1·8
Phosphorus	1·6
Glucose ⎫ Rhamnose ⎬ Galactosamine ⎪ Fucosamine ⎭	[b]

[a] Data for complex purified by using Sephadex G-200 instead of Sepharose 2B.
[b] Present but not determined. Data from Roberts *et al.*, *Microbios*, **2**, 189–208 (1970) Table 6.

components or forms of association cannot be ruled out, the fact that phospholipids, protein and lipopolysaccharide all occur in the outer membrane of the cell envelope makes an artefact seem unlikely. This complex, like the one discussed previously, was apparently heterogeneous in both size and composition: no stable covalent linkages between the components were detected (Roberts *et al.*, 1970).

The extent to which available complex is solubilized by EDTA is not clear, but the material extracted from whole cells constituted at least 13% of the cell dry weight (Roberts *et al.*, 1970). In extractions involving isolated walls, about 35% of the total lipopolysaccharide was solubilized (Gray & Wilkinson, 1965b; Cox & Eagon, 1968; Rogers *et al.*, 1969), together with smaller percentages of the protein and lipid. The results obtained with isolated walls may be misleading, as much lipopolysaccharide may be lost during the preparation of the walls (Roberts *et al.*, 1967). Also, the extent of extraction was much lower if trypsin was not used in 'purification' of the walls, while low values were obtained even with trypsin-treated walls of other EDTA-sensitive pseudomonads (Gray & Wilkinson, 1965b; Wilkinson, 1970). The extent of extraction from the walls of *P. aeruginosa* was less at pH 7·1 than 9·2, and less at 0 °C than at 20 °C (Payne, 1965). Turbidimetric measurements indicated that the action of EDTA was unaffected by acetylation of the walls, by prior extraction from the walls of loosely bound lipids, or by prior treatment of the walls with 10 mM $MgCl_2$ (Payne, 1965). Cox & Eagon (1968) confirmed that the effect of EDTA on isolated walls was considerably enhanced by the presence of tris buffer.

Although comparative studies (Gray & Wilkinson, 1965b) had suggested that the extraction of the lipopolysaccharide-containing complex might be uniquely associated with the toxic action of EDTA on hypersensitive bacteria, the real situation is less simple. Thus, lipopolysaccharide can be released by EDTA from less sensitive organisms under the conditions used to effect non-lethal permeability changes and osmotic shock (Leive, 1965c; Voss, 1967; Leive, Shovlin & Mergenhagen, 1968; Tucker & White, 1970; Winshell & Neu, 1970; Chipley & Edwards, 1972; Chipley, 1974). The release of lipopolysaccharide from strains of *E. coli* occurs rapidly at either 0 °C or 37 °C, but is rather less extensive at the lower temperature (Leive, 1965c; Leive *et al.*, 1968). The amount of lipopolysaccharide released from enterobacteria does not exceed about 50% of the total present, and apparently cannot be increased significantly by raising the EDTA concentration, by retreating the cells with EDTA, or by varying the pH between 6 and 9 (Leive *et al.*, 1968). Both the released and retained fractions of the lipopolysaccharide are equally 'external', in the sense of accessibility to phage (Leive & Lawrence, 1971), and in growing cells the two fractions rapidly attain equilibrium (Levy & Leive, 1968). The fact that newly synthesized lipopolysaccharide resists extraction by EDTA (Levy & Leive, 1968) is consistent with the observation that biosynthesis occurs at the cytoplasmic membrane and is followed by translocation of the lipopolysaccharide to the outer membrane (Osborn, Gander & Parisi, 1972; Mühlradt, Menzel, Golecki & Speth, 1973, 1974).

Although permeability changes induced by EDTA seem to be dependent on the extraction of lipopolysaccharide (e.g. Winshell & Neu, 1970; Chipley & Edwards, 1972), there is evidence that the two effects can be partly dissociated. For example, an almost maximum release of lipopolysaccharide from *E. coli* at pH 6 corresponded to only 30% increase in permeability (Leive *et al.*, 1968), while lipopolysaccharide could be extracted from mutants of two normally EDTA-sensitive strains without obviously altering their permeability (Voll & Leive, 1970). This imperfect correlation has been clarified somewhat by further studies of the EDTA extracts. The high-molecular-weight material from *E. coli* 0111:B4 (85–90% lipopolysaccharide, 5–10% protein, 5% phospholipid) was resolved into two fractions by ultracentrifugation (Leive *et al.*, 1968). A rapidly sedimenting heterogeneous fraction (40–60% of the total material) contained lipopolysaccharide of 'normal' composition, together with most of the protein and phospholipid. The second fraction, having s^0 equal to 5·4, consisted mainly of lipopolysaccharide with a high content of antigenic side-chains. Similar studies of the EDTA extracts from other strains of *E. coli* showed that mutants resistant to the EDTA-induced permeability change released only 60–80% as much lipopolysaccharide as the parent organisms, and that the decrease was in the amount of the slowly sedimenting fraction of lipopolysaccharide (Voll & Leive, 1970). Thus, the effect of EDTA on cell permeability may be related to the amount or the release of this specific fraction of lipopolysaccharide. In further studies of *E. coli* J5 grown in the absence of galactose (which results in an incomplete lipopolysaccharide, lacking antigenic side-chains), 30–40% of the lipopolysaccharide released by EDTA was in the rapidly sedimenting fraction as a complex with phosphatidylethanolamine and galactosyltransferase (Levy & Leive, 1970). The complex was active in transferring galactose from UDP-galactose to the incomplete lipopolysaccharide, and was considered to be the authentic biosynthetic unit. If this is correct, it appears that the damaging effects of EDTA on *E. coli* extend to the cytoplasmic membrane, as in the case of *H. parainfluenzae* (Tucker & White, 1970). As with *P. aeruginosa*, tests using isolated walls or envelopes may underestimate the ability of EDTA to solubilize lipopolysaccharide from *E. coli* (Edwards & Noller, 1964; Gray & Wilkinson, 1965b; Schnaitman, 1971). On the other hand, the lack of effect by EDTA on the isolated walls of *Proteus mirabilis* (Gray & Wilkinson, 1965b) is similar to the results of other studies which show that *Proteus* species are relatively resistant to EDTA (e.g. Repaske, 1958; Neu & Chou, 1967; Winshell & Neu, 1970; Cleeland *et al.*, 1970). *Rhodopseudomonas palustris* and some unrepresentative pseudomonads also seem to be resistant to EDTA (Wilkinson, 1967, 1968; Weckesser, Drews, Fromme & Mayer, 1973).

Dissociation of Cell Envelopes and their Components

As discussed above, the action of EDTA on Gram-negative bacteria characteristically involves solubilization of components of the outer membrane of the cell envelope. Some insight into this dissociative action has come from studies utilizing the techniques of electron microscopy.

Physiologically 'young' (late lag or early logarithmic phase) cells of *E. coli* plasmolysed in 0·5 M sucrose are unusually sensitive to lysozyme, and the treated cells form spheroplasts on 50% dilution of the suspension (Birdsell & Cota-Robles, 1967). Treatment of these spheroplasts with EDTA causes rupture of the outer membrane, much of which peels away from the cytoplasmic membrane as a highly coiled structure: similar observations have been made with *S. typhimurium* (Osborn, Gander, Parisi & Carson, 1972). Although outer membranes weakened by EDTA seem to fragment rather readily (e.g. Miura & Mizushima, 1969), the results of other studies indicate that outer membranes can remain unbroken and superficially unchanged during the preparation of spheroplasts with EDTA–lysozyme, despite the degradation of the peptidoglycan layer of the envelope and the solubilization of lipopolysaccharide (e.g. Murray, Steed & Elson, 1965; De Petris, 1967; Silva & Sousa, 1973). This even appears to be the case with *P. aeruginosa* (Weiss & Fraser, 1973). However, the disruptive effect of EDTA on isolated cell envelopes of *P. aeruginosa* (Stinnett *et al.*, 1973) is very evident in electron micrographs (Figures 2 and 3).

Recently developed methods for the fractionation of cell envelopes and the isolation of purified walls and outer membranes have allowed the effects of EDTA on these structures to be further evaluated. Although EDTA treatment

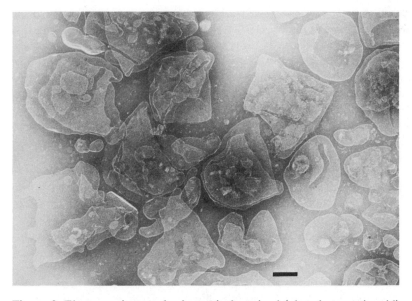

Figure 2. Electron micrograph of negatively stained (phosphotungstic acid) fragments of cell envelopes of *P. aeruginosa*. The marker bar represents 200 nm. Reproduced with permission from Stinnett *et al.*, *J. Bacteriol.*, **114**, 399–407 (1973) Figure 1

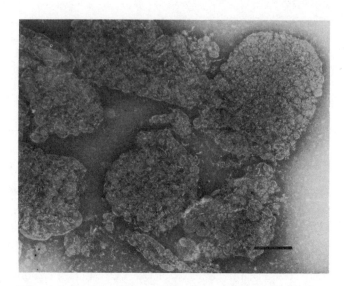

Figure 3. Electron micrograph of negatively stained (phosphotungstic acid) cell envelopes of *P. aeruginosa* treated with EDTA. The marker bar represents 200 nm. Reproduced with permission from Stinnett *et al., J. Bacteriol.*, **114**, 399–407 (1973) Figure 5

was used in most of these fractionation procedures (e.g. Miura & Mizushima, 1968, 1969; DePamphilis, 1971; Schnaitman, 1970a, 1971), no loss of lipopolysaccharide occurred in at least one of them (Osborn, Gander, Parisi & Carson, 1972). The outer membrane from *E. coli* K12, isolated from spheroplasts and treated with Triton X-100 to remove the cytoplasmic membrane, consisted mainly of lipopolysaccharide (55%) and protein (44%) (DePamphilis, 1971). The vesicular preparation was partly dissociated into rodlets (about 7·5 nm × 14–28 nm) and discs (diameter 14–70 nm) by dialysis against EDTA in tris buffer. These sub-structures could be reassociated into vesicles by dialysis against Mg^{2+} in tris buffer. Whereas the Mg^{2+}-containing vesicles were not affected by Triton X-100, the detergent completed the dissociation of outer membrane treated with EDTA. The inference that both cation-bridges and hydrophobic interactions are important for the integrity of the outer membrane (DePamphilis, 1971) is supported by the results of complementary studies by Schnaitman (1971) of 'walls' from *E. coli* J5. These preparations contained all the protein of the cell wall and had a normal morphology (peptidoglycan layer and outer membrane), despite the loss of about 50% of the lipopolysaccharide and 66% of the phospholipid during 'purification' with Triton X-100. EDTA alone had virtually no solubilizing action on the 'walls', but about 50% of the protein and essentially all the remaining lipopolysaccharide and phospholipid were solubilized by EDTA and Triton X-100 together. Evidence that the dissociative effect of EDTA involves chemical as well as physical fractionation of protein–lipopolysaccharide complexes has been obtained by Rogers (1971). Schnaitman (1971) has suggested that the organized structure of the cell wall of *E. coli* is largely dependent on strong hydrophobic interactions between proteins, supported by cation-mediated interactions between protein and lipopolysaccharide. Studies of surface films of a protein–lipopolysaccharide complex from the outer membrane of *P. aeruginosa* have also suggested a stabilizing role for lipopolysaccharide (Suzuki & Goto, 1972), while the degree of association of isolated lipopolysaccharide is markedly influenced by divalent cations (e.g. Olins & Warner, 1967; DePamphilis, 1971; O'Leary, Nelson & MacLeod, 1972). Although phospholipids are considered to play only a minor role in stabilization of the outer membrane (Schnaitman, 1971), treatment of the membrane from a marine pseudomonad with EDTA caused the release of 15% of the phosphorus and facilitated the action of phospholipase C on the phospholipids of the membrane vesicles (Forge, Costerton & Kerr, 1973).

The protein–lipid–lipopolysaccharide complexes of outer membranes constitute the endotoxic O-antigens of Gram-negative bacteria. Both antigenicity and toxicity are properties associated with the lipopolysaccharide components of the complexes (Lüderitz, Westphal, Staub & Nikaido, 1971; Galanos, Rietschel, Lüderitz, Westphal, Kim & Watson, 1972). However, the full expression of these properties (particularly toxicity) depends on the form and composition of the product used, and therefore might be sensitive to the dissociative effects of EDTA. The antigenic properties of EDTA extracts from several species have been demonstrated (Voss, 1967; Leive *et al.*, 1968; Rubio & Lopez, 1971; Chipley, 1972; Pike & Chandler, 1974). In the case of *E. coli*, the EDTA extract was more active than lipopolysaccharide extracted by aqueous phenol (Leive *et al.*, 1968), whereas the reverse was true for *S. enteritidis* (Chipley, 1972). The toxicity for mice of lipopolysaccharide obtained by treatment of *P. aeruginosa* with aqueous diethyl ether was lost after incubation of the lipopolysaccharide with EDTA (Michaels & Eagon, 1966). A recent comparison (Dyke & Berk, 1973a) of the activities of endotoxins extracted from *P. aeruginosa* by various procedures gave similar results. The relatively low toxicity of the product obtained by using EDTA–lysozyme, compared with the activities of products extracted with aqueous phenol or diethyl ether, did not seem to be explained solely by differences in composition between the products. Finally, the 50% decrease in adsorption of a pyocin by a sensitive strain of *P. aeruginosa* after treatment of the cells with EDTA is also consistent with dissociation of the cell envelope and loss of lipopolysaccharide (Stewart & Young, 1971): the solubilization of pyocin receptor sites by EDTA has also been demonstrated by Ikeda & Nishi (1973).

SITE AND MODE OF TOXIC ACTION BY EDTA

On the basis of results already discussed, it seems reasonable to conclude that the permeability changes induced by EDTA and the sensitizing effects of this

compound can be attributed mainly to the dissociation and partial solubilization of the outer membranes of Gram-negative bacteria. Provided that the
conditions of EDTA treatment are not too severe, the viability of most bacteria
is not seriously affected. However, similar treatment of *P. aeruginosa* and other
sensitive species (Table 2) causes lysis and death of the cells: these effects also
seem to be directly related to the effect of EDTA on the cell envelope (Roberts
et al., 1970). Before possible explanations for this high intrinsic sensitivity are
considered, the basis of action by EDTA will be re-examined.

Compelling circumstantial evidence that the antibacterial effects of EDTA
are triggered by the chelation of essential multivalent cations has been
assembled. Persuasive evidence in favour of Mg^{2+} as the cation of primary
importance in *P. aeruginosa* has also been presented. The striking resemblance
between the antibacterial activities of EDTA and polymyxin (e.g. Gray &
Wilkinson, 1965a; Koike, Iida & Matsuo, 1969; Lopes & Inniss, 1969; Brown
& Melling, 1969b; Brown & Watkins, 1970) lends further support to the
hypothesis that EDTA acts by a chelating mechanism (see Chapter 3 for a
comparative discussion of the effects of EDTA and polymyxin). The effect of
Mg limitation on the EDTA-sensitivity of *P. aeruginosa*, (Brown & Melling,
1969a) and the apparently unusual capacity of this organism for Mg^{2+} (Webb,
1966), also tend to implicate Mg as the metal involved. However, two
suggested modes of antibacterial action which do not depend on the chelating
ability of EDTA should be considered briefly. The removal or dissociation of
lipid-containing materials by EDTA was initially attributed to a detergent-like
action on the cell envelope (Colobert, 1958; Noller & Hartsell, 1961a,b).
However, EDTA is not surface-active and should not possess any fat-
solubilizing properties in the pH and concentration ranges used for antibacterial action (e.g. Nezval, 1964). It is just possible that the high activity against
P. aeruginosa of EDTA in borate buffer (pH 9·2) can partly be attributed to the
formation of soaps from free fatty acids present in the cell envelope, which
could assist in the dissociation of the outer membrane. This could not be
counted as a specific property of EDTA, while the borate buffer alone has no
bactericidal action on *P. aeruginosa*. A somewhat more plausible non-
chelating mode of action by EDTA has been considered by Singh (1971). Singh
found that EDTA (used as the ammonium salt at pH 6·1) was superior to KCl
in dissociating complexes formed between oppositely charged ions, including
polyanions and -cations of natural occurrence. However, the concentrations of
EDTA found to be effective seem to be significantly higher than those
necessary for antibacterial activity, while the antibacterial effects of EDTA
cannot in general be mimicked by much higher concentrations of inorganic
salts. Also, it seems doubtful whether coulombic interactions between macro-
ions are of prime importance for the assembly and structural integrity of
bacterial envelopes (Singer, 1971). Thus, lipopolysaccharides contain phosphate residues and are anionic overall, and the common bacterial lipids are
either 'neutral' (e.g. phosphatidylethanolamine) or acidic (e.g. phosphatidylglycerol and free fatty acids). Basic proteins do not seem to predominate in

membranes generally, and although little information is available about the proteins of bacterial outer membranes, the amino acid compositions of the endotoxin proteins from two strains of *P. aeruginosa* (Homma & Suzuki, 1966; Roberts *et al.*, 1970) show molar excesses of acidic over basic amino acids (analyses for glutamine and asparagine were not done). The composition of the (lipo)protein attached to the peptidoglycan of *P. aeruginosa* (Martin, Heilmann & Preusser, 1972) has not yet been determined, but the corresponding lipoprotein from *E coli* is not basic (Braun & Bosch, 1972; Hantke & Braun, 1973). Therefore, it seems safe to conclude that the primary step in EDTA action is chelation of essential metal cations bound in the cell envelope.

The extraction of cations by EDTA is rapidly followed by the partial solubilization of the cell envelopes of sensitive bacteria. Solubilization characteristically involves components of the outer membrane but not peptidoglycan. The cytoplasmic membrane may be affected to some extent, but its permeability function generally seems to be unimpaired. The most commonly accepted explanation for the dissociating effect of EDTA holds that the susceptible cations are not simply counter-ions to the anionic components of the envelope, but have a structural role in forming stabilizing cross-bridges between these components. Solubilization could then be a simple consequence of coulombic repulsion between the polyanions. Complete dissociation of the outer membrane need not be expected, as other forms of association, e.g. hydrophobic interactions and hydrogen bonding, may be more important than cation-mediated bonding. In the case of *P. aeruginosa*, the implication of this interpretation is that the cross-bridges broken by EDTA are between units of the protein–lipid–lipopolysaccharide complex, or between the complex and peptidoglycan–lipoprotein or some part of the outer membrane less dependent on cation-stabilization. A second possible explanation for the dissociating effect could be the activation by EDTA of an autolytic enzyme normally inhibited by metal cations. The outer membranes of Gram-negative bacteria have few known enzymic activities, although phospholipid–degrading enzymes are located in the membranes of *E. coli* and *S. typhimurium* (Machtiger & Fox, 1973). However, these enzymes are *activated* by Ca^{2+}, which makes it unlikely that dissociation of the membranes by EDTA results from the formation of surface active lysophosphatides. Also, the effectiveness of EDTA against isolated, trypsin-treated walls of *P. aeruginosa* and against *E. coli* at both 0 °C and 37 °C makes it unlikely that solubilization is caused primarily by enzymic action.

There remains the problem of accounting for the toxicity of EDTA for *P. aeruginosa*. Firstly, as suggested by Goldschmidt & Wyss (1967), EDTA may attack sensitive sites other than the cell envelope. Such action, which could occur either as a result of dissociation of the outer membrane or independently of it, is probably responsible for the gradual loss of viability of *E. coli* and other Gram-negative bacteria during prolonged exposure to EDTA (e.g. Neu *et al.*, 1967; Leive & Kollin, 1967; Tucker & White, 1970). Although processes such as the degradation of RNA probably occur with *P. aeruginosa* also, e.g. under the conditions used to study the leakage of intracellular solutes, they do not obviously account for the hypersensitivity of the organism to EDTA. One possible explanation (Leive, 1968) for this hypersensitivity would be the presence in the bacteria of an exceptional 'autolysin'. An autolytic system which influenced the action of lysozyme on *P. aeruginosa* was detected by Warren, Gray & Bartell (1955), and an extracellular autolysin was obtained by Collins (1964) from old anaerobic cultures of a different strain of the organism. The autolysin degraded the peptidoglycan component of the cell wall and, not surprisingly, its action was potentiated by EDTA. The apparent decrease in the bactericidal activity of EDTA at low temperature also suggests that enzymic action contributes to the toxic process (Haslam *et al.*, 1969). If autolysis is indeed relevant to the bactericidal action of EDTA on *P. aeruginosa*, the cell envelope is expected to be involved, as the rapid lysis of cells and the release of polynucleotides point to structural failure of the cell envelope as the primary cause of death.

As a separate line of enquiry, attempts have been made to interpret the EDTA-sensitivity of an organism in terms of the composition or structure of its cell wall. This approach was suggested by the correlation between bactericidal action and solubilization of components from isolated walls of organisms differing in sensitivity to EDTA (Gray & Wilkinson, 1965b). Also, the walls of sensitive organisms (*P. aeruginosa* and *P. alcaligenes*—originally described as *Alcaligenes faecalis*) were relatively rich in phosphorus, which suggested that EDTA-sensitivity might be explicable in terms of wall composition only, without the need to invoke autolysis. Thus, the structural integrity of the walls from EDTA-sensitive bacteria may depend to an exceptional degree on cation-stabilization, and this should be reflected in the organic chemistry of the walls. Because lipopolysaccharide contains phosphorus and is the most distinctive component of EDTA extracts, it has received most attention, but studies of other aspects of wall composition and structure for *P. aeruginosa* have also revealed features which may help to explain the toxic effect of EDTA.

Although the cell wall fulfils the major structural role of supporting the cytoplasmic membrane, the source of its mechanical strength is not entirely clear. A vital structural function for the outer membrane has not been conclusively demonstrated (Machtiger & Fox, 1973), and the liberation of its components during the growth of some bacteria may seem to indicate expendability (e.g. Knox *et al.*, 1967; Marsh & Walker, 1968; Rothfield & Pearlman-Kothencz, 1969; Lindsay, Wheeler, Sanderson, Costerton & Cheng, 1973). However, the results of many other studies indicate that both the strength and the rigidity of the cell wall depend on an integrated organization of the various components. Peptidoglycan, which is the primary shape-determining component of the wall, generally constitutes less than 10% by weight of the Gram-negative cell wall (Reaveley & Burge, 1972; Schleiffer & Kandler, 1972), and the amount may be sufficient only for the construction of a monolayer sacculus (Braun, Gnirke, Henning & Rehn, 1973). Provided that autolysis is prevented, the sacculus is 'rigid' and strong enough to maintain its shape and integrity on isolation. However, despite the cross-linking of glycan chains by peptide bridges, the net-like sacculus is probably open enough to allow the passage through it of some macromolecules (e.g. newly synthesized components of the outer membrane). These considerations reinforce the impression that other components must make significant contributions to the strength of the cell wall. It may well be in the nature and relative importance of these contributions that the walls of *P. aeruginosa* and other EDTA-sensitive bacteria differ from those of enterobacteria. Certainly, the peptidoglycan from *P. aeruginosa* OSU 64 seems to have no unusual features. It contains glucosamine, muramic acid, glutamic acid, 2,6-diaminopimelic acid and alanine in molar ratios about $1:1:1:1:1\cdot8$, and about half of the peptide chains are cross-linked via 2,6-diaminopimelic acid and alanine (Heilmann, 1972, 1974). Although the peptidoglycan content of the wall was not determined, the amount was sufficient to form a complete sacculus (Figure 4). As mentioned previously, the sacculus was not degraded by treatment with EDTA. The peptidoglycan from *P. alcaligenes* also has a conventional composition (Martin, Fleck, Mock & Ghuysen, 1973).

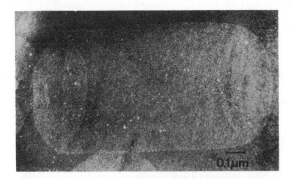

Figure 4. Electron micrograph of negatively stained (phosphotungstic acid) peptidoglycan sacculus of *P. aeruginosa*. Reproduced with permission from Martin *et al.*, *Arch. Mikrobiol.*, **83**, 332–346 Figure 6b

In addition to peptidoglycan, the 'rigid layer' of the wall of *E. coli* contains a substantial quantity of lipoprotein (Braun & Rehn, 1969): similar findings have been made for other enterobacteria (Braun, Rehn & Wolff, 1970; Martin *et al.*, 1972). In electron micrographs, the lipoprotein is visualized as particles (diameter about 10 nm), distributed rather evenly over the surface of the peptidoglycan sacculus (Figure 5). The lipoprotein, of which the structure has been established (Braun & Bosch, 1972; Hantke & Braun, 1973), is covalently attached to the peptidoglycan, with one lipoprotein molecule to about ten disaccharide units of the peptidoglycan. The linkage is a peptide bond between 2,6-diaminopimelic acid and the 6-amino group of the C-terminal lysine residue of the lipoprotein. Apart from such lysine residues, bound lipoprotein

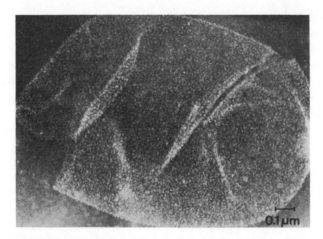

Figure 5. Electron micrograph of negatively stained (phosphotungstic acid) rigid layer of the cell envelope of *E. coli* (peptidoglycan sacculus with covalently attached lipoprotein particles). Reproduced with permission from Martin *et al.*, *Arch. Mikrobiol.*, **83**, 332–346 (1972) Figure 4

can be removed from the rigid layer by treatment with trypsin. Similar treatment of whole cell envelopes causes separation of the cytoplasmic and outer membranes (Braun & Rehn, 1969; Braun *et al.*, 1970). This important observation suggested that the bound lipoprotein had a stabilizing role in the cell envelope and, in particular, that it served to anchor the outer membrane to the peptidoglycan sacculus. The recent discovery of unbound lipoprotein in the outer membrane of *E. coli* supports this inference (Inouye, Shaw & Shen, 1972; Bosch & Braun, 1973; Hirashima, Wu, Venkateswaran & Inouye, 1973). Whereas bound lipoprotein can account for more than 40% by weight of the rigid layer of *E. coli*, it is far less prominent in the corresponding layer of *P. aeruginosa* (Martin *et al.*, 1972). Little or no bound lipoprotein has been detected in the rigid layers of *P. fluorescens* (Braun *et al.*, 1970), *V. foetus* (Winter, Katz & Martin, 1971) or *Sp. serpens* (Martin *et al.*, 1972). Absence of such lipoprotein could partly account for the ready dissociation of the cell envelope of a marine pseudomonad, and for the tendency of the peptidoglycan to associate with the cytoplasmic membrane rather than the outer layers of the cell wall (Forsberg, Rayman, Costerton & MacLeod, 1972). Thus, there are indications that members of the order *Pseudomonadales* may be deficient in the structurally important lipoprotein, which could make these organisms more reliant on other factors which stabilize the outer membrane.

The unusual cation-dependence of the outer membrane of *P. aeruginosa* is apparent both from the extent of solubilization by EDTA and from the fact that—in contrast to *E. coli*—protein is the major component extracted. Recent freeze-etch studies (Lickfeld, Achterrath, Hentrich, Kolehmainen-Seveus & Persson, 1972; Gilleland, Stinnett, Roth & Eagon, 1973) of the cell envelope of *P. aeruginosa* have pointed to the location of the protein-containing complex extracted by EDTA. When glycerol was used as a cryoprotective agent, fracture planes analogous to those for the cell envelope of *E. coli* (e.g. Van Gool & Nanninga, 1971) were obtained. The concave surface (C̃W in Figure 6) exposed by splitting the outer membrane was covered with closely packed spherical units equal in size to those found in EDTA extracts of cell walls and in supernatant fluids obtained during the preparation of osmoplasts. The spherical units were much less closely-packed (Figure 7) on the corresponding concave surface of osmoplasts (Gilleland *et al.*, 1973). When osmoplasts were restored to osmotic stability by the addition of Mg^{2+} in the presence of the EDTA extract, the units were found to have re-aggregated (though in a somewhat disorganized manner) on the concave surface. This was confirmed by analysis of the supernatant fluid for protein before and after the addition of Mg^{2+}. Although no change in the carbohydrate content of the supernatant fluid after the restoration process was detected, this may have been a result of technical difficulties (R. G. Eagon, personal communication). Thus, both protein and lipopolysaccharide were probably re-adsorbed on the cell wall during restoration.

In view of the probable importance of structural protein in maintaining the integrity of the outer membrane (Schnaitman, 1971), the extraction of such protein seems to provide a satisfactory explanation for the toxicity of EDTA for *P. aeruginosa*. However, the fact that the protein is released as a complex with lipid and lipopolysaccharide suggests that the specificity of the action may be determined by other components of the outer membrane. Metal cations participate in the interactions of membrane proteins and lipids (e.g. Razin, 1972), and Mg^{2+} is associated with phospholipids from the cell envelope of *P. aeruginosa* (Gordon & MacLeod, 1966; Bobo & Eagon, 1968; Brown & Watkins, 1970). However, the lipid compositions reported for this organism are unexceptional (e.g. Randle, Albro & Dittmer, 1969; Hancock & Meadow, 1969), while the action of EDTA on lipid-free walls (Payne, 1965) indicates that loosely bound lipids are not responsible for the selective toxicity of EDTA. By contrast, structural studies of lipopolysaccharides from *P. aeruginosa* have revealed several novel features (Meadow, 1975). These lipopolysaccharides are unusually rich in phosphorus, which largely accounts for the rather high phosphorus contents of the cell walls (Gray & Wilkinson, 1965b). The lipopolysaccharide from *P. aeruginosa* NCTC 1999 contains about 4·6% phosphorus (Fenson & Gray, 1969; Chester, Gray & Wilkinson, 1972) and values in the range 3·1–5·6% have been found for similar products extracted with aqueous phenol from other strains (Fensom & Meadow, 1970; Ikeda & Egami, 1973; Chester, Meadow & Pitt, 1973; S. G. Wilkinson, unpublished results). Phosphorus is present in both the lipid A and polysaccharide fractions, but mainly in the latter: the lipid A fraction has a conventional composition and structure (Drewry, Lomax, Gray & Wilkinson, 1973). During the separation of the lipid A and polysaccharide fractions by mild hydrolysis with acetic acid, about half of the total phosphorus in the lipopolysaccharide from *P. aeruginosa*

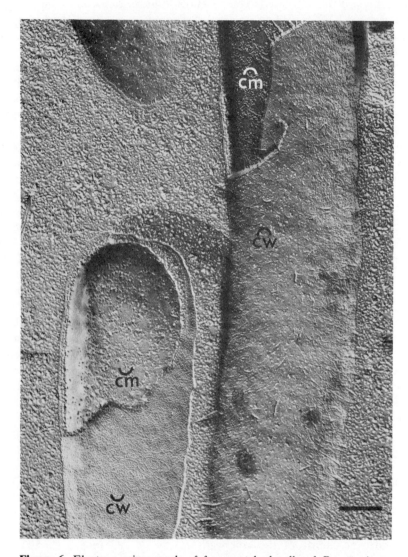

Figure 6. Electron micrograph of freeze-etched cells of *P. aeruginosa* cryoprotected with glycerol. Two pairs of complementary (convex and concave) surfaces are exposed by splitting of the outer membrane of the cell wall (CW) and of the cytoplasmic membrane (CM). The concave cell-wall surface (C̆W) contains closely packed spherical units (diameter about 6 nm) which seem to make up rodlets (length 20–25 nm). The peptidoglycan layer is seen in profile between the two concave surfaces. The marker bar represents 200 nm. Reproduced with permission from Gilleland *et al.*, *J. Bacteriol.*, **113**, 417–432 (1973) Figure 3

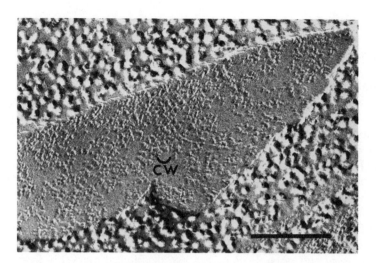

Figure 7. Electron micrograph of freeze-etched osmoplasts of *P. aeruginosa* cryoprotected with glycerol. Compared with whole cells (Figure 6), the concave cell-wall surface (C̆W) is depleted in spherical units as a result of EDTA action. The marker bar represents 200 nm. Reproduced with permission from Gilleland *et al., J. Bacteriol.*, **113**, 417–432 (1973) Figure 8b

NCTC 1999 was released as low-molecular-weight solutes. About 85% of this phosphorus was present in orthophosphate and the balance in pyrophosphate and ethanolamine mono-, di- and triphosphates (Drewry, Gray & Wilkinson, 1971, 1972). Closely similar results have been obtained for the lipopolysaccharides of all other strains of *P. aeruginosa* studied in the author's laboratory (unpublished results). The lability of ethanolamine triphosphate suggests that other fragments are degradation products either of this compound or of higher polyphosphates (possibly lacking ethanolamine in the case of some ortho- and pyrophosphate). Although the origin of the ethanolamine triphosphate has not been proved, it is reasonable to suggest attachment by a pyrophosphate bond to the polysaccharide fraction, which remains rich in phosphorus (5·6% for strain NCTC 1999). As in lipopolysaccharides from enterobacteria, these phosphate groups seem to be mainly or exclusively attached to heptose residues in the inner region of the core polysaccharide (Drewry, 1972). Although ethanolamine diphosphate also occurs in the core polysaccharide of other species (e.g. *Salmonella*), it is ester-bound directly to heptose and is relatively stable to hydrolysis by acetic acid (Lehmann, Lüderitz & Westphal, 1971).

The impression that the lipopolysaccharides of EDTA-sensitive pseudomonads might be characterized by core polysaccharides highly substituted by polyphosphate residues with metal-binding potential is supported by the results of other studies *P. alcaligenes* is even more EDTA-sensitive than *P. aeruginosa* (Wilkinson, 1967), and both the whole lipopolysaccharide and the derived polysaccharide are richer in phosphorus than are the corresponding products from *P. aeruginosa* NCTC 1999 (Key, Gray & Wilkinson, 1970; Lomax, Gray & Wilkinson, 1974). Again, much of the phosphorus is acid-labile: about 55% of the lipopolysaccharide phosphorus was released as orthophosphate by hydrolysis with 1 M HCl at 100 °C for 7 min, and pyrophosphate was also detected after hydrolysis with acetic acid (ethanolamine is absent from the lipopolysaccharide). Analyses of the cell walls of other pseudomonads (Wilkinson, 1968, 1970) also suggested that EDTA-sensitivity could be correlated with the amount or the phosphorus content of the lipopolysaccharide component, and selected species have been studied further (Wilkinson, Galbraith & Lightfoot, 1973). The lipopolysaccharides of EDTA-sensitive species (*P. stutzeri* and *P. syncyanea*) were again relatively rich in phosphorus, but differed from those of *P. aeruginosa* and *P. alcaligenes* in several respects, and the parent cell walls were also unusually susceptible to mechanical comminution. The walls of EDTA-resistant species (*P. diminuta*, *P. pavonacea* and possibly *P. rubescens*) all differed markedly from those of *P. aeruginosa*. Insufficient data are available to indicate whether the lipopolysaccharides of EDTA-sensitive *Vibrio* and *Spirillum* species resemble those of *P. aeruginosa* in relevant respects, but the presence of fructose and the absence of 2-keto-3-deoxyoctonic acid are differentiating features of the lipopolysaccharides of *V. cholerae* (Jackson & Redmond, 1971; Jann, Jann & Beyaert, 1973).

The possible significance of metal-binding polyphosphates in the lipopolysaccharides of EDTA-sensitive pseudomonads is suggested by current models (e.g. Schnaitman, 1971) for the structure of the cell envelope. With the hydrophobic lipid A embedded in the membrane and the antigenic side-chains projecting out from the cell surface, the phosphorylated core polysaccharide would probably be placed at the periphery of the outer membrane, where the binding of other components by cation bridges could be important. Chelation of the cations by EDTA would not only remove the stabilizing bridges but would also create highly anionic regions in the membrane. The consequent repulsive forces could 'open up' the membrane and thereby assist in the dissociative action of EDTA. The notion that lipopolysaccharide might cover diffusion pores of lipoprotein in the outer membrane of *E. coli* has recently been discussed (Inouye, 1974).

The finding of polyamines and basic peptides associated with lipopolysaccharide (Chester *et al.*, 1972; Drewry *et al.*, 1972) also suggests a simple explanation for the loss of EDTA-sensitivity of *P. aeruginosa* grown under conditions of Mg-limitation, if organic cations are then used in place of Mg^{2+}. However, the existence of phenotypic variation in cell-wall composition is now well recognized, and major changes in both the content and composition of wall components can be produced by varying the factors controlling cell growth (Ellwood & Tempest, 1972). Recent observations (Gilleland *et al.*, 1973; Gilleland, Stinnett & Eagon, 1974) indicate that Mg-limitation does indeed cause structural reorganization of the outer membrane of *P. aeruginosa*.

CLINICAL SIGNIFICANCE

As a bactericide, EDTA has severe limitations, including selectivity, ready inactivation by multivalent cations and lack of total toxicity, which seem to preclude its unsupported use in clinical bacteriology. On the other hand, the use of polyphosphates (for other reasons) in food technology seems to carry the fringe benefit of retarding spoilage caused by pseudomonads (Elliott *et al.*, 1964; Hargreaves, Wood & Jarvis, 1972), and there are indications that EDTA might also be useful in this respect (Levin, 1967; Pelroy & Seman, 1969). However, the only clear-cut application of EDTA is in the potentiation of general-purpose antiseptics and disinfectants, and this application has been realized commercially. Although most benefit accrues with *P. aeruginosa*, useful improvements can also be obtained with other Gram-negative bacteria. The disadvantage of EDTA-resistance caused by Mg limitation of *P. aeruginosa* may be more apparent than real, as such cells show enhanced sensitivity to phenolic disinfectants (R. A. Cowen, personal communication). Whilst combinations of EDTA with antibiotics are probably unsuitable for systemic use, their potential for the treatment of surface infections does not yet seem to have been adequately evaluated. *In vitro* studies (e.g. Weiser *et al.*, 1968, 1969) indicate that this form of therapy could be useful for the eradication of *P. aeruginosa*, if not perhaps for enterobacteria (Neu & Winshell, 1970). Some success has been reported in various clinical experiments (e.g. Výmola *et al.*, 1968; Doss, Eissa & El-Hamady, 1969; Nezval, Sedláček, Mráz & Brázdová, 1970; Wilson, 1970; Goldschmidt *et al.*, 1972; Wooley, Schall, Eagon & Scott, 1974).

REFERENCES

Adair, F. W., Geftic, S. G., & Gelzer, J. (1971). Resistance of *Pseudomonas* to quaternary ammonium compounds. II. Cross-resistance characteristics of a mutant of *Pseudomonas aeruginosa*. *Applied Microbiology*, **21**, 1058–1063.

Adhikari, P. C., Raychaudhuri, C. & Chatterjee, S. N. (1969). The lysis of cholera and el Tor vibrios. *Journal of General Microbiology*, **59**, 91–95.

Adhikary, P. & Chatterjee, S. N. (1969). Effect of ethylenediaminetetraacetic acid (EDTA) on cholera and El Tor vibrios. *Bulletin of the Calcutta School of Tropical Medicine*, **17**, 6–8.

Albert, A. (1960). *Selective Toxicity*, 2nd edn., Methuen, London, p. 166.

Alemohammad, M. M. & Knowles, C. J. (1974). Osmotically induced volume and turbidity changes of *Escherichia coli* due to salts, sucrose and glycerol, with particular reference to the rapid permeation of glycerol into the cell. *Journal of General Microbiology*, **82**, 125–142.

Allen, D. E., Baker, D. J. & Gillard, R. D. (1967). Metal complexing by *tris* buffer. *Nature, London*, **214**, 906–907.

Asbell, M. A. & Eagon, R. G. (1966a). The role of multivalent cations in the organization and structure of bacterial cell walls. *Biochemical and Biophysical Research Communications*, **22**, 664–671.

Asbell, M. A. & Eagon, R. G. (1966b). Role of multivalent cations in the organization, structure, and assembly of the cell wall of *Pseudomonas aeruginosa*. *Journal of Bacteriology*, **92**, 380–387.

Benveniste, R. & Davies, J. (1973). Mechanisms of antibiotic resistance in bacteria. *Annual Review of Biochemistry*, **42**, 471–506.

Bernheim, F. (1963). Factors which affect the size of the organisms and the optical density of suspensions of *Pseudomonas aeruginosa* and *Escherichia coli*. *Journal of General Microbiology*, **30**, 53–58.

Bernheim, F. (1969). The effect of cations and certain drugs on the rate of swelling of a strain of *Pseudomonas aeruginosa*. *Microbios*, **1A**, 23–30.

Bernheim, F. (1972). The effect of ethylenediaminetetraacetate and its calcium chelate on the rate of swelling of a strain of *Pseudomonas aeruginosa* in salt solutions. *Canadian Journal of Microbiology*, **18**, 1643–1646.

Bersworth, F. C. & Singer, J. J. (1950). Versene and quaternary compounds. *Proceedings of the Chemical Specialities Manufacturers Association*, 101–103.

Birdsell, D. C. & Cota-Robles, E. H. (1967). Production and ultrastructure of lysozyme and ethylenediaminetetraacetate–lysozyme spheroplasts of *Escherichia coli*. *Journal of Bacteriology*, **93**, 427–437.

Bobo, R. A. & Eagon, R. G. (1968). Lipids of cell walls of *Pseudomonas aeruginosa* and *Brucella abortus*. *Canadian Journal of Microbiology*, **14**, 503–513.

Bosch, V. & Braun, V. (1973). Distribution of murein-lipoprotein between the cytoplasmic and outer membrane of *Escherichia coli*. *FEBS Letters*, **34**, 307–310.

Braun, V. & Bosch, V. (1972). Sequence of the murein-lipoprotein and the attachment site of the lipid. *European Journal of Biochemistry*, **28**, 51–69.

Braun, V., Gnirke, H., Henning, U. & Rehn, K. (1973). Model for the structure of the shape-maintaining layer of the *Escherichia coli* cell envelope. *Journal of Bacteriology*, **114**, 1264–1270.

Braun, V. & Rehn, K. (1969). Chemical characterization, spatial distribution and function of a lipoprotein (murein-lipoprotein) of the *E. coli* cell wall. The specific effect of trypsin on the membrane structure. *European Journal of Biochemistry*, **10**, 426–438.

Braun, V., Rehn, K. & Wolff, H. (1970). Supramolecular structure of the rigid layer of the cell wall of *Salmonella, Serratia, Proteus,* and *Pseudomonas fluorescens*. Number of lipoprotein molecules in a membrane layer. *Biochemistry*, **9**, 5041–5049.

Brown, M. R. W. (1968). Survival of *Pseudomonas aeruginosa* in fluorescein solution. Preservative action of PMN and EDTA. *Journal of Pharmaceutical Sciences*, **57**, 389–392.

Brown, M. R. W. & Foster, J. H. S. (1971). Effect of slime on the sensitivity of *Pseudomonas aeruginosa* to EDTA and polymyxin. *Journal of Pharmacy and Pharmacology*, **23** (Suppl.) 236S.

Brown, M. R. W. & Melling, J. (1969a). Loss of sensitivity to EDTA by *Pseudomonas aeruginosa* grown under conditions of Mg-limitation. *Journal of General Microbiology*, **54**, 439–444.

Brown, M. R. W. & Melling, J. (1969b). Role of divalent cations in the action of polymyxin B and EDTA on *Pseudomonas aeruginosa*. *Journal of General Microbiology*, **59**, 263–274.

Brown, M. R. W. & Richards, R. M. E. (1965). Effect of ethylenediaminetetraacetate on the resistance of *Pseudomonas aeruginosa* to antibacterial agents. *Nature, London*, **207**, 1391–1393.

Brown, M. R. W. & Watkins, W. M. (1970). Low magnesium and phospholipid content of cell walls of *Pseudomonas aeruginosa* resistant to polymyxin. *Nature, London*, **227**, 1360–1361.

Buller, C. S. & Dobbs, K. (1971). T4-Coliphage infection of *Escherichia coli* with defective cell envelopes. *Biochemical and Biophysical Research Communications*, **43**, 658–665.

Campbell, J. J. R., Hogg, L. A. & Strasdine, G. A. (1962). Enzyme distribution in *Pseudomonas aeruginosa*. *Journal of Bacteriology*, **83**, 1155–1160.

Cheng, K.-J., Ingram, J. M. & Costerton, J. W. (1970a). Release of alkaline phosphatase from cells of *Pseudomonas aeruginosa* by manipulation of cation concentration and of pH. *Journal of Bacteriology*, **104**, 748–753.

Cheng, K.-J., Ingram, J. M. & Costerton, J. W. (1970b). Alkaline phosphatase localization and spheroplast formation of *Pseudomonas aeruginosa*. *Canadian Journal of Microbiology*, **16**, 1319–1324.

Chester, I. R., Gray, G. W. & Wilkinson, S. G. (1972). Further studies of the chemical composition of the lipopolysaccharide of *Pseudomonas aeruginosa*. *Biochemical Journal*, **126**, 395–407.

Chester, I. R., Meadow, P. M. & Pitt, T. L. (1973). The relationship between the O-antigenic lipopolysaccharides and serological specificity in strains of *Pseudomonas aeruginosa* of different O-serotypes. *Journal of General Microbiology*, **78**, 305–318.

Chipley, J. R. (1972). Comparison of the antigenicity of phenol and ethylenediaminetetraacetate complexes isolated from cell walls of *Salmonella enteritidis*. *Applied Microbiology*, **23**, 651–653.

Chipley, J. R. (1974). Release of lipopolysaccharide, phospholipids and enzymes from *Salmonella enteritidis* by ethylenediaminetetra-acetic acid. *Microbios*, **10**, 139–150.

Chipley, J. R. & Edwards, H. M. (1972). Permeability increases in cells of *Salmonella enteritidis* induced by ethylenediaminetetraacetate and temperature treatments. *Canadian Journal of Microbiology*, **18**, 1803–1807.

Cleeland, R., Beskid, G. & Grunberg, E. (1970). Effect of Mg^{2+} and ethylenediaminetetraacetate on the *in vitro* activity of coumermycin A_1 and novobiocin against Gram-negative bacteria. *Infection and Immunity*, **2**, 371–375.

Collins, F. M. (1964). Composition of cell walls of ageing *Pseudomonas aeruginosa* and *Salmonella bethesda*. *Journal of General Microbiology*, **34**, 379–388.

Colobert, L. (1958). Étude de la lyse de *Salmonelles* pathogènes provoquée par le lysozyme, après délipidation partielle de la paroi externe. *Annales de l'Institut Pasteur*, **95**, 156–167.

Cox, S. T. & Eagon, R. G. (1968). Action of ethylenediaminetetraacetic acid, tris(hydroxymethyl)aminomethane, and lysozyme on cell walls of *Pseudomonas aeruginosa*. *Canadian Journal of Microbiology*, **14**, 913–922.

DePamphilis, M. L. (1971). Dissociation and reassembly of *Escherichia coli* outer membrane and of lipopolysaccharide, and their reassembly onto flagellar basal bodies. *Journal of Bacteriology*, **105**, 1184–1199.

De Petris, S. (1967). Ultrastructure of the cell wall of *Escherichia coli* and chemical nature of its constituent layers. *Journal of Ultrastructure Research*, **19**, 45–83.

Doss, H., Eissa, H. & El-Hamady, S. (1969). Effect of EDTA on bacterial resistance to antibiotics. (A bacteriological and clinical study.) *Journal of the Egyptian Medical Association*, **52**, 929–941.

Drewry, D. T. (1972). *Structural studies of the lipopolysaccharide of* Pseudomonas aeruginosa. Thesis. University of Hull.

Drewry, D. T., Gray, G. W. & Wilkinson, S. G. (1971). Release of ethanolamine pyrophosphate during mild acid hydrolysis of the lipopolysaccharide of *Pseudomonas aeruginosa*. *European Journal of Biochemistry*, **21**, 400–403.

Drewry, D. T., Gray, G. W. & Wilkinson, S. G. (1972). Low-molecular-weight solutes released during mild acid hydrolysis of the lipopolysaccharide of *Pseudomonas aeruginosa*. Identification of ethanolamine triphosphate. *Biochemical Journal*, **130**, 289–295.

Drewry, D. T., Lomax, J. A., Gray, G. W. & Wilkinson, S. G. (1973). Studies of lipid A fractions from the lipopolysaccharides of *Pseudomonas aeruginosa* and *Pseudomonas alcaligenes*. *Biochemical Journal*, **133**, 563–572.

Dvorak, H. F. (1968). Metallo-enzymes released from *Escherichia coli* by osmotic shock. I. Selective depression of enzymes in cells grown in the presence of ethylenediaminetetraacetate. *Journal of Biological Chemistry*, **243**, 2640–2646.

Dyke, J. W. & Berk, R. S. (1973a). Comparative studies on *Pseudomonas aeruginosa* endotoxin. *Zeitschrift für Allgemeine Mikrobiologie,* **13**, 307–313.

Dyke, J. W. & Berk, R. S. (1973b). Comparative electron microscopic studies on *Pseudomonas aeruginosa* endotoxin. *Zeitschrift für Allgemeine Mikrobiologie,* **13**, 381–393.

Eagon, R. G. (1969). Cell wall-associated inorganic substances from *Pseudomonas aeruginosa. Canadian Journal of Microbiology,* **15**, 235–236.

Eagon, R. G. & Asbell, M. A. (1966). Disruption of activity of induced permeases by tris(hydroxymethyl)aminomethane in combination with ethylenediaminetetraacetate. *Biochemical and Biophysical Research Communications,* **24**, 67–73.

Eagon, R. G. & Carson, K. J. (1965). Lysis of cell walls and intact cells of *Pseudomonas aeruginosa* by ethylenediamine tetraacetic acid and by lysozyme. *Canadian Journal of Microbiology,* **11**, 193–201.

Eagon, R. G., Simmons, G. P. & Carson, K. J. (1965). Evidence for the presence of ash and divalent metals in the cell wall of *Pseudomonas aeruginosa. Canadian Journal of Microbiology,* **11**, 1041–1042.

Edwards, C. D. & Noller, E. C. (1964). Effect of lysozyme-potentiating treatments on *Escherichia coli* cell wall protein. *Proceedings of the Oklahoma Academy of Science,* **44**, 196–200.

Elliott, R. P., Straka, R. P. & Garibaldi, J. A. (1964). Polyphosphate inhibition of growth of pseudomonads from poultry meat. *Applied Microbiology,* **12**, 517–522.

Ellwood, D. C. & Tempest, D. W. (1972). Effects of environment on bacterial wall content and composition. *Advances in Microbial Physiology,* **7**, 83–117.

Ennis, H. L. (1967). Bacterial resistance to the synergistic antibiotics of the PA 114, streptogramin, and vernamycin complexes. *Journal of Bacteriology,* **93**, 1881–1887.

Farrell, J. & Rose, A. H. (1968). Cold shock in a mesophilic and a psychrophilic pseudomonad. *Journal of General Microbiology,* **50**, 429–439.

Fensom, A. H. & Gray, G. W. (1969). The chemical composition of the lipopolysaccharide of *Pseudomonas aeruginosa. Biochemical Journal,* **114**, 185–196.

Fensom, A. H. & Meadow, P. M. (1970). Evidence for two regions in the polysaccharide moiety of the lipopolysaccharide of *Pseudomonas aeruginosa* 8602. *FEBS Letters,* **9**, 81–84.

Findley, J. E. & Akagi, J. M. (1968). Lysis of *Desulfovibrio vulgaris* by ethylenediaminetetraacetic acid and lysozyme. *Journal of Bacteriology,* **96**, 1427–1428.

Forge, A., Costerton, J. W. & Kerr, K. A. (1973). Biophysical examination of the cell wall of a Gram-negative marine pseudomonad. The effects of various treatments on the isolated double-track layer. *Canadian Journal of Microbiology,* **19**, 451–459.

Forsberg, C. W., Rayman, M. K., Costerton, J. W. & MacLeod, R. A. (1972). Isolation, characterization, and ultrastructure of the peptidoglycan layer of a marine pseudomonad. *Journal of Bacteriology,* **109**, 895–905.

Franklin, T. J. (1973). Antibiotic transport in bacteria. *CRC Critical Reviews in Microbiology,* **2**, 253–272.

Franklin, T. J. & Snow, G. A. (1971). *Biochemistry of Antimicrobial Action,* Chapman and Hall, London.

Galanos, C., Rietschel, E. Th., Lüderitz, O., Westphal, O., Kim, Y. B. & Watson, D. W. (1972). Biological activities of lipid A complexed with bovine-serum albumin. *European Journal of Biochemistry,* **31**, 230–233.

Garrard, W. T. (1971). Selelective release of proteins from *Spirillum itersonii* by tris(hydroxymethyl)aminomethane and ethylenediaminetetraacetate. *Journal of Bacteriolgy,* **105**, 93–100.

Gilleland, H. E., Stinnett, J. D. & Eagon, R. G. (1974). Ultrastructural and chemical alteration of the cell envelope of *Pseudomonas aeruginosa* associated with resistance to ethylenediaminetetraacetate resulting from growth in a Mg^{2+}-deficient medium. *Journal of Bacteriology,* **117**, 302–311.

Gilleland, H. E., Stinnett, J. D., Roth, I. L. & Eagon, R. G. (1973). Freeze-etch study of *Pseudomonas aeruginosa:* localization within the cell wall of an ethylenediaminetetraacetate-extractable component. *Journal of Bacteriology,* **113**, 417–432.

Glauert, A. M. & Thornley, M. J. (1969). The topography of the bacterial cell wall. *Annual Review of Microbiology,* **23**, 159–198.

Goldschmidt, M. C. & Wyss, O. (1966). Chelation effects on *Azotobacter* cells and cysts. *Journal of Bacteriology,* **91**, 120–124.

Goldschmidt, M. C. & Wyss, O. (1967). The role of tris in EDTA toxicity and lysozyme lysis. *Journal of General Microbiology,* **47**, 421–431.

Goldschmidt, M. C., Goldschmidt, E. P. & Wyss, O. (1967). Differences in toxicity of EDTA + Tris among mating types of *Escherichia coli. Canadian Journal of Microbiology,* **13**, 1401–1407.

Goldschmidt, M. C., Kuhn, C. R., Perry, K. & Johnson, D. E. (1972). EDTA and lysozyme lavage in the treatment of *Pseudomonas* and bladder infections. *Journal of Urology,* **107**, 969–972.

Gordon, R. C. & Macleod, R. A. (1966). Mg^{2+} phospholipids in cell envelopes of a marine and a terrestrial pseudomonad. *Biochemical and Biophysical Research Communications,* **24**, 684–690.

Gorrill, R. H. & McNeil, E. M. (1960). The effect of cold diluent on the viable count of *Pseudomonas pyocyanea. Journal of General Microbiology,* **22**, 437–442.

Gray, G. W. & Wilkinson, S. G. (1965a). The action of ethylenediaminetetra-acetic acid on *Pseudomonas aeruginosa. Journal of Applied Bacteriology,* **28**, 153–164.

Gray, G. W. & Wilkinson, S. G. (1965b). The effect of ethylenediaminetetra-acetic acid on the cell walls of some Gram-negative bacteria. *Journal of General Microbiology,* **39**, 385–399.

Grossowicz, N. & Ariel, M. (1963). Mechanism of protection of cells by spermine against lysozyme-induced lysis. *Journal of Bacteriology,* **85**, 293–300.

Haque, H. & Russell, A. D. (1974). Effect of ethylenediaminetetraacetic acid and related chelating agents on whole cells of Gram-negative bacteria. *Antimicrobial Agents and Chemotherapy,* **5**, 447–452.

Hamilton-Miller, J. M. T. (1965). Effect of EDTA upon bacterial permeability to benzylpenicillin. *Biochemical and Biophysical Research Communications,* **20**, 688–691.

Hamilton-Miller, J. M. T. (1966). Damaging effects of ethylenediaminetetra-acetate and penicillins on permeability barriers in Gram-negative bacteria. *Biochemical Journal,* **100**, 675–682.

Hancock, I. C. & Meadow, P. M. (1969). The extractable lipids of *Pseudomonas aeruginosa. Biochimica et biophysica acta,* **187**, 366–379.

Hanlon, D. P., Watt, D. S. & Westhead, E. W. (1966). The interaction of divalent metal ions with tris buffer in dilute solution. *Analytical Biochemistry,* **16**, 225–233.

Hantke, K. & Braun, V. (1973). Covalent binding of lipid to protein. Diglyceride and amide-linked fatty acid at the N-terminal end of the murein-lipoprotein of the *Escherichia coli* outer membrane. *European Journal of Biochemistry,* **34**, 284–296.

Hargreaves, L. L., Wood, J. M. & Jarvis, B. (1972). The antimicrobial effect of phosphates with particular reference to food products. Scientific and Technical Survey No. 76. The British Food Manufacturing Industries Research Association.

Haslam, D. F., Best, G. K. & Durham, N. N. (1969). Activation of autolytic enzyme(s) in *Pseudomonas aeruginosa* by ethylenediaminetetraacetate treatment. *Bacteriological Proceedings,* 136.

Haslam, D. F., Best, G. K. & Durham, N. N. (1970). Quantitation of the action of ethylenediaminetetraacetic acid and tris(hydroxymethyl)aminomethane on a Gram-negative bacterium by vancomycin adsorption. *Journal of Bacteriology,* **103,** 523–524.

Hatch, E. & Cooper, P. (1948). Sodium hexametaphosphate in emulsions of Dettol for obstetric use. *Pharmaceutical Journal,* **161,** 198–199.

Heilmann, H.-D. (1972). On the peptidoglycan of the cell walls of *Pseudomonas aeruginosa. European Journal of Biochemistry,* **31,** 456–463.

Heilmann, H.-D. (1974). On the peptidoglycan of the cell walls of *Pseudomonas aeruginosa.* Structure of the peptide side chains. *European Journal of Biochemistry,* **43,** 35–38.

Heppel, L. A. (1971). In *Structure and Function of Biological Membranes,* (Ed. L. I. Rothfield), Chapter 5, Academic Press, New York.

Hirashima, A., Wu, H. C., Venkateswaran, P. S. & Inouye, M. (1973). Two forms of a structural lipoprotein in the envelope of *Escherichia coli.* Further characterization of the free form. *Journal of Biological Chemistry,* **248,** 5654–5659.

Homma, J. Y. & Suzuki, N. (1966). The protein moiety of the endotoxin of *Pseudomonas aeruginosa. Annals of the New York Academy of Sciences,* **133,** 508–526.

Humphrey, B. & Vincent, J. M. (1962). Calcium in cell walls of *Rhizobium trifolii. Journal of General Microbiology,* **29,** 557–561.

Ikeda, K. & Egami, F. (1973). Lipopolysaccharide of *Pseudomonas aeruginosa* with special reference to pyocin R receptor activity. *Journal of General and Applied Microbiology,* **19,** 115–128.

Ikeda, K. & Nishi, Y. (1973). Interaction between pyocin R and pyocin R receptor. *Journal of General and Applied Microbiology,* **19,** 209–219.

Inouye, M. (1974). A three-dimensional molecular assembly model of a lipoprotein from the *Escherichia coli* outer membrane. *Proceedings of the National Academy of Sciences of the United States of America,* **71,** 2396–2400.

Inouye, M. & Yee, M.-L. (1973). Homogeneity of envelope proteins of *Escherichia coli* separated by gel electrophoresis in sodium dodecyl sulfate. *Journal of Bacteriology,* **113,** 304–312.

Inouye, M., Shaw, J. & Shen, C. (1972). The assembly of a structural lipoprotein in the envelope of *Escherichia coli. Journal of Biological Chemistry,* **247,** 8154–8159.

Jackson, G. D. F. & Redmond, J. W. (1971). Immunochemical studies of the O-antigens of *Vibrio cholerae.* The constitution of a lipopolysaccharide from *V. cholerae* 569B (Inaba). *FEBS Letters,* **13,** 117–120.

Jann, B., Jann, K. & Beyaert, G. O. (1973). 2-Amino-2,6-dideoxy-D-glucose (D-quinovosamine): a constituent of the lipopolysaccharides of *Vibrio cholerae. European Journal of Biochemistry,* **37,** 531–534.

Key, B. A., Gray, G. W. & Wilkinson, S. G. (1970). Purification and chemical composition of the lipopolysaccharide of *Pseudomonas alcaligenes. Biochemical Journal,* **120,** 559–566.

Kleber, H.-P. & Sorger, H. (1970). Einfluss von EDTA auf die induzierbare Carnitinpermease bei *Pseudomonas aeruginosa. Acta Biologica et Medica Germanica,* **24,** 209–213.

Knowles, C. J. (1971). Salt-induced changes of turbidity and volume of *E. coli. Nature New Biology, London,* **229,** 154–155.

Knox, K. W., Cullen, J. & Work, E. (1967). An extracellular lipopolysaccharide-phospholipid–protein complex produced by *Escherichia coli* grown under lysine-limiting conditions. *Biochemical Journal,* **103,** 192–201.

Koike, M., Iida, K. & Matsuo, T. (1969). Electron microscopic studies on mode of action of polymyxin. *Journal of Bacteriology,* **97,** 448–452.

Lehmann, V., Lüderitz, O. & Westphal, O. (1971). The linkage of pyrophosphorylethanolamine to heptose in the core of *Salmonella minnesota* lipopolysaccharides. *European Journal of Biochemistry,* **21,** 339–347.

Leive, L. (1965a). Actinomycin sensitivity in *Escherichia coli* produced by EDTA. *Biochemical and Biophysical Research Communications*, **18**, 13–17.

Leive, L. (1965b). A nonspecific increase in permeability in *Escherichia coli* produced by EDTA. *Proceedings of the National Academy of Sciences*, **53**, 745–750.

Leive, L. (1965c). Release of lipopolysaccharide by EDTA treatment of *E. coli*. *Biochemical and Biophysical Research Communications*, **21**, 290–296.

Leive, L. (1968). Studies on the permeability change produced in coliform bacteria by ethylenediaminetetraacetate. *Journal of Biological Chemistry*, **243**, 2373–2380.

Leive, L. & Kollin, V. (1967). Controlling EDTA treatment to produce permeable *Escherichia coli* with normal metabolic processes. *Biochemical and Biophysical Research Communications*, **28**, 229–236.

Leive, L. & Lawrence, D. (1971). On the location of lipopolysaccharide releasable by EDTA treatment of coliform bacteria, as tested by accessibility to phage. *Federation Proceedings*, **30**, 1173 Abs.

Leive, L., Shovlin, V. K. & Mergenhagen, S. E. (1968). Physical, chemical, and immunological properties of lipopolysaccharide released from *Escherichia coli* by ethylenediaminetetraacetate. *Journal of Biological Chemistry*, **243**, 6384–6391.

Levin, R. E., (1967). The effectiveness of EDTA as a fish preservative. *Journal of Milk and Food Technology*, **30**, 277–283.

Levy. S. B. & Leive, L. (1968). An equilibrium between two fractions of lipopolysaccharide in *Escherichia coli*. *Proceedings of the National Academy of Sciences*, **61**, 1435–1439.

Levy, S. B. & Leive, L. (1970). Release from *Escherichia coli* of a galactosyltransferase complex active in lipopolysaccharide synthesis. *Journal of Biological Chemistry*, **245**, 585–594.

Lickfeld, K. G., Achterrath, M., Hentrich, F., Kolehmainen-Seveus, L. & Persson, A. (1972). Die Feinstrukturen von *Pseudomonas aeruginosa* in ihrer Deutung durch die Gefrierätztechnik, Ultramikrotomie und Kryo-Ultramikrotomie. *Journal of Ultrastructure Research*, **38**, 27–45.

Lindsay, S. S., Wheeler, B., Sanderson, K. E., Costerton, J. W. & Cheng, K.-J. (1973). The release of alkaline phosphatase and of lipopolysaccharide during the growth of rough and smooth strains of *Salmonella typhimurium*. *Canadian Journal of Microbiology*, **19**, 335–343.

Lomax, J. A., Gray, G. W. & Wilkinson, S. G. (1974). Studies of the polysaccharide fraction from the lipopolysaccharide of *Pseudomonas alcaligenes*. *Biochemical Journal*, **139**, 633–643.

Lopes, J. & Inniss, W. E. (1969). Electron microscopy of effect of polymyxin on *Escherichia coli* lipopolysaccharide. *Journal of Bacteriology*, **100**, 1128–1130.

Lüderitz, O., Westphal, O., Staub, A. M. & Nikaido, H. (1971). In *Microbial Endotoxins*, (Ed. G. Weinbaum, S. Kadis and S. J. Ajl), Chapter 4, Academic Press, New York.

Lusk, J. E., Williams, R. J. P. & Kennedy, E. P. (1968). Magnesium and the growth of *Escherichia coli*. *Journal of Biological Chemistry*, **243**, 2618–2624.

MacGregor, D. R. & Elliker, P. R. (1958). A comparison of some properties of strains of *Pseudomonas aeruginosa* sensitive and resistant to quaternary ammonium compounds. *Canadian Journal of Microbiology*, **4**, 499–503.

Machtiger, N. A. & Fox, C. F. (1973). Biochemistry of bacterial membranes. *Annual Review of Biochemistry*, **42**, 575–600.

MacKelvie, R. M., Gronlund, A. F. & Campbell, J. J. R. (1968). Influence of cold-shock on the endogenous metabolism of *Pseudomonas aeruginosa*. *Canadian Journal of Microbiology*, **14**, 633–638.

Malamy, M. H. & Horecker, B. L. (1964). Release of alkaline phosphatase from cells of *Escherichia coli* upon lysozyme spheroplast formation. *Biochemistry*, **3**, 1889–1893.

Marquis, R. E. (1968). Salt-induced contraction of bacterial cell walls. *Journal of Bacteriology*, **95**, 775–781.

Marsh, D. G. & Walker, P. D. (1968). Free endotoxin and non-toxic material from Gram-negative bacteria: electron microscopy of fractions from *Escherichia coli*. *Journal of General Microbiology*, **52**, 125–130.

Martin, H. H., Heilmann, H. D. & Preusser, H. J. (1972). State of the rigid-layer in cell walls of some Gram-negative bacteria. *Archiv für Mikrobiologie*, **83**, 332–346.

Martin, J. P., Fleck, J., Mock, M. & Ghuysen, J. M. (1973). The wall peptidoglycans of *Neisseria perflava, Moraxella glucidolytica, Pseudomonas alcaligenes* and *Proteus vulgaris* strain P18. *European Journal of Biochemistry*, **38**, 301–306.

Matula, T. I. & MacLeod, R. A. (1969). Penetration of *Pseudomonas aeruginosa* by sodium chloride and its relation to the mechanism of optical effects. *Journal of Bacteriology*, **100**, 411–416.

Meadow, P. M. (1975). In *The Biochemistry and Genetics of Pseudomonas,* (Ed. P. H. Clark and M. H. Richmond), John Wiley, London.

Michaels, G. B. & Eagon, R. G. (1966). The effect of ethylenediaminetetraacetate and of lysozyme on isolated lipopolysaccharide from *Pseudomonas aeruginosa*. *Proceedings of the Society for Experimental Biology and Medicine*, **122**, 866–868.

Miura, T. & Mizushima, S. (1968). Separation by density gradient centrifugation of two types of membranes from spheroplast membrane of *Escherichia coli* K12. *Biochimica et biophysica acta*, **150**, 159–161.

Miura, T. & Mizushima, S. (1969). Separation and properties of outer and cytoplasmic membranes in *Escherichia coli*. *Biochimica et biophysica acta*, **193**, 268–276.

Mühlradt, P. F., Menzel, J., Golecki, J. R. & Speth, V. (1973). Outer membrane of *Salmonella*. Sites of export of newly synthesised lipopolysaccharide on the bacterial surface. *European Journal of Biochemistry*, **35**, 471–481.

Mühlradt, P. F., Menzel, J., Golecki, J. R. & Speth, V. (1974). Lateral mobility and surface density of lipopolysaccharide in the outer membrane of *Salmonella typhimurium*. *European Journal of Biochemistry*, **43**, 533–539.

Murray, R. G. E., Steed, P. & Elson, H. E. (1965). The location of the mucopeptide in sections of the cell wall of *Escherichia coli* and other Gram-negative bacteria. *Canadian Journal of Microbiology*, **11**, 547–560.

Murti, C. R. K. & Gupta, A. S. (1960). Lysis of *Vibrio cholerae (V. comma)* by lysozyme. *Journal of Scientific and Industrial Research (India)*, **19C**, 83–87.

Muschel, L. H. & Gustafson, L. (1968). Antibiotic, detergent, and complement sensitivity of *Salmonella typhi* after ethylenediaminetetraacetic acid treatment. *Journal of Bacteriology*, **95**, 2010–2013.

Nagata, Y., Mizuno, S. & Maruo, B. (1966). Preparation and properties of active membrane systems from various species of bacteria. *Journal of Biochemistry*, **59**, 404–410.

Neu, H. C. (1969). The role of amine buffers in EDTA toxicity and their effect on osmotic shock. *Journal of General Microbiology*, **57**, 215–220.

Neu, H. C., Ashman, D. F. & Price, T. D. (1967). Effect of ethylenediaminetetraacetic acid-tris(hydroxymethyl)aminomethane on release of the acid-soluble nucleotide pool and on breakdown of ribosomal ribonucleic acid in *Escherichia coli*. *Journal of Bacteriology*, **93**, 1360–1368.

Neu, H. C. & Chou, J. (1967). Release of surface enzymes in *Enterobacteriaceae* by osmotic shock. *Journal of Bacteriology*, **94**, 1934–1945.

Neu, H. C. & Heppel, L. A. (1965). The release of enzymes from *Escherichia coli* by osmotic shock and during the formation of spheroplasts. *Journal of Biological Chemistry*, **240**, 3685–3692.

Neu, H. C. & Winshell, E. B. (1970). Lack of synergy of EDTA with antimicrobials in resistant Enterobacteriaceae. *Nature, London*, **225**, 763.

Nezval, J. (1964). Some aspects of the enhancing effect of ethylenediaminetetraacetic acid on the bactericidal activity of the quaternary ammonium compound Septonex. *Journal of Hygiene, Epidemiology, Microbiology and Immunology,* **8**, 457–465.

Nezval, J. & Halačka, K. (1967). The enhancing effect of EDTA on the antibacterial activity of nalidixic acid against *Pseudomonas aeruginosa. Experientia,* **23**, 1043–1044.

Nezval, J. & Ritzerfeld, W. (1969a). Die Bedeutung der Äthylen–diamino-tetraessigsäure (EDTA) in der mikrobiologischen Forschung. *Archiv für Hygiene und Bakteriologie,* **153**, 438–446.

Nezval, J. & Ritzerfeld, W. (1969b). Zur antibakteriellen Wirkung der Kombination Rifampicin-EDTA auf *Pseudomonas* und *Proteus. Archiv für Hygiene und Bakteriologie,* **153**, 548–551.

Nezval, J. & Ritzerfeld, W. (1970). Zur Kombinationswirkung von EDTA und antibiotischen Substanzen auf *Pseudomonas aeruginosa. Zentralblatt für Bakteriologie, Parasitenkunde, Infektionskrankheiten und Hygiene* (Abteilung I, Originale), **212**, 526–530.

Nezval, J., Sedláček, J., Mráz, J. & Brázdová, K. (1970). The first phase of pseudomonadal pneumonia influenced by the administration of ampicillin + EDTA *in vivo. Internationale Zeitschrift für Klinische Pharmakologie, Therapie und Toxikologie,* **3**, 152–156.

Nezval, J., Smékal, E., Skotáková, M. & Rýc, M. (1965). A contribution to studies on the influence of EDTA and Ca^{2+} on the antibacterial activity of neomycin on *Pseudomonas aeruginosa. Scripta Medica* (*Brno*), **38**, 311–316.

Noller, E. C. & Hartsell, S. E. (1961a). Bacteriolysis of *Enterobacteriaceae.* I. Lysis by four lytic systems utilizing lysozyme. *Journal of Bacteriology,* **81**, 482–491.

Noller, E. C. & Hartsell, S. E. (1961b). Bacteriolysis of *Enterobacteriaceae.* II. Pre- and co-lytic treatments potentiating the action of lysozyme. *Journal of Bacteriology,* **81**, 492–499.

Norton, J. E., Bulmer, G. S. & Sokatch, J. R. (1963). The oxidation of D-alanine by cell membranes of *Pseudomonas aeruginosa. Biochimica et biophysica acta,* **78**, 136–147.

O'Leary, G. P., Nelson, J. D. & MacLeod, R. A. (1972). Requirement for salts for the isolation of lipopolysaccharide from a marine pseudomonad. *Canadian Journal of Microbiology,* **18**, 601–606.

Olins, A. L. & Warner, R. C. (1967). Physicochemical studies on a lipopolysaccharide from the cell wall of *Azotobacter vinelandii. Journal of Biological Chemistry,* **242**, 4994–5001.

Osborn, M. J., Gander, J. E. & Parisi, E. (1972). Mechanism of assembly of the outer membrane of *Salmonella typhimurium.* Site of synthesis of lipopolysaccharide. *Journal of Biological Chemistry,* **247**, 3973–3986.

Osborn, M. J., Gander, J. E., Parisi, E. & Carson, J. (1972). Mechanism of assembly of the outer membrane of *Salmonella typhimurium.* Isolation and characterization of cytoplasmic and outer membrane. *Journal of Biological Chemistry,* **247**, 3962–3972.

Ou, L.-T. & Marquis, R. E. (1970). Electromechanical interactions in cell walls of Gram-positive cocci. *Journal of Bacteriology,* **101**, 92–101.

Patel, R. P. & Shah, A. B. (1965). Disodium salt of EDTA as an antimicrobial agent. *Indian Journal of Pharmacy,* **27**, 147–148.

Payne, J. W. (1965). The action of ethylenediaminetetra-acetic acid on the cell wall of *Pseudomonas aeruginosa.* Thesis. University of Hull.

Pechey, D. T. & James, A. M. (1974). Surface properties of cells of gentamicin-sensitive and gentamicin-resistant strains of *Pseudomonas aeruginosa. Microbios,* **10A**, 111–126.

Pelroy, G. A. & Seman, J. P. (1966). Effect of EDTA treatment on spoilage characteristics of petrale sole and ocean perch fillets. *Journal of the Fisheries Research Board of Canada,* **26**, 2651–2657.

Pike, R. M. & Chandler, C. H. (1974). The spontaneous release of somatic antigen from *Vibrio cholerae*. *Journal of General Microbiology*, **81**, 59–67.

Post, F. J., Krishnamurty, G. B. & Flanagan, M. D. (1963). Influence of sodium hexametaphosphate on selected bacteria. *Applied Microbiology*, **11**, 430–435.

Randle, C. L., Albro, P. W. & Dittmer, J. C. (1969). The phosphoglyceride composition of Gram-negative bacteria and the changes in composition during growth. *Biochimica et biophysica acta*,. **187**, 214–220.

Rawal, B. D. & Owen, W. R. (1971). Combined action of sulfamethoxazole, trimethoprim, and ethylenediaminetetraacetic acid on *Pseudomonas aeruginosa*. *Applied Microbiology*, **21**, 367–368.

Raza Nasir, M. M. & Ghatak, S. (1970). Effect of different reagents on lysis of *Salmonella typhosa*. *Indian Journal of Medical Research*, **58**, 1–10.

Razin, S. (1972). Reconstitution of biological membranes. *Biochimica et biophysica acta*, **265**, 241–296.

Reaveley, D. A. & Burge, R. E. (1972). Walls and membranes in bacteria. *Advances in Microbial Physiology*, **7**, 1–81.

Reid, P. & Speyer, J. (1970). Rifampicin inhibition of RNA and protein synthesis in normal and EDTA treated *Escherichia coli*. *Journal of Bacteriology*, **104**, 376–389.

Repaske, R. (1956). Lysis of Gram-negative bacteria by lysozyme. *Biochimica et biophysica acta*, **22**, 189–191.

Repaske, R. (1958). Lysis of Gram-negative organisms and the role of Versene. *Biochimica et biophysica acta*, **30**, 225–232.

Reybrouck, G. & van de Voorde, H. (1969). Effect of ethylenediamine tetraacetate on the germicidal action of disinfectants against *Pseudomonas aeruginosa*. *Acta Clinica Belgica*, **24**, 32–41.

Ringbom, A. (1954). Volumetric determination of metals with the aid of complexing agents. *Svensk Kemisk Tidskrift*, **66**, 159–172.

Roberts, N. A., Gray, G. W. & Wilkinson, S. G. (1967). Release of lipopolysaccharide during the preparation of cell walls of *Pseudomonas aeruginosa*. *Biochimica et biophysica acta*, **135**, 1068–1071.

Roberts, N. A., Gray, G. W. & Wilkinson, S. G. (1970). The bactericidal action of ethylenediaminetetra-acetic acid on *Pseudomonas aeruginosa*. *Microbios*, **2**, 189–208.

Rodwell, A. W. (1965). The stability of *Mycoplasma mycoides*. *Journal of General Microbiology*, **40**, 227–234.

Rogers, D. (1971). Release of a lipopolysaccharide–protein complex from *Escherichia coli* by warm-water treatment. *Biochimica et biophysica acta*, **230**, 72–81.

Rogers, S. W., Gilleland, H. E. & Eagon, R. G. (1969). Characterization of a protein–lipopolysaccharide complex released from cell walls of *Pseudomonas aeruginosa* by ethylenediaminetetraacetic acid. *Canadian Journal of Microbiology*, **15**, 743–748.

Rothfield, L. & Pearlman-Kothencz, M. (1969). Synthesis and assembly of bacterial membrane components. A lipopolysaccharide–phospholipid–protein complex excreted by living bacteria. *Journal of Molecular Biology*, **44**, 477–492.

Rubio, N. & Lopez, R. (1971). Purification of *Pseudomonas aeruginosa* endotoxin by gel filtration on Sepharose 4B. *Journal of Chromatography*, **57**, 148–150.

Rubio, N. & Lopez, R. (1972). Purification of *Pseudomonas aeruginosa* endotoxin by membrane partition chromatography. *Applied Microbiology*, **23**, 211–213.

Russell, A. D. (1967). Effect of magnesium ions and ethylenediamine tetra-acetic acid on the activity of vancomycin against *Escherichia coli* and *Staphylococcus aureus*. *Journal of Applied Bacteriology*, **30**, 395–401.

Russell, A. D. (1971). In *Inhibition and Destruction of the Microbial Cell*, (Ed. W. B. Hugo), Chapter 3G, Academic Press, London.

Schleiffer, K. H. & Kandler, O. (1972). Peptidoglycan types of bacterial cell walls and their taxonomic implications. *Bacteriological Reviews,* **36**, 407–477.

Schnaitman, C. A. (1970a). Protein composition of the cell wall and cytoplasmic membrane of *Escherichia coli. Journal of Bacteriology,* **104**, 890–901.

Schnaitman, C. A. (1970b). Comparison of the envelope protein compositions of several Gram-negative bacteria. *Journal of Bacteriology,* **104**, 1404–1405.

Schnaitman, C. A. (1971). Effect of ethylenediaminetetraacetic acid, Triton X-100, and lysozyme on the morphology and chemical composition of isolated cell walls of *Escherichia coli. Journal of Bacteriology,* **108**, 553–563.

Sellin, H. G., Srinivasan, P. R. & Borek, E. (1966). Studies of a phage-induced DNA methylase. *Journal of Molecular Biology,* **19**, 219–222.

Shively, J. M. & Hartsell, S. E. (1964a). Bacteriolysis of the pseudomonads. I. Agents potentiating lysis. *Canadian Journal of Microbiology,* **10**, 905–909.

Shively, J. M. & Hartsell, S. E. (1964b). Bacteriolysis of the pseudomonads. II. Chemical treatments affecting the lytic response. *Canadian Journal of Microbiology,* **10**, 911–915.

Silva, M. T. & Sousa, J. C. F. (1973). Ultrastructure of the cell wall and cytoplasmic membrane of Gram-negative bacteria with different fixation techniques. *Journal of Bacteriology,* **113**, 953–962.

Singer, S. J. (1971). In *Structure and Function of Biological Membranes,* (Ed. L. I. Rothfield), Chapter 4, Academic Press, New York.

Singh, C. (1971). A non-chelating property of EDTA and some of its biochemical and biological implications. *Indian Journal of Biochemistry and Biophysics,* **8**, 45–49.

Slein, M. W. & Logan, G. F. (1967). Lysis of *Escherichia coli* by ethylenediamine-tetraacetate and phospholipases as measured by β-galactosidase activity. *Journal of Bacteriology,* **94**, 934–941.

Smith, G. (1970). Ethylene diamine tetra-acetic acid and the bactericidal efficiency of some phenolic disinfectants against *Pseudomonas aeruginosa. Journal of Medical Laboratory Technology,* **27**, 203–206.

Socolofsky, M. D. & Wyss, O. (1961). Cysts of *Azotobacter. Journal of Bacteriology,* **91**, 946–954.

Spicer, A. B. & Spooner, D. F. (1974). The inhibition of growth of *Escherichia coli* spheroplasts by antibacterial agents. *Journal of General Microbiology,* **80**, 37–50.

Stewart, D. J. & Young, H. (1971). Factors affecting the adsorption of a pyocin by cells of *Pseudomonas aeruginosa. Microbios,* **3**, 15–22.

Stinnett, J. D. & Eagon, R. G. (1973). Outer (cell wall) membrane proteins of *Pseudomonas aeruginosa. Canadian Journal of Microbiology,* **19**, 1469–1471.

Stinnett, J. D., Gilleland, H. E. & Eagon, R. G. (1973). Proteins released from cell envelopes of *Pseudomonas aeruginosa* on exposure to ethylenediaminetetraacetate: comparison with dimethylformamide-extractable proteins. *Journal of Bacteriology,* **144**, 399–407.

Stothart, S. N. H. & Beecroft, G. C. (1961). British patent 858, 030 (*Chemical Abstracts,* **55**, 12783d).

Suzuki, A. & Goto, S. (1972). Surface films of protein and a protein-lipopolysaccharide complex extracted from *Pseudomonas aeruginosa. Biochimica et biophysica acta,* **255**, 734–743.

Then, R. (1972). Versuche zur Wirkungssteigerung der Kombination Sulfamethoxazol/Trimethoprim durch EDTA und Levallorphan an *Escherichia coli. Experientia,* **28**, 1118–1119.

Tucker, A. N. & White, D. C. (1970). Release of membrane components from viable *Haemophilus parainfluenzae* by ethylenediaminetetraacetic acid-tris(hydroxymethyl)aminomethane. *Journal of Bacteriology,* **102**, 498–507.

Vakil, J. R., Chandan, R. C., Parry, R. M. & Shahani, K. M. (1969). Susceptibility of several microorganisms to milk lysozymes. *Journal of Dairy Science,* **52**, 1192–1197.

Van Gool, A. P. & Nanninga, N. (1971). Fracture faces in the cell envelope of *Escherichia coli*. *Journal of Bacteriology*, **108**, 474–481.

Voll, M. J. & Leive, L. (1970). Release of lipopolysaccharide in *Escherichia coli* resistant to the permeability increase induced by ethylenediaminetetraacetate. *Journal of Biological Chemistry*, **245**, 1108–1114.

Voss, J. G. (1964). Lysozyme lysis of Gram-negative bacteria without production of spheroplasts. *Journal of General Microbiology*, **35**, 313–317.

Voss, J. G. (1967). Effects of organic cations on the Gram-negative cell wall and their bactericidal activity with ethylenediaminetetra-acetate and surface active agents. *Journal of General Microbiology*, **48**, 391–400.

Výmola, F., Nezval, J., Rýc, M., Táborský, I., Pillich, J. & Páčová, Z. (1968). Prevention of the emergence of drug resistance in *Pseudomonas aeruginosa* by EDTA. *Scripta Medica (Brno)*, **41**, 411–422.

Warren, G. H., Gray, J. & Bartell, P. (1955). The lysis of *Pseudomonas aeruginosa* by lysozyme. *Journal of Bacteriology*, **70**, 614–619.

Webb, M. (1966). The utilization of magnesium by certain Gram-positive and Gram-negative bacteria. *Journal of General Microbiology*, **43**, 401–409.

Weckesser, J., Drews, G., Fromme, I. & Mayer, H. (1973). Isolation and chemical composition of the lipopolysaccharides of *Rhodopseudomonas palustris* strains. *Archiv für Mikrobiologie*, **92**, 123–138.

Weiser, R., Asscher, A. W. & Wimpenny, J. (1968). *In vitro* reversal of antibiotic resistance by ethylenediamine tetraacetic acid. *Nature, London*, **219**, 1365–1366.

Weiser, R., Wimpenny, J. & Asscher, A. W. (1969). Synergistic effect of edetic-acid/antibiotic combinations on *Pseudomonas aeruginosa*. *Lancet*, **ii**, 619–620.

Weiss, R. L. & Fraser, D. (1973). Surface structure of intact cells and spheroplasts of *Pseudomonas aeruginosa*. *Journal of Bacteriology*, **113**, 963–968.

Wilkinson, S. G. (1967). The sensitivity of pseudomonads to ethylenediaminetetra-acetic acid. *Journal of General Microbiology*, **47**, 67–76.

Wilkinson, S. G. (1968). Studies on the cell walls of *Pseudomonas* species resistant to ethylenediaminetetra-acetic acid. *Journal of General Microbiology*, **54**, 195–213.

Wilkinson, S. G. (1970). Cell walls of *Pseudomonas* species sensitive to ethylenediaminetetraacetic acid. *Journal of Bacteriology*, **104**, 1035–1044.

Wilkinson, S. G., Galbraith, L. & Lightfoot, G. A. (1973). Cell walls, lipids, and lipopolysaccharides of *Pseudomonas* species. *European Journal of Biochemistry*, **33**, 158–174.

Wilson, L. A. (1970). Chelation in experimental *Pseudomonas* keratitis. *British Journal of Ophthalmology*, **54**, 587–593.

Winshell, E. B. & Neu, H. C. (1970). Relation of lipopolysaccharide and fatty acid ester release to the ethylenediaminetetraacetic acid alteration of permeability in *Enterobacteriaceae*. *Journal of Bacteriology*, **102**, 537–539.

Winter, A. J., Katz, W. & Martin, H. H. (1971). Murein (peptidoglycan) structure of *Vibrio fetus*. Comparison of a venereal and an intestinal strain. *Biochimica et biophysica acta*, **244**, 58–64.

Wolin, M. J. (1966). Lysis of *Vibrio succinogenes* by ethylenediaminetetraacetic acid or lysozyme. *Journal of Bacteriology*, **91**, 1781–1786.

Wooley, R. E., Schall, W. D., Eagon, R. G. & Scott, T. A. (1974). The efficacy of EDTA-tris-lysozyme lavage in the treatment of experimentally induced *Pseudomonas aeruginosa* cystitis in the dog. *American Journal of Veterinary Medicine*, **35**, 27–29.

Yu, K. K.-Y. & Jordan, D. C. (1971). Cation content and cation-exchange capacity of intact cells and cell envelopes of viomycin-sensitive and -resistant strains of *Rhizobium meliloti*. *Canadian Journal of Microbiology*, **17**, 1283–1286.

Zemjanis, R. & Hoyt, H. H. (1960). The effect of enzyme inhibitors on *Vibrio fetus*, *Proteus vulgaris*, and *Pseudomonas aeruginosa*. *American Journal of Veterinary Research*, **21**, 1066–1074.

CHAPTER 6

Epidemiological Typing of
Pseudomonas aeruginosa

TOM BERGAN

Department of Microbiology, Institute of Medical Biology, University of Tromsø, Tromsø now at Microbiology Department, University of Oslo, Blindern, PO Box 1108, Oslo 3, Norway.

INTRODUCTION

The rise in infections due to *Pseudomonas aeruginosa* has been commented upon frequently during the past decade (Bergan, 1967, 1968; Finland, 1971; Shooter, 1971, 1972–1973 and see Chapter 7). In Finland's experience, during the period 1935–1965 the frequency of pseudomonas rose from 3–4 to 9% of all isolates from blood cultures.

Pseudomonas infections are mainly a consequence of modern hospitalization. The mechanisms responsible for this change are discussed elsewhere (Lowbury, 1974; Lowbury & Jones, this volume, Chapter 7).

Clinical aspects of pseudomonas* infections have been detailed by Forkner (1960) and Caselitz (1966). Most common are infections of the urinary tract, respiratory tract—particularly in the aged, in premature babies, and in tracheostomized patients—and burn wounds (Bergan, 1968a). To a considerable extent, patients with infections maintain the nosocomial situation since they constitute reservoirs from which spread may occur to the environment. It is also significant that there are healthy carriers of pseudomonas (Shooter *et al.*, 1966) and that it spreads rapidly. Because of the extensive resistance to antibiotics, these pseudomonas infections are particularly serious.

In such a situation, it is desirable to identify the sources and follow the routes of transmission. As means to this end epidemiological methods of pyocine, serological and bacteriophage typing have been developed. Physical and chemical properties of phages and pyocines are described in detail elsewhere (Holloway & Krishnapillai, 1975). This chapter will discuss methods of typing, their physiological or physical basis, techniques and results of their application and the relative value and performance of each method.

BACTERIOPHAGE TYPING

Phage–Host Interaction

Pseudomonas phages may be isolated from sewage or from lysogenic strains. Among *P. aeruginosa*, 90–100% are lysogenic (Alföldi, 1957b; Feary *et al.*, 1963; Hamon *et al.*, 1961; Meitert & Meitert, 1961; Paterson, 1965). A single bacterial cell may be polylysogenic, i.e. contain several antigenically different phages (Holloway *et al.*, 1960; Feary *et al.*, 1963).

Phage action is dependent upon specific receptors for phage attachment to the bacterial surface. Phage receptor structures appear either to overlap with part of the pyocine receptors (Homma & Shionoya, 1967) or to be identical with them (Ito & Kageyama, 1970). Bacterial trichloroacetic acid extracts inhibit the action of phages on strains sensitive to them (Mead & van den Ende, 1953).

The characteristics of pseudomonas phages have been subjected to many studies (Alföldi, 1957a; Bradley & Robertson, 1968; Feary *et al.*, 1964; Goepfert & Naylor, 1964; Kelln & Warren, 1971; Minamishima *et al.*, 1968;

---

* In the following, the term 'pseudomonas' is used synonymously with *P. aeruginosa*.

O'Callaghan *et al.*, 1969; Olsen *et al.*, 1968; Shionoya *et al.*, 1967; Takeya *et al.*, 1959).

Historical Development

The early studies on pseudomonas phages often confused true phage plaques with the plaque-like autolytic phenomenon characteristic for *P. aeruginosa* (Bergan, 1972g; Govan, 1968; Vieu, 1969). Warner (1950) and Don & van den Ende (1950) demonstrated the differences in phage susceptibility patterns of pseudomonas that is the basis of phage typing. Terry (1952) developed the first set for phage typing of pseudomonas and later Potel (1957), Yamada (1960), Grogan & Artz (1961), Hoff & Drake (1961), Postic & Finland (1961) and Grün *et al.* (1967) developed their own typing sets. The usefulness of pseudomonas phage typing was thereby demonstrated, but all these sets were only used locally.

During the 1960s, several more elaborate sets were developed: Gould & McLeod (1960), Pavlatou & Kaklamani (1961), Graber *et al.* (1962), Lindberg *et al.* (1963, 1964), Feary *et al.* (1963), Zanen & van den Berge (1963), Meitert (1965), Sutter *et al.* (1965), Jedlicková & Pillich (1968), and Herrmann (1970) each with their own typing sets examined the spread of pseudomonas hospital infections. Each set was developed locally except that the Lindberg *et al.* set was a further development of the Graber *et al.* set. Approximately 50% of the Lindberg *et al.* phages came from the Hoff & Drake study. Sutter *et al.* included 12 phages from Postic & Finland, 10 from Pavlatou & Kaklamani, and five phages which had at one time been used with the Pavlatou & Kaklamani set at the Central Public Health Laboratory at Colindale, London. The Zanen & van den Berge set used phages from Colindale, London, together with an equal number isolated by Zanen.

The number of alternate phage typing methods is therefore large. Unfortunately, none of them has been promulgated as a reference or international typing system as is the case with *Staphylococcus aureus*.

The only typing sets apparently in current use are those of Lindberg *et al.*, of Meitert & Meitert, and of Bergan (1972). The first two have been examined together with the sets of Sutter *et al.*, Zanen & van den Berge; and Pavlatou & Kaklamani (Bergan, 1972a,b,c,d,g). The Sutter *et al.* and the Lindberg *et al.* sets appear qualitatively to be the most useful ones with the latter being the most widely distributed of the two. Key characteristics of previous sets are shown in Table 1.

Interpretation

The interpretation of results has mainly followed the conventions used for staphylococcal phage typing (Blair & Williams, 1961) i.e. the phage susceptibility pattern has been recorded.

The Meitert & Meitert set is interpreted differently. There, each of the first 10 phages defines a distinct phage group. Each group is further subdivided

Table 1. Key characteristics of performance of phage typing sets as reported by first authors

	No. of phages	No. of bact. used for testing set	% Typable	% Lysed by phage	Reproducibility	No. of patterns
Potel (1957)	7	150	—	—	—	—
Yamada (1960)	6	34	—	—	—	6
Grogan & Artz (1961)	8	—	—	—	Same focus yields same strain in 72%. Cultures from more foci of same patient are same in 59%	—
Hoff & Drake (1961)	20	ca. 300	—	—	—	—
Postic & Finland (1961)	13	161	89	—	Satisfactory	—
Feary et al. (1963)	12	95	70	1–37	—	—
Grün et al. (1967)	10	130	97	19–87	—	—
Gould & McLeod (1960)	16	286	92	—	Little smaller than for phage typing of *S. aureus*	19
Meitert (1965)	13	652	93	—	—	64
Pavlatou & Kaklamani (1961)	12	174	79	—	10% change sensit. pattern after 6 months	12
Graber et al. (1962)	21	508	88	—	—	6
Lindberg et al. (1963)	15	1100	92	—	—	—
Zanen & van den Berge (1963)	13	—	—	—	—	—
Sutter et al. (1965)	18	317	86	0·3–65	Studied	87
Jedličková & Pillich (1968)	9	—	—	—	—	15
Herrmann (1970)	11	372	67	—	—	—
Bergan (1972d)	24	486	96	1–44	ca. 90% showed diff. in only one or less reaction upon retyping within a week	240

according to the susceptibility to the other phages. For instance, strains of lysogroup 1 are all sensitive to phage number 1 which consists of the subgroups 1a, 1b, 1c, etc., each with a different susceptibility pattern to the phages 2–10. Group 2 pseudomonas strains are resistant to phage 1 but sensitive to phage 2 and are subdivided according to their sensitivity to the phages 3–10. Group 3 strains are resistant to phages 1 and 2, but sensitive to phage 3 and so on. Three phages are used in addition for subdivision of pseudomonas strains not lysed by the first 10 phages. A similar group concept was used by Graber *et al.* (1962) and Pavlatou & Kaklamani (1961, 1962). However, the usefulness of this approach is debatable as it puts too much emphasis on the reaction of one single phage. In the Meitert & Meitert system, as much as 16% of the bacteria show a different lysotype after only two months storage.

New Typing Set

In an attempt to establish a phage typing system that was better than any of the previous ones, Bergan (1972c,d,g) recently compared 113 internationally available phages from previous sets. On the basis of numerical analyses of lytic activity on some 500 bacterial strains, a new phage typing set was developed (Bergan, 1972a,b). The bacteria employed for the comparison of phages were partly isolated at a local hospital and partly obtained from abroad. Eight of the 16 previous typing sets, including all the more elaborate ones, were covered by the examination, some indirectly by virtue of their inclusion in the sets of Lindberg *et al.*, and of Sutter *et al.* (Table 2).

Table 2. Key characteristics of 6 sets studied simultaneously (Bergan, 1972d). Performance on 486 pseudomonas strains

	% Typed	No. of patterns	Mean no. of reactions per plate
Pavlatou & Kaklamani (1961, 1962)	70	78	2·0
Lindberg *et al.* (1964)	86	224	3·9
Zanen & van den Berge (1963)	75	219	3·1
Meitert (1965)	74	158	4·0
Sutter *et al.* (1965)	86	278	3·9
Bergan (1972d)	96	240	2·6

The Pavlatou & Kaklamani set used lacked phage 11. The Sutter *et al.* set was modified by Sutter in relation to the set published, *vide* (Bergan, 1972d). The Lindberg *et al.* set comprised 2 more phages added by Lindberg after their first publication.

The new set consists of 19 phages with a lower percentage of lysis (lytic to a mean of 12·0 ± 8·6%), the primary set and an additional set of 5 phages lytic to more strains (mean 31·3 ± 11·0%), the auxiliary set. The pattern obtained by the auxiliary set is only considered for isolates resistant to the primary set. The primary set alone lyses 88% of the strains (Bergan, 1972d). The less discriminatory, more avid phages of the auxiliary set reduce the fraction of non-typable strains to 4%.

Some may prefer the method of considering the sensitivity pattern of all 24 phages. The lytic pattern codes, however, would thereby be much longer, since each of the 5 auxiliary phages lyses approximately one-third of the isolates. Consequently, the auxiliary phages would appear in a large number of phage pattern codes, thereby biasing similarly between isolates.

Comparison of Sets

The key characteristics for usefulness of a phage typing set are
(a) the percentage of typable strains,
(b) ability to split up a collection of bacterial strains,
(c) mean number of reactions per isolate, and
(d) the reproducibility of the typing results.

In Tables 1 and 2 these characteristics have been listed for various sets. It appears from (i) the results reported in the original report of each previous set and (ii) those obtained in the comparative study (Bergan 1972d,e) that the new typing set has favourable characteristics compared to the previous sets. The former had a higher number of typable strains, a high number of different reaction patterns combined with a more convenient, lower, number of reactions per plate. The reason why some of the other typing sets have longer pattern codes is that they consist of phages with more overlapping lytic activity. The figures shown in Table 3 also include plates without reactions, such that the number of reactions per plate was often much longer than that appearing in the table. The explanation for the improved balance of lytic activities in the new set is that numerical analysis preceded phage selection. This allowed better comparison and reduced to a minimum the simultaneous occurrence of lysis by more phages.

The new phage typing set has been compared with that of Lindberg *et al.* The former had several advantages rendering shorter pattern codes and variation in the patterns of related strains. The longer typing patterns of the Lindberg *et al.* set could fortuitously indicate a greater relationship even in strains which were different in pyocine type and serogroup. Kozaczek *et al.* (1973), who compared the Lindberg *et al.* set with the new typing set together with serogrouping and pyocine typing by Bergan's modification (1968b), reached the same conclusions. Further work at other centres is needed to evaluate and compare the new set with previous ones.

Method of bacteriophage typing

For phage typing, the method developed by the author may be used (Bergan, 1972c); the techniques for cultivation, controlling phage suspensions and scoring results resemble the procedures used internationally for *Staph. aureus* (Blair & Williams, 1961).

Bacteriophages

The designations of the phages included in the new set are 73, F7, M6, Me13, 113, F116, Px3, Clc, C4, C13, C21, H249, P10, VII, XVI, Z2, Z3, Z19, Z20—all in the primary set. The auxiliary set consists of the phages 21B, 68, Col 11, K9, C15. In recording results, these are indicated by simple numerals from 1–24 in the order listed, such that, for example, phage Z20 is denoted by 19.

Other sets have other designations. That of Lindberg *et al.* (1963a–c) employs the phages 2, 7, 16, 21, 24, 31, 44, 68, 73, 109, 119x, 352, 1214, F7, F8, F10, M4, M6, Col 11, Col 18, Col 21 (the last three phages being added by the Cross-Infection Reference Laboratory, Colindale, London). Sutter *et al.*'s (1965) set employs Clc, Clt, C3, C4, C7, C9, C13, C15, C16, C19, C21, C22, H95, H116, H249, P2, P6, P7, P8, P9, P10, P12.

Culture Medium

For propagation of phages and typing the following medium is used:

Tryptone Difco	10 g
Yeast Extract Difco	5 g
NaCl	5 g
CaCl	0·4 g
$MgSO_4.7H_2O$	0·2 g
Glucose	4 g
0·2 M tris	250 ml
0·2 M HCl	225 ml
Distilled water to	1000 ml

pH adjustment to 7·1, prior to autoclaving at 121 °C for 15 min. Typing plates contain 1·4% Agar Difco.

Propagation

Propagation is preferably done in larger, flat-bottom 2 litre Erlenmeyer flasks with 250 ml broth. The initial number of bacteria should be 10^7 cells per ml taken from an overnight broth culture of the propagation strain. Phage is added to a multiplicity of infection of one plaque forming unit (PFU) per 100 viable cells. After inoculation, the flasks are incubated in a gyratory shaker at 37 °C for 5 hr. Subsequently, the culture is centrifuged at 7000 r.p.m. (MSE High Speed Centrifuge) and filtered by Millipore membrane filter of 0·45 μm pores. The filtrates may be stored at +4 °C.

Typing Procedure

The strength of the phage suspension is determined by titration to determine the routine test dilution (RTD (Figure 1). The typing procedure otherwise followed the conventions used for staphylococcal phage typing (Blair & Williams, 1961). Typing of *P. aeruginosa*, however, is only performed at RTD notwithstanding the recommendation of Bernstein-Ziv *et al.* (1973) to use 100 × RTD.

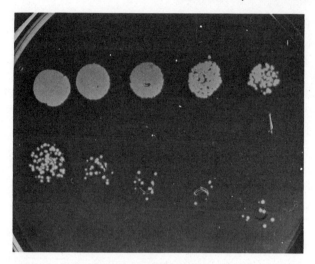

Figure 1. Example showing titration of a phage stock
suspension to determine the routine test dilution (RTD)

The plates are inoculated by flooding with evenly suspended cells from an
overnight blood agar culture (mixers or shakers such as Vortex or Whirlmixer
are recommended) to render an O.D. of 0·1–0·2 as measured on a Beckman
Colorimeter D.B. The recommendation to use agar cultures rather than broth
cultures follows the findings of Smith (1948) that agar cultures of staphylococci
render more reproducible results than broth cultures. Figure 2 shows a
phage typing plate with pseudomonas.

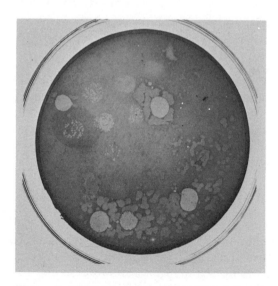

Figure 2. Phage typing results of a strain of
Pseudomonas aeruginosa

PYOCINE TYPING

Nomenclature

The bacteriocine of *P. aeruginosa*, pyocine, was first studied by Jacob (1954). Besides having priority, the term pyocine has gained universal acceptance. Tagg & Mushin (1971), however, pointed out that logically it should be renamed 'aeruginocine', since the species epithet is *aeruginosa* instead of *pyocyaneus* which has now been referred to the list of *nomina rejicienda*. Still, the term pyocine causes no confusion and is likely to remain the chosen term.

Physiological basis

Pyocine production may be governed by an episome linked to a tryptophane marker (Kageyama, 1970a) and may be transferred by transduction (Kageyama, 1970b). Physiochemical properties are reported elsewhere (Higerd *et al.*, 1967; Holloway & Krishnapillai, 1974).

Pyocines resembling phage tails have been studied in the electron microscope (Higerd *et al.*, 1967, 1969; Ito *et al.*, 1970) and pyocines of proteinous nature have been found. Heavy pyocines, R-types, have MW of 1×10^7 and lightweight pyocines, S-types, MW of 1×10^5 (Ito *et al.*, 1970). These occur together in the same bacterium, but the S-type has not been demonstrated by electron microscopy and the R- and S-type pyocine have not been shown together in the same phage particle. To what extent the kinetics of adsorption and kill of the lightweight pyocine is similar to that of the R-type has not been clarified. The R-type is not dialysable, but diffuses slowly in agar. R-type pyocines resembling phage tails have been sensitive to trypsin (Rampling, personal communication 1973), but trypsin-resistant S-types may exist (Govan, personal communication 1973).

Like bacteriophages, pyocines exert their activity only after adsorption to specific receptors on the cell surface of sensitive bacteria (Ito & Kageyama, 1970). Base-plate appendages and fibres that might play a role in the adsorption of pyocine have been described (Higerd, 1969). Pyocines cross-react immunologically with certain pseudomonas phages (Ito & Kageyama, 1970). Adsorption of pyocine to the bacteria occurs rapidly and is nearly completed within 5–15 min depending on the concentration of bacteria (Stewart & Young, 1971).

Various treatments of the bacterial surface reduce pyocine adsorption. This includes removal of cell lipids and EDTA treatment which causes release of lipopolysaccharide, the building material of the receptors (Stewart & Young, 1971). Various agents interfering with proteins and mucopeptides, such as trypsin, pronase, lysozyme and heat of 100 °C, have not affected adsorption. Calcium and magnesium are required for optimal receptor function. The receptors consist of lipopolysaccharide, which is capable of inactivating pyocine even in solution (Ikeda & Egami, 1969).

Pyocines have bactericidal action (Hamon, 1956; Holloway & Krishnapillai, 1974; Jacob, 1954). Cells are most sensitive in the logarithmic growth phase (Kaziro & Tanaka, 1965a). A reduction in metabolism occurs without any latent period, but it takes a while before complete elimination of respiration (Jacob, 1954) and synthesis of RNA, DNA and protein (Kaziro & Tanaka, 1965a). The protein synthesis is probably interfered with at the ribosomal level. R-type pyocines apparently remain outside the cells and do not attach to the ribosomes (Kaziro & Tanaka, 1965b). This resembles the action of colicine K or megacine C. Pyocines may also cause release of cytoplasmic material and with a large excess, they cause outright cell lysis. Unlike colicine E2 or megacine, the pyocines studied have not induced temperate phage of lysogenized strains or caused DNA degradation. It appears that R-type pyocines act more rapidly than bacteriophages (Jacob, 1954).

Higerd *et al.* (1967) have found that pyocine consists of a contractile sheath and an inner core reminiscent of T-even coliphage tails. The pyocine activity in a preparation was proportional to the number of contracted or relaxed forms.

On the basis of the morphological similarity between relaxed pyocines and phage tails (Higerd *et al.*, 1969) and the immunological cross-reactivity between phages and pyocines (Ito & Kageyama, 1970; Homma et al., 1967) the possibility of a relationship between pyocines and pseudomonas phage tails has been discussed.

Differentiation in S- and R-type pyocines has been interpreted to indicate the existence of two entirely different classes of pyocines. The possibility that the two forms may in some way be integrated has not previously been discussed. However, in the light of all available information it would seem entirely possible.

We know that morphologically the R-type consists of cylinders which contract upon contact with the cell surface and are orientated with a cylinder 'head' and a cylinder 'tail'. It is tempting to submit the hypothesis that the S-form may be contained within the R-form and is injected after contact with the cell surface.

This hypothesis is compatible with (i) the finding that both S- and R-forms are produced simultaneously as has been shown by separative gel filtration and ultracentrifugation. It would (ii) also explain why the R-form cylinders contract after contact with the bacterial cell surface, being similar to phage tail contraction and injection of phage nucleic acid. (iii) This would also explain the puzzle of why R-type pyocines may be *reversibly adsorbed* to the surface receptors of sensitive bacteria (Kageyama *et al.*, 1964) in spite of the fact that attempts to reverse the pyocine *action* have been unsuccessful (Kaziro & Tanaka, 1965a). When both the action and the *adsorption* are reversed, as occurs for colicine K, the agent is thought to act from without (Kaziro & Tanaka, 1965b). (iv) Hitherto, the transmitter substances of the pyocines have been unknown, but since the R-type pyocines remain outside the cell wall, an intracellular mediator substance has been suggested. The S-form being proteinous, it may itself act as an intracellular inhibitor blocking the ribosome RNA templates. A hypothetical amplification principle (Kaziro & Tanaka, 1965b) would thereby become redundant.

Paterson (1965) found that pyocines generally have wider host spectra (of activity) than bacteriophages, although pyocines with narrow spectra may also be found. There is no relationship between the activity of phages and pyocines produced by the same strain.

Pyocine Typing Systems

Pyocines from different producer strains act differently on a given set of indicator strains. This is the very basis of pyocine typing. A producer strain is resistant to its own pyocine.

Holloway (1960) was the first to suggest that this could be utilized for typing purposes; Papavassilou (1961) was the first to try pyocine typing. Darrell & Wahba (1964) (see also Wahba, 1965a,b) used 12 indicator strains and let the producer strain grow overnight at 37 °C. They noted that reactions were not always clear-cut; others have considered the reproducibility of this pyocine typing method quite unsatisfactory (Bergan, 1968b; Gillies & Govan, 1966).

Bergan (1968b) thought that the major problem was a concomitant production of pyocine inactivators and tried to improve the Darrell & Wahba procedure by excision of the agar with producer strain growth. Inhibition of indicator strains was then due to pyocines that had diffused into the agar. The results were better, but still not considered entirely satisfactory and the technique became more elaborate. This modification, though, has been used with success by Kozaczek *et al.* (1973). They selected other indicators than the Darrell & Wahba strains used originally in the Bergan modification.

Gillies & Govan (1966) attacked the problem of pyocine typing reproducibility with more success. They selected new indicator strains and redefined growth conditions. Their method has since been distributed to many centres (Bergan, 1973a; Booth, 1969; Csiszár & Lányi, 1970; Deighton *et al.*, 1971; Neussel, 1971; Rose *et al.* 1971; Ziv *et al.*, 1971) and used with excellent results. This method appears at present to be the most suitable alternative for pyocine typing.

Other pyocine typing approaches have been tried. Lewis (1967) examined the susceptibility of unknown strains to seven fixed pyocines. The producer strains were first grown on agar at 30 °C for 18 hr. Then the unknown strains were incorporated in a soft agar layer poured on top. Growth inhibition in the top layer appeared, corresponding to the position of active pyocines. Among 169 strains, 17 types were distinguished.

Another variant is to invert the agar after growth of the producer strain instead of killing the producer with chloroform (Kékessy & Piguet, 1970). The previous (sterile) bottom of the agar then becomes exposed and is used for the growth of the indicators.

An entirely different method is the employment of pyocine preparations (Osman, 1965): this uses liquid pyocine dropped on to the surface of an agar inoculated with the unknown strains. The result resembles phage typing with lack of growth corresponding to active pyocines. Jacob *et al.* (1973) found that the pyocine preparations must have fixed strength in this procedure to make reproducibility acceptable. A similar procedure has been described by Farmer & Herman (1969); Jones *et al.*, (1973). The results of Bobo *et al.* (1973), however, indicate that epidemiologically more stable results are obtained with the method of Gillies & Govan (1966).

The difficulty with such procedures is that phages are also present in some pyocine preparations and drawing the distinction between the action of phage and pyocine may be complicated. Pyocine preparations are generally not diluted as much as phages to reach RTD. These pyocin drop procedures appear to have less discrimination than a new technique worked out by Rampling (personal communication, 1973). This procedure examines the sensitivity to phage-free pyocine preparations of standardized strength. The pyocines have been prepared by treatment of broth cultures (grown for 16–18 hr at 32 °C) with mitomycin-C followed by chloroform to kill bacteria and u.v. radiation to inactivate phages. The preparations have been stored at 4 °C for at least 6 months. Cultures to be typed are overlayered in 5 ml 0·7% agar on nutrient agar plates and a set of 25 pyocines applied to it by a multi-inoculator contrivance.

The Rampling procedure has several advantages over other pyocine drop methods. One is that the pyocines are selected on the basis of numerical analysis of their activity. This is similar to the procedure used by Bergan (1972a,b,c,d) in the selection of phages for his typing set and vouches for a balance of activities of the components of the set. Because of the u.v. treatment, there is no confusion with phage activity. The standardization of the liquid pyocine preparations might be more accurate than the determination of phage RTD, since a turbidimetric calibration may be used (Young & Stewart, 1971).

The reproducibility of the Rampling procedure is possibly somewhat higher than that observed by Govan (1968), but this point still needs further evaluation by others. This procedure typed more strains than the Gillies & Govan typing method, the Habs serogrouping or the Lindberg *et al.* phage typing set as modified by the Cross-Infection Reference Laboratory at Colindale, London.

The new procedure has been applied to nosocomial outbreaks in a renal unit with good results. Modes of transmission and environment reservoirs were determined and the Rampling results were confirmed by phage typing and serogrouping. The number of different patterns was of the same order as observed with phage typing used simultaneously, and far better than with the Gillies & Govan pyocine typing procedure or the Habs serogrouping. The Rampling method typed 98%, whereas the Gillies & Govan procedure typed

97% of the same material, lysotyping 97% and serogrouping 89%. Another advantage of pyocine dropping methods is that the results are obtained one day earlier than with the indicator strain streaking techniques.

The main disadvantage of the Rampling method is the instability of the pyocines studied and the fact that their behaviour is somewhat inconsistent. However, after a number of improvements, this method has more recently been used for typing several hundreds of hospital strains of *P. aeruginosa* and has compared favourably with phage typing in terms of both discrimination between isolates and reproducibility of patterns (Rampling, personal communication, 1973).

The discrimination of the streaking procedures is fair. With his 12 indicators, Wahba (1965b) was able to subdivide 1849 strains from various sources into only 11 types, including one group for non-typable strains.

Four types contributed more than 70%. Others have obtained better differentiation (Caroli *et al.*, 1968), but on the whole the Gillies & Govan set has rendered only a few types (Bergan, 1973a; Gillies & Govan, 1966). Particularly frequent, both in human and animal strains, is the pyocine type 1, p1, which contributes about $\frac{1}{3}$of the strains (Bergan, 1973a; Gillies & Govan, 1966; Heckman *et al.*, 1972; Mushin & Ziv, 1973), The only way to circumvent this is by retyping with another set. With the Gillies & Govan set some 95–97% are typable (Bergan, 1973a; Gillies & Govan, 1966).

Due to the predominance of p1 strains, Govan & Gillies (1969) have subtyped them with a second set of 5 indicator strains. In this way 8 subtypes are obtained (Table 3) including one subtype without inhibition, i.e. in reality

Table 3. Subtypes of Gillies & Govan (1966) pyocine type 1

| Subtype | Inhibition of indicator strains | | | | |
	A	B	C	D	E
a	+	+	+	+	+
b	−	+	+	+	+
c	−	−	+	+	+
d	+	−	+	+	+
e	−	+	+	−	+
f	−	−	−	−	−
g	−	−	+	−	+
h	−	+	−	+	+

+ = Inhibition of indicator strain.
− = No influence on indicator strain.

non-typability by subgrouping. Zabransky & Day (1969), using the Wahba method, proposed a similar approach.

Another problem with these methods is non-typability (Table 4). In a

Table 4. Pyocine typable strains in various materials

Darrell & Wahba typing set		Gillies & Govan typing set	
Report	% Typable	Report	% Typable
Caroli *et al.* (1968)	38	Bodey (1970)	69
Matsumoto *et al.* (1968)	81	Booth (1969)	88
Sjöberg & Lindberg (1968)	88	Mushin & Ziv (1973b)	88
Wahba (1965a)	88	Gillies & Govan (1966)	88
Darrell & Wahba (1964)	92	Heckman *et al.* (1972)	89
Zabransky & Day (1969)	93	Ziv *et al.* (1971)	90
Kominos *et al.* (1972b)	ca.98	Csiszár & Lányi (1970)	91
		Govan & Gillies (1969)	92
		Tagg & Mushin (1971)	94
		Mushin & Ziv (1973a)	95
		Greible *et al.* (1970)	96
		Deighton *et al.* (1971)	97
		Bergan (1973a)	97
		Merrikin & Terry (1972)	98
		Mushin & Ziv (1973b)	98

number of strains, this may be solved by pyocine induction with mitomycin-C. Only after such induction, for instance, were Williams & Govan (1973) able to pyocine-type mucoid pseudomonas strains. Following such modifications of the method, results should be interpreted with caution since some strains may change from one pyocine type to another. An increment in the number of typable strains has also been achieved by adding locally isolated indicator strains to the standard set (Tagg & Mushin, 1971). In this way the most frequent pyocine types can be subdivided.

Method for Pyocine Typing

Indicator Strains

The pyocine typing method of Gillies & Govan (1966) employs 8 indicator strains designated by the numerals 1 to 8. In addition, p1 is subdivided by a subsequent typing with a set of 5 indicators, designated A to E.

Culture Medium

Tryptone Soya Agar (Oxoid) (TSA) with a supplement of 0·08% $CaCl_2$ and 5% whole, defibrinated horse blood is used for typing. The indicator strains are grown in broth (e.g. infusion broth) for 3–4 hr (gyratory shaker at 37 °C) and diluted 1:100 before streaking. Stationary broth cultures need 4–6 hr for development.

Typing Procedure

A *P. aeruginosa* isolate to be typed is streaked out as a 0·5 cm wide band across the diameter of a TSA plate. Subsequently, the plate is incubated at 32 °C for 14 hr. The temperature and time of pyocine production are critical (Bergan, 1973a, Govan, 1968). Wahba (1965a) demonstrated pyocine-inactivating agents after longer growth.

After incubation, the bacterial material is scraped off with a glass slide with cellophane self-adhesive tape attached to the edge to make it less acute.* After removal of most of the growth, the remaining bacteria are killed by 3–5 ml chloroform poured into the lid of the Petri dish after which the bottom is replaced (with the lid down) for 15 min. This is followed by exposure to air for 30 min to evacuate $CHCl_3$. Since the $CHCl_3$ dissolves plastic, glass dishes are mandatory.

Subsequently, indicator strains are streaked in parallel at a right-angle across the plate diameter where the producer strain was grown. For convenience, several loops may be fixed on a piece of India rubber 1 cm apart, thereby allowing all streaks to be made simultaneously (Brown, 1973). Five indicators are streaked on one side, the remaining 3 on the other side of the producer strain diameter. In the subtyping of p1, all 5 indicators are streaked clear across the producer strain line. The positions of the indicator streaks and the appearance of the results are illustrated in Figure 3.

Strict adherence to a time schedule is recommended for reproducible results.

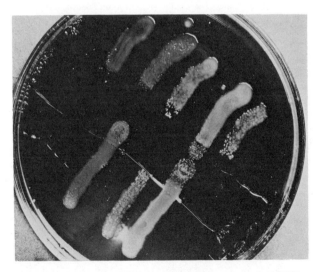

Figure 3. Pyocine typing results with the method of Gillies & Govan (1966)

* Experiments have been made with producer strain growth on cellulose acetate laminates placed on the agar surface. The bacterial culture may thereby be easily and fully removed, but inconsistent results have been obtained (Govan, 1968; MacPherson & Gillies, 1969).

The producer strain is removed in the morning and, after CHCl₃ treatment, the plates are put in the refrigerator until the indicators are streaked towards the end of the day. The indicator strains are allowed to grow for 14–18 hr.

The pyocines have diffused into the medium and inhibit the appropriately sensitive indicators. Different pyocine types are recognized according to which indicators are inhibited (Table 5); The subtype patterns of p1 are discernible from Table 3.

Table 5. Pyocine types encountered with the Gillies & Govan method

Pyocine type	Inhibition of indicator strains							
	1	2	3	4	5	6	7	8
1	+	+	+	+	+	−	+	+
2	−	+	−	−	−	−	−	−
3	+	+	+	−	+	−	+	−
4	+	+	+	+	+	−	−	+
5	−	−	−	−	+	−	−	−
6	+	+	+	+	+	−	+	−
7	+	+	+	−	−	−	+	+
8	−	+	+	+	−	−	+	−
9	−	−	−	−	+	−	+	−
10	+	+	+	+	+	+	+	+
11	+	+	+	−	−	−	+	−
12	+	+	−	+	+	−	−	+
13	−	−	−	+	−	−	−	+
14	−	−	+	−	+	−	+	−
15	−	+	−	−	+	−	+	−
16	+	−	+	+	−	−	+	+
17	−	−	+	−	−	−	+	−
18	+	−	+	+	+	−	+	+
19	−	−	+	+	−	−	+	−
20	−	−	−	−	+	+	−	−
21	−	+	−	+	+	−	−	−
22	+	+	+	−	+	+	+	−
23	+	−	−	−	+	−	+	−
24	−	−	+	+	+	−	+	+
25	+	−	+	−	−	−	+	−
26	+	−	−	−	−	−	+	−
27	+	−	+	−	+	−	+	−
28	−	−	−	+	−	−	+	−
29	−	+	−	−	+	−	−	−
30	−	+	+	−	−	−	−	−
31	−	−	−	−	−	−	+	−
32	−	−	−	+	+	−	−	+
33	+	+	+	+	+	+	+	−
34	−	−	−	−	−	−	−	+
35	+	+	−	−	+	−	+	−
36	−	+	−	+	−	−	−	+
37	−	+	+	+	+	−	+	−
38	−	+	+	−	−	−	+	−

Table 5—*cont.*

Pyocine type	Inhibition of indicator strains							
	1	2	3	4	5	6	7	8
39	−	+	+	+	−	−	+	+
40	+	+	−	−	+	−	−	−
41	−	+	+	−	+	−	+	−
42	−	−	+	−	−	−	+	+
43	−	+	+	+	+	−	+	+
44	+	+	+	−	+	−	−	−
45	+	+	+	−	+	−	+	+
46	+	+	+	+	−	−	+	−
47	−	−	+	−	−	+	+	−
48	+	+	−	−	+	+	+	−
49	−	−	+	−	+	−	−	−
50	−	−	+	−	−	−	−	−
51	+	+	+	+	−	−	−	+

+ = Inhibition of indicator strain.
− = No influence on indicator strain.

Instead of classifying each pyocine inhibition pattern as a distinct type, it may be useful to regard pattern codes as in phage typing. It has also been suggested that sets of three reactions be given individual scores. This has been termed mnemonic reporting and is an alternative (Farmer, 1970), although seemingly more complicated.

SEROLOGICAL TYPING

Serological Approaches

Serological examinations of *P. aeruginosa* have been carried out since the beginning of this century. Plehn & Trommsdorff (1916) separated 24 isolates into 5 serogroups. The number of distinct groups seems high considering the few strains examined. Other pioneers were Aoki (1926) and Kanzaki (1934). There is no agglutinogen common to all *P. aeruginosa* strains, but there are many cross-reactions among minor antigens. The evolution of *P. aeruginosa* serology has also been discussed by Caselitz (1966), Köhler (1957) and by Govan (1968).

Instead of starting from previous results, the tendency has often been to build up independent serogrouping systems from the bottom. This has hampered comparison of results but the situation might now change. Several independent serogrouping systems have been established (Christie, 1948; van den Ende, 1952; Fisher *et al.*, 1969; Habs, 1957; Homma *et al.*, 1971; Lányi, 1966/1967, 1970; Sandvik, 1960a,b; Verder & Evans, 1961) (see Table 6). The most widely distributed O-grouping system is the Habs schema. This has been compared to other schemas (Bergan 1973a; Liu, personal communication, 1973; Matsumoto *et al.*, 1968; Muraschi *et al.*, 1966).

Table 6. Key characteristics of serogrouping schemas for *Pseudomonas aeruginosa*

		Typing results with individual sets		
Serogrouping system	No. of O-antigens	Publication	% Typed	Self-agglu-tinable
Habs (1957)	12	Kleinmaier & Quincke (1959)	84	5
		Wokatsch (1964)	62	0
		Borst & deJong (1970)	86	?
		Wahba[a] (1965b)	99·7	0
		Mikkelsen (1970)	87	12
		Bergan (1973a)	86	7
International schema	16			
Fisher *et al.* (1969)	7	Fisher *et al.* (1969)	94	?
		Adler & Finland (1971)	88	0
		Moody *et al.* (1972)	99	0
Chia-Ying (1963)	5	Chia-Ying (1963)	96	?
Homma (Pers comm., 1973)	16	Maruyama *et al.* (1971)	73	0
		Yoshioka *et al.* (1970)	81	0
Lányi (1966/67)	27 (supple-mented by 7 H-antigens, 1970)	Lányi (1966/67)	88[b]	1
Meitert (1965)	10	Meitert & Meitert (1966)	85	?
Sandvik (1960a and personal comm., 1971)	8	Sandvik (1960a,b)	98	2
Verder & Evans (1961)	13 (supple-mented by 10 H-antigens)	Verder & Evans (1961)	100	0
Wokatsch[c] (1964)	25	Wokatsch (1964)	100	0

[a] With 2 additional O-antigens such that a total of 14 O-groups was included.
[b] Twentysix were self-agglutinable and 236 poly-agglutinable (Lányi, personal communication 1973).
[c] Used Habs's 12 serogroups extended with 13 O-sera to type animal strains. The latter 13 sera were probably not factor sera since many bacteria reacted with 2–4 of them.

Under the auspices of the Subcommittee of *Pseudomonadaceae* and Related Organisms of the International Committee on Systematic Bacteriology of the International Association of Microbiological Societies, Professor P. V. Liu,

Louisville Ky., WA., is heading an International Cooperative Study Group (ICSG) of *P. aeruginosa* which is attempting to establish an International Antigenic Typing Schema (IATS).

This has been based on the first 12 O-groups of the Habs schema. Working in Habs's laboratory, Kleinmaier & Quincke (1959) identified 3 additional O-groups, but these have never been studied by other workers. Group O:13 in the future international schema is identical to the Sandvik O:II and corresponds to what has been designated O:13 by Wahba (1965a,b), Bergan, (1973a) and Mikkelsen (1970). The group O:14 of the IATS corresponds to the Verder & Evans O:V and Meitert O:10. This is different from the O:14 group used by Wahba (1965b) and Bergan (1970a). The latter O:14 cross-reacts with Habs O:6, but also has distinct antigenic determinants not found on the O:6 type strain. Mikkelsen (1970) used a different serogroup O:14. The O:15 in the IATS corresponds to Lányi's O:12 and Homma's O:11. The O:16 equals Homma's O:13.

Lipopolysaccharides are responsible for O-group specificity (Ádám *et al.*, 1971; Boivin, 1937). In pseudomonas, the O-antigen may be separated from the endotoxin which is of proteinous nature (Homma, 1968).

The major and minor antigenic determinants of the corresponding type-strains of different serogrouping schemas are not fully identical. Differences in cross-reactions of the same serogrouping schema (Habs' method) have been noted from one investigator to another (Bergan, 1973a). Consequently, a balance table (Table 7) of comparable groups in different schemas based on the results of various workers (Bergan, 1973a; Liu, personal communication, 1973; Homma, personal communication, 1972; Matsumoto & Tazaki, 1969; Muraschi *et al.*, 1966a,b) only gives an indication of correspondence in major group antigens.

Typing by thermolabile antigens, (Kleinmaier *et al.*, 1958; Lányi, 1970; Verder & Evans, 1961), has not gained wide recognition. The thermolabile antigens are considered by Lányi (1970) to be flagellar antigens, analogous to the H-antigens of *Salmonella*. Pseudomonas has only one polar flagellum; some consider that, in this species, the heat labile determinants may be surface antigens not restricted to the flagellum (Liu, personal communication, 1973). Antibody against purified flagellar preparations would resolve this, but such a study has not yet been carried out. Non-motile strains may have a thermolabile antigen (Lányi, 1970; Liu, personal communication, 1973). There are two distinct thermolabile antigens, each subdivided into minor components leading to a total of 8 determinants (Lányi, 1970). The thermolabile antigens are valuable supplements to O-grouping and should be determined more often. By combining the two, Lányi distinguished 58 types; Verder & Evans (1961) similarly found 29 serotypes.

Other serological methods have also been investigated. Fluorescent antibody technique has distinguished the Habs's agglutinogens (Nishimura *et al.*, 1973). Köhler (1957) made extensive studies with precipitation of HCl and formamide extracts in capillary tubes and found clear-cut results. Formamide

Table 7. Correspondence of major O-group antigens within different serogrouping systems

Inter-national schema	Habs	Sandvik	Bergan[a] Mikkelsen[a] Veron[a] Wahba	Lányi Strain[b]	Lányi Group	Meitert	Homma	Verder & Evans	Fisher et al.
1	1	VII	1	14	6	9	10	IV	4
2	2	—	2	4, 6	3	2	7	I(X)	3
3	3	III	3	1	1	5	1	VI	—
4	4	IV	4	21	11	—	6	—	7
5	5	—	5	3, 5, 7	3	6	2	X(I)	1
6	6	I	6	8, 9, 10	4	1 or 4	8	II	—
7	7	—	7	(11)	(5)	—	—	—	6
8	8	VIII	8	13, 15	5	3	3	VIII	—
9	9	V	9	19, 20	10	—	4	IX	5
10	10	—	10	2	2	8	9	—	2
11	11	VI	11	15, 16	7	7	5	III	—
12	12	—	12	23	13	—	14	VII	—
13	—	II	13	—	—	—	12	—	—
14	—	—	—	—	—	10	—	V	—
15	—	—	—	22	12	—	11	—	—
16	—	—	—	—	—	—	13	—	—

[a] Bergan and Wahba had an O:14 group which cross-reacted with O:6. This was different from the O:6 used by Mikkelsen. None of these O:14 are identical to the O:14 of the International Antigenetic Typing Schema (IATS).

[b] Lányi type strains 170001–170009 are indicated by numbers 1–9; the strains 170010–170023 are indicated by the numbers 10–23. The strains 170017 and 170018, representing Lányi's groups, O:8 and O:9 are serolabile.

The O:2–O:5–O:16 complex of the IATS has cross-reactions of major and minor antigens; the antigens found in these strains may be differently represented by individual isolates. This commonly encountered entity (15% of strains, Bergan, 1973a) may therefore be considered a complex. Véron (1961) has subdivided the O:2–O:5 complex of Habs in subgroups O:2ab and O:5cd. As a consequence of these varying cross-reactions, the balance table between individual groups of the different serogrouping schemas is to be interpreted as reactions of major antigens only. Further strains within this complex will be agglutinated by one or more factor sera produced against either strain and adsorbed by the other two determinant carriers of the complex. Accordingly, Lányi (personal communication, 1973) considers the corresponding group specificity in his system (Lányi O:3) to be represented by his strains 170003, 170004, 170005, 170006 and 170007. The following antigenic determinants are recognized within the complex (3abcdf):

170003   ab
170004   c
170005   ad
170006   adc
170007   df

The Lányi O:3 complex was represented by 26·0% (Lányi, 1966/67). To the same complex belong the Verder–Evans O:I and O:X; Homma O:7, O:4 (the O:4-relationship found by Lányi, personal communication, 1973), O:2, and O:13; Fisher *et al.* O:3 and O:7; and Meitert O:2 and O:6. In the Sandvik schema, which was based on animal strains, this complex was not included.

extracts rendered a better subdivision than cell agglutination. This was debated by Kleinmaier & Müller (1958).

The group specific substances of Köhler were carbohydrates. Nucleoproteins participated in cross-reactions between groups. These were shared by most strains of *P. aeruginosa* and were found in *P. fluorescens*. Kleinmaier & Müller found that the precipitation reactions were related to the O-groups of Habs, a finding which was also made by van den Ende (1952).

Gel precipitation by the Ouchterlony technique with antigens prepared by sonication of live cells has also demonstrated cross-reactions between O-groups of Habs without cross-agglutination (Bergan, unpublished results). The more complex antigenic structure suggested by these findings could be ascribed to the obviously more antigenically complex nature of whole-cell preparations. Kleinmaier & Müller (1958), with boiled extracts and gel precipitation, concluded likewise that each O-group antigen was a composite of several antigenic components. Similarly, van Eeden (1967), using trichloroacetic acid extracts, distinguished at least 12 antigens among 5 O-groups.

Frequency of Serogroups

The frequencies of the serogroups are very different. The Habs O:6 usually contributes some 10–20%. Among strains from cattle O:6 was found in 37%. Next in frequency are the cross-reacting O:2 and O:5 which together contribute 10–20% among human strains, but are infrequent among animal strains (Bergan, 1972f). Group O:3 is also frequent and O:6 also dominates among mucoid strains (Diaz *et al.*, 1970).

Self-agglutination is a problem with pseudomonas (Table 7) (Bergan, 1972f; Homma *et al.*,.1951; Lányi, 1966/67; Meitert, 1964; Mikkelsen, 1968; Sandvik, 1960a,b).

Homma's schema with 12 O-groups (Homma *et al.*, 1971) yielded 95% typable strains. Two of the serogroups contributed 52% of the typable strains. The Meitert & Meitert set typed 91% human and 98% animal strains (Meitert & Meitert, 1973). The Habs schema has typed 86% Norwegian human strains, 71% among Polish hospital strains and as much as 97% among animal strains (Bergan, 1972g, 1973a). Achromogenic and melaninogenic *P. aeruginosa* strains appear to be less typable (Yabuuchi *et al.*, 1971).

Conversion of Serogroups by Lysogenization

Serogroup specificity is generally thought to be a stable character. However, the serogroups of pseudomonas have changed upon subcultivation and storage of cultures at room temperature (Homma *et al.*, 1971). Seroconversion has been induced *in vitro* by lysogenization (Bergan & Midtvedt, 1975; Holloway & Cooper, 1962; Liu, 1969). Phage-induced seroconversion has also been noted *in vivo* in rats monocontaminated with one strain of pseudomonas which had first been subcultivated repeatedly to ensure purity before introduction in the gnotobiotic system (Bergan & Midtvedt, 1975). Clinically, spontaneous changes of serogroups have been reported, but are rare (Liu, 1969); differentiation between seroconversion, i.e. change of serogroup specificity caused by lysogenization of a persisting bacterial clone (Liu, 1969; Bergan & Midtvedt, 1975), and bacterial superinfection may be difficult in the clinical situation.

O-antigen specificity is determined at least in part by a gene (or genes) located near the *leu* locus on the linkage map of Holloway *et al.* (1971) (Matsumoto, personal communication 1973).

International Antigenic Typing Schema (IATS)

The IATS at present consists of 16 serogroups, part of which cross-react (Table 8). Cross-reacting groups should perhaps have subgroup status with a common numerical designation as in the system of Lányi. For instance, IATS groups O:2, O:5 and O:16 correspond to Lányi's 3abcdf complex. The Lányi procedure resembles the system conveniently used in almost all genera of the *Enterobacteriaceae* and allows a finer separation of minor antigenic determinants within the framework of each group. The terminology of the IATS is currently being discussed by the ICSG.

Table 8. Cross-reactions between O-groups of *Pseudomonas aeruginosa* in the international schema

Antiserum	Antigen 1	2	3	4	5	6	7	8	9	10	11	12	13	14	15	16
1	·															
2		·			×											×
3			·													
4				·												
5		×			·											×
6						·										
7							·	×								
8							×	·								
9									·	×						
10									×	·						
11											·					
12												·				
13													·	×		
14													×	·		
15															·	
16		×			×											·

· = Homologous reaction.
× = Cross-reaction.

Method of Serogrouping

Immunization

The immunization must yield specific sera with high titres and limited cross-reactions. Based on Mikkelsen's (1968, 1970) systematic comparisons of different immunization procedures, the following procedure is recommended.

(i) Antigen is prepared from an aerated culture of the reference strain (infusion broth, 37 °C, 18 hr) followed by boiling for $2\frac{1}{2}$ hrs and two washings with physiological saline. A suspension of density 5×10^{10} cells per ml is suitable for immunization.

(ii) Injections are made intravenously with increasing volumes of 0·25–0·5–1·0–1·5 ml every 4 days. Titre controls should be made on the second day after the third (or subsequent) injection and bleeding made when a titre of at least 1/800 against the homologous strain has been reached. Mikkelsen (1970) recommended pooling of sera from 2–7 rabbits immunized with the same antigen.

Commercial distribution of the IATS type sera is planned in cooperation with the Difco Laboratories, but they are not yet generally available.

Agglutination

Serogrouping may be done by tube or slide agglutination with standard techniques (Bergan, 1973a; Habs, 1957; Kleinmaier, 1957; Lányi, 1967). Higher titres are generally obtained with live antigens than with antigens boiled for $2\frac{1}{2}$ hr. The slide procedure has given just as reliable and specific results as tube procedures (Kleinmaier, 1957; Lányi, 1966/67).

Grouping is first done with three pools of partly cross-reacting unabsorbed sera followed by the factor sera for each component of the reacting pool. The Habs schema with the IATS extension is the typing schema of choice. The following composition of pools has been found suitable:

           Pool I: 1, 3, 9, 10, 11, 15
           Pool II: 6, 7, 8, 13, 14
           Pool III: 2, 4, 5, 12, 16

To obtain factor sera, mutual absorption with standard technique needs to be carried out with the following groups: 2,5 and 16; 7 and 8; 9 and 10; 13 and 14 (Table 8). For typing purposes, working concentrations should be 5 times more concentrated than the homologous titres and should render clear-cut reactions within 1 min.

REPRODUCIBILITY OF TYPING METHODS

Phage Typing

Proper evaluation of the various typing procedures requires assessment of reproducibility and as yet only limited studies have been carried out.

The new phage typing set has been carefully evaluated (Bergan, 1972a). As much as 11% of individual isolates upon retyping showed a gain or loss of more than one major reaction (+ or ++ reaction strength at RTD). With these criteria, 4% received different patterns by two independent observers. When re-examined, the same plates differed by 2% for one observer and by 4% for another, the figures indicating the degree of individual inconsistency.

An idea of the reproducibility of the phage typing results is also obtainable from strains isolated from the same site of one patient throughout the period of hospitalization. With a mean observation period of 49 days (ranging from 1 to 247 days) 1/3 of the isolates from one single source were serologically identical. Among such isolates, 38% varied in more than one reaction and 19% in only one phage reaction.

In these evaluations, both + and ++ reactions were combined. In considering ++ reactions only, the reproducibility of results would appear more favourable. However, the difference between the two reaction scores in pseudomonas seems too feeble to justify the distinction used e.g. for staphylococci. Nevertheless, our results with pseudomonas would appear to indicate a lower reproducibility than is desirable for all the important phage typing sets.

Grogan & Artz (1961) made detailed evaluations of serial isolates from the same sources and obtained identical phage patterns in 72%. Only 59% were identical among strains from different sites of the same individuals.

Pavlatou & Kaklamani (1962) subjected the reproducibility of their typing set to quite extensive studies. They confirmed the Grogan & Artz findings that cultures considered pure often consisted of several strains. When kept at 4 °C for 6 months, 10% changed lysotype. Changes in phage patterns were also observed after passage through rabbits.

Sutter *et al.* (1965) found a 2% variation in duplicate cultures tested on the same day. When typed after storage in 0·1% nutrient agar for 1–3 months, 6% showed a loss or gain of one strong reaction. Variation in minor reactions was observed in 26–42%. On 2–10 subcultures, a loss or gain of one strong reaction was observed in 13%, and more than one reaction in 14%. In 2–22 sequential cultures from the same sites, 17% showed a variation of 1 strong reaction and 28% more variation. The difference was less when several sites of the same patient were examined simultaneously: then 4% varied in one major reaction, 13% in more. One-fifth of the strains showed pattern variation in less than one strong reaction. If the variation margin used in staphylococcal phage typing were adopted (permitting a variation of one strong reaction), there are indications that more than one lysotype may exist simultaneously in the same patient.

Details of the performance of pilot sets like those of Hoff & Drake (1961) and Postic & Finland (1961) are not available, but the impressions of the two groups were described as 'stable' and 'satisfactory'. Gould & McLeod (1960) described reproducibility in general terms as being a little smaller than in staphylococcal typing.

Applied on actual outbreaks, Kozaczek *et al.* (1973) showed that the reproducibility of the new phage typing set of Bergan (1972d) was satisfactory and better than a modification of the set of Lindberg *et al.* Bennet & Grogan (1962) and Grogan (1966) showed that cultures from several sites of the same patient exhibited the same phage types.

The results with the set of Lindberg *et al.* have varied considerably on collections of strains from different sources. Piguet & Kékessy (1972), for instance, with the phage Col 21, noted lysis with ca. 60% of the isolates from Geneva, whereas the same modified strain in London lysed some 5%, the same order as seen in Norway (Bergan, 1972c). Beumer *et al.* (1972), with the phage typing set of Lindberg *et al.*, noted variation in 23% upon retyping, in more than one reaction of 3%. Lyophilization between the first and second typing increased the figures, 38% of the strains differing in at least one reaction, 15% in more than one reaction. With the examination of more colonies from the same culture, a difference of more than one strong reaction occurred in 45% and of one reaction in 24%. Rabin *et al.* (1961) reported identical phage patterns in repeated blood cultures from all but one of nine patients with severe burns.

The variation of phage typing being large for pseudomonas, it is important that variation is also sizable for phage typing of other species. For instance, the international phage typing set for *S. aureus* rendered identical lysotype patterns in only 46% of simultaneous duplicate typings from the same broth and in a mere 21% when some days elapsed before retyping (Williams & Rippon, 1952). The variation may be due to (i) technical variation, (ii) changes arising during storage of cultures or (iii) the simultaneous existence within the same culture of more than one strain. Bergan & Midtvedt (1975) have noted that phage mediated conversion may occur *in vivo*; consequently, the impact of (ii) should not be underestimated.

Pyocine Typing

Much effort has gone into the elucidation of the stability of pyocine types. Retyping the same strains with the Gillies & Govan method (Deighton *et al.*, 1971; Gillies & Govan, 1966; Govan, 1968) usually leads to the same types. When stored at room temperature for periods from 3 months to 4 years, 6% show differences in pyocine types (Govan & Gillies, 1969; Merrikin & Terry, 1972).

Variation having been reduced by the improved conditions of Gillies & Govan (1966), one source of error in pyocine typing is variation in density of pyocine indicator suspensions (Merrikin & Terry, 1972). Bergan (1968b) improved the Wahba technique by introducing a fixed density of the indicator strain suspension rendering densely situated, but discrete colonies. This approach was considered superior to other methods by Kozaczek *et al.* (1973).

More variation has been noted for the Darrell & Wahba procedure (Naito *et al.*, 1972, 1973). In one instance, 19% of the strains showed varying pyocine sensitivity (Merrikin & Terry, 1972). Cultures have been described as having 'fluctuation of pyocine pattern' (Mushin & Ziv, 1973a,b). Serial subcultivation of strains has shown a type variation of 2·2% (Zabransky & Day, 1967).

When several colonies from the same plates have been tested, more than one type has been noted in 12–17% (Deighton *et al.*, 1971; Mushin & Ziv, 1973a,b). In serial cultures from the same foci, 15–19% variation has occurred (Deighton *et al.*, 1971; Merrikin & Terry, 1972). When different foci of the same patients are examined 25% differences occur.

The number of pyocine types in the same patient increases proportionally to the length of hospitalization. The variation in hospitalized patients is approximately twice that in domiciliary practice (Govan, 1968; Govan & Gillies, 1969). These phenomena indicate the existence of mixed infections rather than an instability of the method as such. If more indicator strains were employed, the variability of pyocine typing would conceivably increase.

When pyocine types are more reproducible than phage type patterns, this factor is partly associated with the existence of fewer pyocine types. However, better type reproducibility would also be desirable for pyocine typing.

Serogrouping

The variability for serogrouping is also higher than is desirable. Eleven strains of different serotypes, on multiple subcultures, in four instances produced different serogroups (Homma, 1971; Homma *et al.*, 1971). Variations have also been noted among different colonies of the same culture. Kawaharajo (1973), after subcultivation and storage at room temperature for 85 days, demonstrated that only 96% of his strains maintained their serogroup.

Conversely, Kleinmaier (1957) has not noted any serogroup changes after storage for periods of 3 months. In the experience of the author, (Bergan, 1973c), the serogroup is a stable character. Seropyocine types in urinary tract infection also tend to be stable (Matsumoto *et al.*, 1968).

Shionoya & Homma (1968) suggest that serovariation may be at least partly due to colony dissociation, an experience paralleled by phage typing (Zierdt & Smith, 1964). Another explanation may be lysogenic specificity of the bacterium (Liu, 1969; Bergan & Midtvedt, 1975).

INTERRELATIONSHIP BETWEEN TYPING METHODS

The interrelationships between different classes of typing methods have been studied. Gould & McLeod (1960) and Gould (1963) combined serogrouping and lysotyping on a small number of nosocomially related strains. Three phage sensitivity patterns alone comprised 85% of the 286 isolates examined. This also explains why only a few serogroups were identified and a relationship between serological and phage typing was suggested. The conclusion of Meitert & Meitert (1966) on 364 isolates was quite different. Each lysotype was divisible into more serogroups and lysotyping subdivided each serogroup, rendering a differentiation adequate for a detailed assessment of a nosocomial situation.

Recently, the possibility of a correlation between serogrouping and pyocine typing has been studied (Bergan, 1973a). Comparatively few strains were epidemiologically related but, nonetheless, a tendency for a relationship between a few pyocine types and serogroups was suggested. Thus, whereas pyocine type 1 (p1) occurred in $\frac{1}{5}$ of the total material, $\frac{4}{5}$ of the strains of the cross-reacting serogroups O:2 and O:5, and group O:6 were all of p1; 14% of the total material was p5, but p5 contributed 54% of the group O:3 strains. Whereas the group O:6 contributed 18% of the total, among the p3 strains 57% were O:6. Similarly, 18% of the total were O:3, but among the p5 strains as much as 72% were O:3. Wahba (1965a,b) who combined the Darrel & Wahba pyocine typing system with the Habs serogrouping schema, and Csiszár & Lányi (1970) with the Gillies & Govan pyocine system and Lányi serogrouping schema, all concluded that some relationship exists between pyocine type and serogroup.

It is interesting to note in this connection that Homma & Suzuki (1961) found pyocine activity to be associated with the protein component of the cell wall lipopolysaccharide–protein complex.

It may seem surprising that serogroup and phage susceptibility do not show more overlapping since both are determined by surface structures. The possibility of a relationship between lysotype and serogroup was an axiom in *S. aureus* until Oeding & Williams (1958) found no absolute interdependence between the two. Also in *P. aeruginosa*, phages do not appear to have a preference for certain serogroups (Bergan, 1973b; Meitert & Meitert, 1966; Edmonds *et al.*, 1972b). Lantos *et al.* (1969) on pseudomonas isolates from a water supply found many lysotypes among each serogroup according to the serogroup schema of Lányi. In one instance the pseudomonas isolates from a particular water supply were all of the same serogroup and phage type indicating that water pollution originated from one single source. Such a tendency (Bergan, 1973b) was only disclosed for a few phages, and the tendency was so feeble that generally no relationship exists between lysosensitivity and serogroup. Jedličková & Pillich (1968) thought that there might be a slight tendency towards a relationship between serogroups and lysosensitivity, but the results show that serogroups are efficiently subdivided by phages and that individual phages lyse strains of several serogroups. Yamada (1960) with 6 phages and 6 O-sera typed a very limited material of only 34 strains and concluded that the two methods rendered almost the same subdivision.

Similarly, pyocine (indicator strain streaking technique) and phage typing are not correlated (Bergan, 1973b; Sjöberg & Lindberg, 1967, 1968; Farmer & Herman, 1969). Since pyocine typing examines the ability to *produce* a substance and phage typing the *sensitivity* to an agent produced elsewhere, this is not surprising. There is a definite relationship, however, between the pyocines and phages, i.e. between the agents (Homma & Shionoya, 1967; Ito & Kageyama, 1970). Antisera against bacteriophages also inhibit the activity of pyocines and antipyocine sera neutralize phage activity. Such results would, of course, be obtained if the immunizing antigens contained both pyocines and phages. Purifications were carried out by various procedures and, as evidenced by electron microscopy, the antigen preparations were pure with either phages or pyocines. Still, it is difficult to exclude completely the possibility that there could have been impurities, in concentrations below the sensitivity level of the control methods. The relationship also concerns the function of the two agents. Sensitivity to certain phages was accompanied by sensitivity to given pyocines (Ito & Kageyama, 1970). Indeed, Ito & Kageyama concluded that phage and pyocine receptors were identical.

BIOLOGICAL PROPERTIES OF EPIDEMIOLOGICAL TYPES

One may ask whether epidemiological typing methods may have other functions than to aid in the elucidation of epidemiological problems. Are certain types for instance more pathogenic or resistant to antibiotics; is there any preference for particular sites or types of infection?

On the whole, it appears that no biological properties are concordant with given serogroups, phage patterns or pyocine types. The deviations from overall frequency data found in some instances are very difficult to interpret with confidence.

Neussel (1971) found that p1 in some patients with urinary tract infections contributed only 18% of the strains as contrasted with 32–34% reported elsewhere for p1 (Bergan, 1973b; Gillies & Govan, 1966). It was suggested that p1 strains have a 'preference' for the urinary tract. However, the reason for the lower frequency in Neussel's study is probably associated with a larger number of non-typable strains and rare types in that study. The frequency of p1 strains relative to the other pyocine types is not markedly different from that in other materials.

Nord *et al.* (1972) reported that a single serogroup, Habs O:1, and phage type, 21, 44, 1214, 109, F8, dominated in oral infections associated with poor oral hygiene. Fifteen patients out of 29 had O:1, which was a higher percentage of O:1 than usual. For comparison, Bergan (1972g) reported an overall frequency for O:1 of 32%. The number of patients with oral infections was small, such that the rate differences may be coincidental. On this basis, no fundamental biological properties can be pin-pointed for given pseudomonas types. The possibility of nosocomial reasons for a preponderance of certain types could be discussed, although Nord *et al.* considered this possible only for two of the 29 strains.

A nosocomial association was the obvious explanation in a study on sputum made by Sutter *et al.* (1966). They found one single phage type in 13 out of 19 patients who had required endotracheal suctioning. The same type was recovered in a lubricating solution for the suction catheters. This model clearly demonstrated nosocomial reasons for a predominance of a certain epidemiological type among strains from a single kind of infection.

Moody *et al.* (1972) studied cancer patients and concluded that particular foci have predominance of certain serogroups. The Fisher *et al.* serogroups O:1

and O:2 were retrieved from blood cultures more often than from other sources. Group O:4 and O:5 occurred more often in wounds. It was concluded that a particular serogroup was more 'capable of establishing persisting colonization' than others.

The group frequencies were evaluated statistically. It is, however, doubtful whether evaluation of a small portion of the data in a large table can proceed by standard statistical procedures, since they would be constrained by all the other data. It is obvious that e.g. an epidemic of O:7-wound infections will make O:7 more frequent in wounds than in urines and thus influence the apparent frequency of any other group. A predilection of a certain epidemiological type among patients with a similar clinical picture from the same environment may have a nosocomial explanation. Although differences in the relative frequencies of different types may be obvious, these *per se* are not indicative of fundamental biological differences between certain types. In the Moody *et al.* (1972) study, the types found in wounds were also encountered in the hospital environment, although the primary event is open to speculation. No data are available to suggest whether most of the septicaemia patients, for instance, come from the same hospital environment which had a distinct nosocomial predominance of the O:1 or O:2 strains from blood. At present it is best to regard the question of biological differences between epidemiological types with an open mind.

Edmonds *et al.* (1972a) found no difference between serogroup, pyocine type, or phage type for burn wound septicaemia compared to non-fatal infections from the same environment. Bodey (1970), in the same patients, recovered identical pyocine types at the site of infection and other parts of the body. Bergan (1967, 1973c, unpublished results) has observed the same phage and serological types in various clinical manifestations within the same departments. The types have varied from one ward to another.

Southern *et al.* (1970) differentiated *P. aeruginosa* according to rapidity of disappearance from mouse lungs, but noted no relationship to serogroup, pyocine type or bacteriophage type. Likewise, Meitert & Meitert (1971) found no association between virulence and lysotype or serogroup. Kobayashi (1971a,b) found no particular serogroup among virulent strains, but higher virulence was noted for non-typable isolates. Wretlind *et al.* (1973) could not detect any correlation between serogroups or phage type and the production of enzymes or toxins.

Others have failed to see correlation between pyocine type and antibiotic resistance or pathogenicity. No association has been revealed between serogroups and susceptibility to antibiotics, pathogenicity, site of infection, or biochemical or cultural characteristics (Adler & Finland, 1971; Bergan, 1972f,g; Klyhn, 1967; Köhler, 1957; Lányi, 1968, 1969).

In bovine mastitis, predominance of certain pyocine types (Mushin & Ziv, 1973a) or serogroups has been noted, but this has been due to epidemic spread of the strains (Bergan, 1972f; Sandvik, 1960a,b; Thörne & Kyrkebø, 1966).

APPLICATION OF TYPING METHODS

Epidemiological typing methods have special uses such as differentiation between relapse and re-infection of urinary tract infection (Neussel, 1971), but their chief merit is the elucidation of nosocomial outbreaks of infection, determination of sources, reservoirs and vectors of infectious agents.

A constant source of pseudomonas is healthy people who have a faecal carrier rate of 4–6% (Shooter *et al.*, 1966; Stoodley & Thom, 1970). The frequency of individual serogroups of pseudomonas in water reflects their incidence in the healthy people living in the same area (Lantos *et al.*, 1969). Usually, a large number of bacteria are needed (more than 10^6 bacteria) for colonization, and the duration of excretion is short. Buck & Cooke (1969) recovered pseudomonas for a maximum of 6 days, and only when more than 10^6 bacteria were ingested. The interplay between microbe and host is such that disease favours colonization. Healthy hospital personnel had a sixfold lesser frequency in stool than patients (Shooter *et al.*, 1966), this in spite of the close contact which nursing personnel often have with a large number of patients. Eleven to 14% have pseudomonas in the stool at admission and an additional 10–17% acquire it during hospitalization (Arseni & Doxiadis, 1967; Shooter *et al.*, 1966). Among leukaemia patients, $\frac{1}{4}$ exhibit pseudomonas in the bowel at admission; again, approximately the same number acquire the organism during their stay in hospital. The influence of the hospital milieu and disease is also reflected in the finding that out-patients have a threefold lesser probability of faecal pseudomonas carriage than warded patients (Shooter *et al.*, 1966). Previous hospitalization, antibiotic treatment and enterostomias were some factors associated with increased occurrence.

Shooter *et al.* (1966) used phage, pyocine and serological typing to substantiate that in a number of cases pseudomonas was spread from the bowel of one patient to another. Strains were only considered related when similar phage patterns were combined with identity in serogroup and pyocine type.

Colonization of the gut has been followed by auto-infection in a number of instances (Deighton *et al.*, 1971; Shooter *et al.*, 1971). Pseudomonas in the bowel may derive from infested foods. Clinical isolates have been traced by pyocine typing to vegetables in the hospital kitchens (Kominos *et al.*, 1972b; Shooter *et al.*, 1971). Even pharmaceutical products have been incriminated (Shooter *et al.*, 1971). Pseudomonas may be found in drinking water; Lantos *et al.* (1969) observed an episode of grossly polluted municipal water.

Nosocomial pseudomonas infections usually spread in one of three ways.

1. They may be transmitted directly between patients, as frequently occurs in burn units and surgical wards.
2. An inanimate object may be involved as reservoir or vector.
3. In a number of cases, autoinfection follows colonization of the bowel.

Spread from the bowel to the hospital environment is inevitable both among adults and newborns (Shooter *et al.*, 1966; Maruyama *et al.*, 1971). Shooter *et al.* recovered patient strains from water jugs, draw sheets, table tops and floors;

sluices and bathrooms were frequent sources. Whitby & Rampling (1972) made an interesting comparison of the level of pseudomonas contamination in hospital and domestic milieu. Although only hospital staff were involved, pseudomonas was rarely observed in private homes. None of the domestic strains were identical to pyocine types found simultaneously in the hospital.

Staff probably is a rare *source* of pseudomonas infections, but nurses and physicians play an important role in the spread of microbes. This has been amply documented by epidemiological typing (Bergan, 1967; Deighton *et al.*, 1971; Jellard & Churcher, 1967; Kominos *et al.*, 1972a; Lowbury *et al.*, 1970). A study by Deighton *et al.* (1971) demonstrated many typical facets of nosocomial pseudomonas infections. By pyocine typing, serogrouping and phage typing, the recognition of isolates was easy. Both objects and persons in the surroundings of the infected patients became contaminated. Cross-infection was repeatedly demonstrated. Infected hands of health personnel contributed decisively to the spread of infection. The potential danger of healthy carriers was shown in an instance when a nurse became contaminated during the bathing of a child and subsequently transmitted the organism to another child.

Whereas hands are very important factors, in a few instances the role of inanimate objects has been proven. Ayliffe *et al.* (1965) observed a series of cases with pseudomonas meningitis after neurosurgery. The causative organism was typed by phage, pyocine and serological typing and was found to come from a shaving brush used for depilation prior to surgery. The typing methods were very useful in pointing out the relationship and in eliminating as potential cause a number of isolates from staff, hand creams, sinks, soaps, trays, aseptic bottles, urine bottles and another depilation brush.

Ayliffe *et al.* (1966) in another study noted that intraocular pseudomonas infections arising after eye operations were caused by a contaminated saline solution used to moisten the cornea during operations. This had been contaminated from the sink used to wash the bottles.

Rouques *et al.* (1969) studied a series of pseudomonas infections in haemodialysis patients. The same phage type was recovered in benzalkonium solution used with the intent of sterilizing (sic!) the equipment used for extracorporeal circulation.

Bodey (1970) found that the frequency of pseudomonas septicaemia was high in leukaemia patients, reflecting a high carrier rate of 54% in the stool of this particular group. Parallel isolates from the same patients (blood, stool, throat) were always of the same pyocine types, but in some instances the pyocine type was not reproducible. In the inanimate milieu, pseudomonas was found in sinks, in the air and on the floors. Sixtyeight % of the strains belonged to p1.

When cross-infections are common, the number of predominant epidemiological types may be small. Grogan (1966) demonstated 3 dominant phage types among surgical patients where environment isolates only reflected the patient strains to a minor degree.

Typing methods have been instrumental in the elucidation of nosocomial patterns of infection in paediatric departments. Knights *et al.* (1968) employed all three typing methods to characterize the epidemiology within a neonatal unit. Pseudomonas infections had been a problem in the unit for some time. Several strains had been isolated from the wards and a nosocomial spread suspected, but only with typing methods could the reservoirs and modes of spread be definitely determined. Subsequently, four distinct groups of strains, each with common serological, pyocine and phage types were found. Then, cross-infections implicating several wards were distinguished. Epidemic strains colonized nursery washbasins, sinks and sluices. Cleaning equipment was always infested. In these outbreaks, humidifiers, resuscitation equipment and suction tubes, which often have been the sources in nurseries, were not involved. Measures instituted to eradicate pseudomonas from potential reservoirs and vectors, i.e. disinfection, were successful in that no milieu or patient specimen rendered pseudomonas during a subsequent 8-month period. Dexter (personal communication, 1973) eliminated cross-infection by combatting pseudomonas in moist areas.

Jellard & Churcher (1967) studied the pseudomonas situation in a baby unit for $1\frac{1}{2}$ years. During this period, isolates of a uniform phage type repeatedly appeared in routine stool cultures. Sixtyfive of 66 cultures had the same lysotype. Infections of many types occurred: nose, throat, eye, ear, vagina and skin. Episodes of nosocomial outbreaks were followed, but the epidemic types were never obtained from healthy personnel, inanimate objects or an operation theatre. The babies themselves constituted the main reservoir and source of infection. The usefulness of phage typing was clear, since without it many isolates of other types could falsely have been incriminated as sources.

Whereas pseudomonas is eliminated rapidly from the bowel of healthy adults (Buck & Cooke, 1969), in infants pseudomonas excretion may continue for more than 2 months. Clearing is more efficient in full-term normal babies than in premature or sick infants.

In burns representing large, exposed areas with excellent growth conditions for bacteria, colonization by pseudomonas is a serious problem. Colonization may partly be a consequence of autoinfection (Sutter & Hurst, 1966) from the bowel, but usually is a consequence of cross-infection. Liljedahl *et al.* (1972) found a single phage type, 1214, 109/F8, in $\frac{1}{3}$ of a group of burn patients, clearly indicating a nosocomial pattern.

The infection may come directly from other patients as was demonstrated when cross-infection was reduced by segregation in infected and non-infected patients and of nurses tending either category of patients (Dexter, 1971). The role of the inanimate environment is important. Patient strain types have often been found in large numbers on inanimate objects (Dexter, 1971). Although pseudomonas may persist in the environment for a long time before colonization of burns (Linjedahl *et al.*, 1972; Malmborg *et al.*, 1969), the organisms may also remain long after discharge of the patients. Hurst & Sutter (1966) thus recovered patient phage types from the floor for more than 8 weeks. In other cases, pseudomonas has disappeared more rapidly after patient discharge (Dexter, 1971). On many occasions, modern technology efficiently assists in the spread of infection. In one instance pseudomonas discharged from infected burns during dressing was carried to remote parts of a burns unit by a positive pressure ventilation system. This spread was eliminated only after negative pressure and a positive air pressure had been applied to the entrance of the dressing suite (Dexter, 1971).

The importance of bacteria from the environment has been indicated by the circumstance that the number of different phage types in a burn wound increases with prolonged hospitalization (Sutter & Hurst, 1966). Superinfection was also shown during topical treatment with Sulfamylon (*p*-amino-methyl-benzenesulphonamide-HCl) when the appearance of resistant organisms was accompanied by the emergence of new phage types (Lindberg *et al.*, 1966, 1970).

Pseudomonas infections are also a prominent problem of the respiratory tract in respirator-treated and tracheostomized patients (Greible *et al.*, 1970). Mucoid strains of *P. aeruginosa* have been noted particularly frequently in cystic fibrosis. When mucoid and non-mucoid strains occurred at the same time they often belonged to identical pyocine types indicating that they were indeed variants of the same strain (Williams & Govan, 1973). Mucoid variation may be due to lysogenization (Martin, 1973). The organisms may be traced to the environment or staff (Losonczy *et al.*, 1971). Epidemic types may be found on the hands of staff and parents visiting their children (Bergan, 1967), occasionally derived from infested cloth towels. The respirators and/or their humidifier units may carry organisms from one patient to another. Serogrouping and lysotyping have shown that bronchial infections may be derived from infected lubrication fluid for bronchoscopes or suction tubes (Meitert *et al.*, 1971; Phillips, 1966; Rubbo *et al.*, 1966). Autoinfection has also been demonstrated in a number of cases (Darrell & Wahba, 1964; Lowbury *et al.*, 1970). Autoinfection has often been preceded by bowel colonization.

Faecal carriers among the staff may also be a hazard to the patients, as was shown in a nursery where a staff strain was recovered in a number of infants with diarrhoea caused by the same pyocine type (Falcão *et al.*, 1972).

Important to the elimination of pseudomonas infections is adherence to rigorous aseptic techniques and good nursing procedures (Lowbury *et al.*, 1970). Pharmaceuticals, instruments, utilities and the environment (sinks and other objects) must be free from pseudomonas. Good hand hygiene is perhaps the one single most decisive factor. It is recommended to monitor the carrier rate of patients and staff by routine stool cultures on selective media and to follow a nosocomial surveillance programme with epidemiological typing as an adjunct to reduce and control the animate reservoir of pseudomonas.

INTERNATIONAL STANDARDIZATION

For several bacteria such as *Salmonella*, pneumococci, streptococci, meningococci and *Pasteurella* there exist serological, bacteriocine or phage-typing methods that are internationally recognized. For *P. aeruginosa*, there is little uniformity of typing methods. The organism has been a popular scientific object, but most works on typing methods have been started from scratch instead of improving on existing schemas.

This has often made it impossible to compare results, but the situation has now led to a reaction among the involved microbiologists. Formal pleas for standardization of procedures have been made (Herman & Farmer, 1970). A '*Pseudomonas Typing Newsletter*' is available from Dr. J. R. Farmer, University of Alabama. An International Cooperative Study Group is at present comparing existing serogrouping schemas; it attempts to establish an International Antigenic Typing Schema (IATS) that may receive international approval.

For pyocine typing, the Gillies & Govan system (1966) would appear to be the most internationally acceptable method. It is reasonably reproducible (Bergan, 1973a,c; Gillies & Govan, 1966; Govan & Gillies, 1969) and has been distributed to a large number of laboratories.

For phage typing, among the 17 sets proposed, only three are in current use, the sets of Meitert & Meitert (1965), of Lindberg *et al.* (1963, 1964) with several modifications, and of Bergan (1972e). The last mentioned was selected by numerical grouping analysis of all internationally available phages; it has favourable characteristics compared to previous typing sets (Tables 2 and 3) (Bergan, 1972d,e,g, 1973c; Kozaczek *et al.*, 1973), but further evaluation at more centres would be preferable. Before a phage set is used at several centres, it would be useful, in conjunction with a central reference laboratory for *P. aeruginosa* typing, to ensure phage pattern stability in a way similar to the central control exercised for the international phage typing set of *S. aureus*.

PREFERENCE OF PARTICULAR TYPING METHOD

Comparison

Each of the epidemiological typing methods of *P. aeruginosa* has its assets and its disadvantages. Pyocine typing by the Gillies & Govan method (1966) is simple and relatively quite reproducible (Bergan, 1973a; Govan, 1968; Govan & Gillies, 1969; Kasomson, 1970). With three pyocine types comprising $\frac{3}{4}$ of the isolates, the method has a fair differentiation. It is difficult at present to compare the Gillies & Govan method and the Rampling procedure, but two disadvantages of the latter are obvious: (i) instability of the pyocine preparations which only maintain activity for 2–6 months (Edmonds *et al.*, 1972a; Rampling, personal communication, 1973); (ii) the labour involved in typing is comparable to phage typing. Gillies & Govan recommend that pyocine typing should be the initial method of characterizing *P. aeruginosa* isolates (Govan, personal communication, 1973).

The number of serogroups depends on the serological schema, but a few groups dominate. In the International Antigenic Typing Schema, 16 groups are currently recognized, but the serogroups O:2, O:5, O:6 comprise about half of the isolates. By combining O-grouping and H-typing, a larger number evolves (Lányi, 1970).

Phage typing divides pseudomonas into a considerably larger number of categories than the other methods. This advantage is counterbalanced by the much more laborious and intricate nature of phage typing. Its reproducibility is lower than with the other methods, but if a difference in one strong reaction is tolerated as is customary for phage typing of other species, the method is of considerable assistance.

Another aspect to consider is typability. Phage typing by the method of Bergan (1972e) appears to lyse more strains than the other phage typing methods. This method and the Gillies & Govan pyocine typing procedure are comparable in this respect. Serogrouping by the Habs schema types fewer strains, approximately 71–97%.

Usually each of the three typing approaches is used in its own right—on all strains of *P. aeruginosa*. In analogy with the salmonellae where e.g. phage typing is only applied to strains of the same serotype, some consider a hierarchical arrangement of these typing systems also more appropriate for pseudomonas (Liu, personal communication, 1973). This would entail that serogrouping should be carried out as a first step and that phage typing or pyocine typing should be used to differentiate strains of identical serogroup specificity, rather than using these methods on the species as a whole. At the moment, either way of considering different classes of typing procedures is a matter of philosophy.

Conclusion

It is recommended that at least one of the *P. aeruginosa* typing methods should be used at larger, central laboratories. Since pseudomonas usually occurs sporadically with a few isolates at a time, most laboratories would find pyocine or serogrouping suitable. Serogrouping or pyocine typing alone, however, cannot render sufficient discrimination. An adequate distinction is achieved by combining these two methods (Bergan, 1973c; Bassett *et al.*, 1965; Wahba, 1965a,b; Csiszár & Lányi, 1970). An alternative is the Lányi serotyping system with O- and H-antigen determinations. A combination of serogrouping and pyocine typing results in a differentiation comparable to phage typing (Bergan, 1973c).

Due to the variability of phage typing, it is an advantage to combine it with serogrouping (Bergan, 1973c; Edmonds *et al.*, 1972). Bernstein-Ziv *et al.* (1973) favoured a combination of phage and pyocine typing.

Used alone, phage typing is the method with the greatest power to discriminate between isolates, i.e. with the greatest number of subgroups. Ayliffe *et al.* (1966) found that, used alone, only phage typing had the necessary discrimination to pin-point a source of infection. Due to the time consumed for maintenance of the system and for setting up the method with adequate controls, phage typing is recommended only for larger laboratories with sufficient resources and a relatively large number of pseudomonas cultures.

REFERENCES

Ádám, M. M., Kontrohr, T. & Horváth, E. (1971). Serological studies on *Pseudomonas aeruginosa* O group lipopolysaccharides. *Acta microbiol. Acad. Sci. Hung.*, **18**, 307–317.

Adler, J. L. & Finland, M. (1971). Susceptibility of recent isolates of *Pseudomonas aeruginosa* to gentamicin, polymyxin, and five penicillins, with observations on the pyocin and immunotypes of the strains. *Appl. Microbiol.* **22**, 870–875.

Alföldi, L. (1957a). Isolation and characterisation of some *Pseudomonas pyocyanea* bacteriophages. *Acta. Microbiol. hung.*, **4**, 107–118.

Alföldi, L. (1957b). Frequency of lysogenic strains in *Pseudomonas pyocyanea. Acta. Microbiol. hung.*, **4**, 119–122.

Aoki, K. (1926). Agglutinatorische Einteilung von *Pyocyaneus*—Bazillen. *Zbl. Bakt., I. Abt. Orig.*, **98**, 186–195.

Arseni, A. E. & Doxiadis, S. A. (1967). Faecal carriage of pseudomonas. *Lancet*, **i**, p. 787.

Ayliffe, G. A. J., Lowbury, E. J. L., Hamilton, J. G., Small, J. M., Asheshov, E. A. & Parker, M. T. (1965). Hospital infection with *Pseudomonas aeruginosa* in neurosurgery. *Lancet*, **ii**, 365–369.

Ayliffe, G. A. J., Barry, D. R., Lowbury, E. J. L., Roper-Hall, M. J. & Walker, W. M. (1966). Postoperative infection with *Pseudomonas aeruginosa* in an eye-hospital. *Lancet*, **i**, 1113–1117.

Bassett, D. C. J., Thompson, S. A. S. & Page, B. (1965). Neonatal infections with *Pseudomonas aeruginosa* associated with contaminated resuscitation equipment. *Lancet*, **i**, 781–784.

Bennett, J. C., Grogan, J. B. & Welch, L. J. (1962). Further information on pseudomonas infections using an improved technique. *Surg. Forum*, **13**, 45–47.

Bergan, T. (1967). Nosokomielle Pseudomonas-infeksjoner. *Farmakoterapi (Oslo)*, **23**, 72–86.

Bergan, T. (1968a). *Pseudomonas aeruginosa*—typemetoder og sykehusinfeksjoner. *Nord. Med.*, **79**, 505–509.

Bergan, T. (1968b). Typing of *Pseudomonas aeruginosa* by pyocine production *Acta path. microbiol. scand.*, **72**, 401–411.

Bergan, T. (1971). Influence of cultural milieu on the replication of *Pseudomonas* bacteriophages. *Acta path. microbiol. scand.*, **79 B**, 841–849.

Bergan, T. (1972a). Comparison of numerical procedures for grouping pseudomonas bacteriophages according to lytic spectra. *Acta path. microbiol. scand.* **80 B**, 55–70.

Bergan, T. (1972b). A transformed Yule correlation coefficient employed in numerical grouping procedures on bacteriophage lytic spectra. *Acta path. microbiol. scand.*, **80 B**, 89–100.

Bergan, T. (1972c). A new bacteriophage typing set for *Pseudomonas aeruginosa*. 1. Selection procedure. *Acta. path. microbiol. scand.*, **80 B**, 177–188.

Bergan, T. (1972d). A new bacteriophage typing set for *Pseudomonas aeruginosa*. 2. Characterization and comparisons of new and previous typing sets. *Acta. path. microbiol. scand.*, **80 B**, 189–201.

Bergan, T. & Lystad, A. (1972e). Reproducibility in bacteriophage sensitivity pattern of *Pseudomonas aeruginosa. Acta path. microbiol. scand.*, **80 B**, 345–350.

Bergan, T. (1972f). Bacteriophage typing and serogrouping *Pseudomonas aeruginosa* from animals. *Acta path. microbiol. scand.*, **80 B**, 351–361.

Bergan, T. (1972g). Bacteriophage Typing of *Pseudomonas aeruginosa*. Universitetsforlaget, Oslo.

Bergan, T. (1973a). Epidemiological markers for *Pseudomonas aeruginosa*. 1. Serogrouping, pyocine typing—and their interrelations. *Acta path. microbiol. scand.*, **81 B**, 70–80.

Bergan, T. (1973b). Epidemiological markers for *Pseudomonas aeruginosa*. 2. Relationship between bacteriophage susceptibility and serogroup or pyocine type. *Acta path. microbiol. scand.*, **81 B**, 81–90.

Bergan, T. (1973c). Epidemiological markers for *Pseudomonas aeruginosa*. 3. Comparison of bacteriophage typing, serogrouping, and pyocine typing on a heterogeneous clinical material. *Acta path. microbiol. scand.*, **81 B**, 91–101.

Bergan, T. & Midtvedt, T. (1975). Epidemiological markers for *Pseudomonas aeruginosa*. 4. Change of ½-antigen and phage sensitivity after phage infection *in vitro* and *in vivo* of *Pseudomonas aeruginosa*. *Acta path. microbiol. scand.* **83B**. In press.

Bernstein-Ziv, R., Mushin, R. & Rabinowitz, K. (1973). Typing of *Pseudomonas aeruginosa*: comparison of the phage procedure with the pyocine technique. *J. Hyg.*, **71**, 403–410.

Beumer, J., Cotton, E., Delmotte, A., Millet, M., von Grünigen, W. & Yourassowsky, E. (1972). Ampleur des modifications du lysotype provoquées par la lyophilisation chez des souches de 'Pseudomonas aeruginosa'. *Ann. Inst. Pasteur*, **122**, 415–423.

Blair, J. E. & Williams, R. E. O. (1961). Phage typing of staphylococci. *Bull. Wld Hlth Org.*, **24**, 771–784.

Bobo, R. A., Newton, E. J., Jones, L. F., Farmer, L. H. & Farmer, J. J. (1973). Nursery outbreak of *Pseudomonas aeruginosa*: epidemiological conclusions from five different typing methods. *Appl. Microbiol*, **25**, 414–420.

Bodey, G. P. (1970). Epidemiological studies of *Pseudomonas* species in patients with leukemia. *Amer. J. med. Sci.*, **260**, 82–89.

Boivin, A. & Mesrobeanu, L. (1937). Sur l'antigène O; endotoxine des pyocyaniques. *C.R. Soc. Biol. (Paris)*, **125**, 273–275.

Booth, E. V. (1969). Methods for studying the epidemiology of *Pseudomonas aeruginosa* in the hospital environment. *Canad. J. med. Technol.* **33**, 214–223.

Borst, J. & de Jong, J. H. L. (1970). Serological typing of *Pseudomonas aeruginosa*. *Antonie v. Leeuwenhoek*, **36**, p. 190.

Bradley, D. E. & Robertson, D. (1968). The structure and infective process of a contractile *Pseudomonas aeruginosa* bacteriophage. *J. gen. Virol.*, **3**, 247–254.

Brown, D. O. (1973). Multiple loop inoculator as an aid in bacteriocine typing techniques. *Med. Lab. Technol.*, **30**, 351–353.

Buck, A. C. & Cooke, E. M. (1969). The fate of ingested *Pseudomonas aeruginosa* in normal persons. *J. med. Microbiol.*, **2**, 521–525.

Caroli, G., Levré, E. & Lauro, P. (1968). Sui metodi de tipizzazione di "*Pseudomonas aeruginosa*" a fini epidemiologici. *Quad. Sclavo diagn.*, **4**, 547–566.

Caselitz, F.-H. (1966). Pseudomonas-Aeromonas *und ihre Humanmedizinische Bedeutung*, Fischer, Jena.

Chia-Ying, W. (1963). A study on the typing of *Pseudomonas aeruginosa*. *Chin. med. J.*, **82**, 358–362.

Christie, R. (1948). Observations on the biochemical and serological characteristics of *Pseudomonas aeruginosa*. *Aust. J. exp. Biol.*, **26**, 425–437.

Csiszár, K. & Lányi, B. (1970). Pyocine typing of *Pseudomonas aeruginosa*: association between antigenic structure and pyocine type. *Acta microbiol. Acad. Sci. hung.*, **17**, 361–370.

Darrell, J. H. & Wahba, A. H. (1964). Pyocine-typing of hospital strains of *Pseudomonas pyocyanea*. *J. clin. Path.*, **17**, 236–242.

Deighton, M. A., Tagg, J. R. & Mushin, R. (1971). Epidemiology of *Pseudomonas aeruginosa* infection in hospitals. 2 'Fingerprinting' of *Pseudomonas aeruginosa* strains in a study of cross-infection in a children's hospital. *Med. J. Aust.*, **i**, 892–896.

Dexter, F. (1971). *Pseudomonas aeruginosa* in a regional burns centre. *J. Hyg.*, **69**, 179–186.

Diaz, F., Mosovich, L. L. & Neter, E. (1970). Serogroups of *Pseudomonas aeruginosa* and the immune response of patients with cystic fibrosis. *J. infect. Dis.*, **121**, 269–274.

Don, P. A. & van den Ende, M. (1950). A preliminary study of the bacteriophages of *Pseudomonas aeruginosa. J. Hyg.*, **48**, 196–214.

van Eeden, D. (1967). The antigens of *Pseudomonas aeruginosa* studied by the Ouchterlony technique and immuno-electrophoresis. *J. gen. Microbiol.*, **48**, 95–105.

Edmonds, P., Suskind, R. R., MacMillan, B. G. & Holder, I. A. (1972a). Epidemiology of *Pseudomonas aeruginosa* in a burns hospital: evaluation of serological, bacteriophage, and pyocine typing methods. *Appl. Microbiol.*, **24**, 213–218.

Edmonds, P., Suskind, R. R., MacMillan, B. G. & Holder, I. A. (1972b). Epidemiology of *Pseudomonas aeruginosa* in a burns hospital: surveillance by a combined typing system. *Appl. Microbiol.*, **24**, 219–225.

van den Ende, M. (1952). Observations on the antigenic structure of *Pseudomonas aeruginosa. J. Hyg.*, **50**, 405–414.

Falcão, D. P., Mendonça, C. P., Scrassolo, A. & de Almeida, B. B. (1972). Nursery outbreak of severe diarrhoea due to multiple strains of *Pseudomonas aeruginosa. Lancet,* **ii**, 38–40.

Farmer, J. J. (1970). Mnemonic for reporting bacteriocin and bacteriophage types. *Lancet,* **ii**, p. 96.

Farmer, J. J. & Herman, L. G. (1969). Epidemiological fingerprinting of *Pseudomonas aeruginosa* by the production of and sensitivity to pyocin and bacteriophage. *Appl. Microbiol.*, **18**, 760–765.

Feary, T. W., Fisher, E. & Fisher, T. N. (1963). Lysogeny and phage resistance in *Pseudomonas aeruginosa. Proc. Soc. exp. Biol. (N.Y.),* **113**, 426–430.

Feary, T. W., Fisher, E. & Fisher, T. N. (1964). Isolation and preliminary characteristics of three bacteriophages associated with a lysogenic strain of *Pseudomonas aeruginosa. J. Bact.*, **87**, 196–208.

Finland, M. (1971). Changing prevalence of pathogenic bacteria in relation to time and the introduction and use of new antimicrobial agents. In *Bacterial Infections. Changes in Their Causative Agents, Trends and Possible Basis,* (Eds. M. Finland, W. Marget & K. Bartmann), Springer Verlag, Berlin, Heidelberg, New York, pp. 4–18.

Fisher, M. W., Devlin, H. B. & Gnabasik, F. J. (1969). New immunotype schema for *Pseudomonas aeruginosa* based on protective antigens. *J. Bact.*, **98**, 835–836.

Forkner, C. E. (1960). Pseudomonas aeruginosa *Infections. Modern Medical Monographs,* Grune & Stratton, New York, London.

Gillies, R. R. & Govan, J. R. W. (1966). Typing of *Pseudomonas pyrocyanea* by pyocine production. *J. Path. Bact.*, **91**, 339–345.

Goepfert, J. M. & Naylor, H. B. (1964). Purification and properties, of a bacteriophage included enzyme. *Bact. Proc.*, p. 142.

Gould, J. C. & McLeod, J. W. (1960). A study of the use of agglutinating sera and phage lysis in the classification of strains of *Pseudomonas aeruginosa. J. Path. Bact.*, **79**, 295–311.

Gould, J. C. (1963). *Pseudomonas pyocyanea* infections in hospital. In *Infection in Hospitals, Epidemiology and Control,* (Eds. R. E. O. Williams & R. A. Shooter), Blackwell Scientific Publications, Oxford, pp. 119–130.

Govan, J. R. W. (1968). *The pyocines of* Pseudomonas pyocyanea. Department of Bacteriology, University of Edinburgh. Thesis presented for the Degree of Doctor of Philosophy. Edinburgh.

Govan, J. R. W. & Gillies, R. R. (1969). Further studies in the pyocine typing of *Pseudomonas pyocyanea. J. med. Microbiol.*, **2**, 17–25.

Graber, C. D., Latta, R., Vogel, E. H. & Brame, R. (1962). Bacteriophage grouping of *Pseudomonas aeruginosa* with special emphasis on lysotypes occurring in infected burns. *Amer. J. clin. Path.*, **37**, 54–62.

Greible, H. G., Colton, F. R., Bird, T. J., Toigo, A. & Griffith, L. G. (1970). Fine-particle humidifiers. Source of *Pseudomonas aeruginosa* infections in a respiratory-disease unit. *New Engl. J. Med.*, **282**, 531–535.

Grogan, J. B. (1966). *Pseudomonas aeruginosa* carriage in patients. *J. Trauma*, **6**, 639–643.

Grogan, J. B. & Artz, C. P. (1961). Studies of *Pseudomonas* infections by a new bacteriophage typing technique. *Surg. Forum*, **12**, 26–28.

Grün, L., Pillich, J. & Heyn, U. (1967). Zur Metodik der Differenzierung von *Pseudomonas pyocyanea* mittels Bakteriophagen. *Arch. Hyg.* (*Berl.*), **151**, 640–646.

Habs, I. (1957). Untersuchungen über die O-Antigene von *Pseudomonas aeruginosa*. *Z. Hyg. Infekt.-Kr.*, **144**, 218–228.

Hamon, Y. (1956). Contribution a l'étude des pyocines. *Ann. Inst. Pasteur*, **91**, 82–90.

Hamon, Y., Véron, M. & Peron, Y. (1961). Contribution à l'étude des propriétés lysogènes et bacteriocinogènes dans le genre *Pseudomonas*. *Ann. Inst. Pasteur*, **101**, 738–753.

Heckman, M. G., Babcock, J. B. & Rose, H. D. (1972). Pyocine typing of *Pseudomonas aeruginosa*: clinical and epidemiologic aspects. *Amer. J. clin. Path.*, **57**, 35–42.

Herman, L. G. & Farmer, J. J. (1970). Pyocin typing of *Pseudomonas aeruginosa*—a plea for international standardization. Abstracts. *Tenth International Congress for Microbiology.* **8**, p. 98.

Herrmann, H. (1970). Untersuchungen zur Lysotypie von *Pseudomonas aeruginosa*. *Z. ges. Hyg.*, **16**, 876–879.

Higerd, T. B., Baechler, C. A. & Berk, R. S. (1967). *In vitro* and *in vivo* characterization of pyocin. *J. Bact.*, **93**, 1976–1986.

Higerd, T. B., Baechler, C. A. & Berk, R. S. (1969). Morphological studies on relaxed and contracted forms of purified pyocin particles. *J. Bact.*, **98**, 1378–1389.

Hoff, J. C. & Drake, C. H. (1961). Bacteriophage typing of *Pseudomonas aeruginosa*. *Amer. J. publ. Hlth.*, **51**, p. 918.

Holloway, B. W. (1960). Grouping *Pseudomonas aeruginosa* by lysogenicity and pyocinogenicity. *J. Path. Bact.*, **80**, 448–450.

Holloway, B. W. & Cooper, G. N. (1962). Lysogenic conversion in *Pseudomonas aeruginosa*. *J. Bact.*, **84**, 1321–1324.

Holloway, B. W. & Krishnapillai, V. (1975). Bacteriophages and bacteriocines. In *Genetics and Biochemistry of* Pseudomonas, (Eds. P. H. Clarke and M. H. Richmond), John Wiley, London.

Holloway, B. W., Krishnapillai, V. & Stanisich, V. (1971). *Pseudomonas* genetics. *Ann. Rev. Genet.*, **5**, 425–446.

Holloway, B. W., Egan, J. B. & Monk, M. (1960). Lysogeny in *Pseudomonas aeruginosa*. *Aust. J. exp. Biol. med. Sci.*, **38**, 321–329.

Homma, J. Y. (1971). Recent investigations on *Pseudomonas aeruginosa*. *Jap. J. exp. Med.*, **41**, 387–400.

Homma, J. Y. (1968). The protein moiety of the endotoxin of *Pseudomonas aeruginosa*. *Z. Allg. Mikrobiol.*, **8**, 227–248.

Homma, J. Y., Sagehashi, K. & Hosoya, S. (1951). Serological types of *Pseudomonas aeruginosa*. *Jap. J. exp. Med.*, **21**, 375–379.

Homma, J. Y. & Shinoya, H. (1967). Relationship between pyocine and temperate phage of *Pseudomonas aeruginosa*. III. Serological relationship between pyocines and temperate phage. *Jap. J. exp. Med.*, **37**, 395–421.

Homma, J. Y., Shionoya, H., Mequero, M. & Tanabe, Y. (1967). A short communication on pyocine 28 produced by *Pseudomonas aeruginosa*. *Jap. J. exp. Med.*, **37**, 511–513.

Homma, J. Y. & Suzuki, N. (1961). A simple protein with pyocine activity isolated from the cell wall of *Pseudomonas aeruginosa* and its close relation to endotoxin. *Jap. J. exp. Med.,* **31**, 209–213.

Homma, J. Y., Watabe, H. & Tanabe, Y. (1968). The temperate phages having serological relationship with the 'phage bound pyocine'. *Jap. J. exp. Med.,* **38**, 213–224.

Homma, J. Y., Kim, K. S., Yamada, H., Ito, M., Shionoya, H. & Kawabe, Y. (1970). Serological typing of *Pseudomonas aeruginosa* and its cross-infection. *Jap. J. exp. Med.,* **40**, 347–359.

Homma, J. Y., Shionoya, H., Yamada, H. & Kawabe, Y. (1971). Production of antibody against *Pseudomonas aeruginosa* and its serological typing. *Jap. J. exp. Med.,* **41**, 89–94.

Homma, J. Y., Shionoya, H., Yamada, H., Enomoto, M. & Miyao, K. (1972). Changes in serotype of *Pseudomonas aeruginosa. Jap. J. exp. Med.,* **42**, 171–172.

Hurst, V. & Sutter, V. L. (1966). Survival of *Pseudomonas aeruginosa* in the hospital environment. *J. infect. Dis.,* **116**, 151–154.

Ikeda, K. & Egami, F. (1969). Receptor substance for pyocin R. I. Partial purification and chemical properties. *J. Biochem. (Tokyo),* **65**, 603–609.

Ikeda, K. & Egami, F. (1973). Lipopolysaccharide of *Pseudomonas aeruginosa* with special reference to pyocin R receptor activity. *J. gen. appl. Microbiol. (Tokyo),* **19**, 115–128.

Ito, S. & Kageyama, M. (1970). Relationship between pyocins and a bacteriophage in *Pseudomonas aeruginosa. J. gen. appl. Microbiol. (Tokyo),* **16**, 231–240.

Ito, S., Kageyama, M. & Egami, F. (1970). Isolation and characterization of pyocine from several strains of *Pseudomonas aeruginosa. J. gen. appl. Microbiol. (Tokyo),* **16**, 205–214.

Jacob, F. (1954). Biosynthèse induite et mode d'action d'une pyocine, antibiotique de *Pseudomonas pyocyanea. Ann. Inst. Pasteur,* **86**, 149–160.

Jacob, F., Blobel, H. & Scharmann, W. (1973). Die Typisierung von *Pseudomonas aeruginosa* mit titrierten Pyocinen. *Zbl. Bakt., I. Abt. Orig.,* **224**, 472–477.

Jedličková, Z. & Pillich, J. (1968). Versuch einer serologischen und phagotypisieren-den Klassifizierung der aus pathologischem Material gewonnenen *Pseudomonas aeruginosa*-Stämme. *Zschr. inn. Med.,* **23**, 21–25.

Jellard, C. H. & Churcher, G. M. (1967). An outbreak of *Pseudomonas aeruginosa* (*pyocyanea*) infection in a premature baby unit, with observations on the intestinal carriage of *Pseudomonas aeruginosa* in the newborn. *J. Hyg.,* **65**, 219–228.

Jones, L. F., Pinto, B. V., Thomas, E. T. & Farmer, J. J. (1973). Simplified method for producing pyocin from *Pseudomonas aeruginosa. Appl. Microbiol.,* **26**, 120–121.

Kageyama, M. (1970a). Genetic Mapping of a bacteriocinogenic factor in *Pseudomonas aeruginosa.* I. Mapping of pyocin R2 factor by conjugation. *J. gen. appl. Microbiol. (Tokyo),* **16**, 523–530.

Kageyama, M. (1970b). Genetic mapping of a bacteriocinogenic factor in *Pseudomonas aeruginosa.* II. Mapping of pyocin R2 factor by transduction with phage F116. *J. gen. appl. Microbiol. (Tokyo),* **16**, 531–535.

Kageyama, M., Ikeda, K. & Egami, F. (1964). Studies of a pyocin. III. Biological properties of the pyocin. *J. Biochem. (Tokyo),* **55**, 59–64.

Kanzaki, K. (1934). Immunisatorische Studien au Pyozyaneusbazillen. I. Mitteilung Immunisatorische Einteilung von Pyozyaneusbazillen. *Zbl. Bakt., I. Abt. Orig.,* **133**, 89–94.

Kasomson, T., Roberts, C. E. & Panas-Ampol, K. (1970). Pyocine typing: a simple, precise epidemiologic tool. *South-East Asian J. trop. Med. publ. Hlth.,* **1**, 391–400.

Kawaharajo, K. (1973). Changes in serotype of *Pseudomonas aeruginosa. Jap. J. exp. Med.,* **43**, 225–226.

Kaziro, Y. & Tanaka, M. (1965a). Studies on the mode of action of pyocin. I. Inhibition of macromolecular synthesis in sensitive cells. *J. Biochem.* (*Tokyo*), **57**, 689–695.

Kaziro, Y. & Tanaka, M. (1965b). Studies on the mode of action of pyocin. II. Inactivation of ribosomes. *J. Biochem.* (*Tokyo*), **58**, 357–363.

Kékessy, D. A. & Piguet, J. D. (1970). New method for detecting bacteriocin production. *Appl. Microbiol.*, **20**, 282–283.

Kelln, R. A. & Warren, R. A. J. (1971). Isolation and properties of a bacteriophage lytic for a wide range of pseudomonads. *Canad. J. Microbiol.*, **17**, 677–682.

Kleinmaier, H. (1957). Die O-Gruppenbestimmung von *Pseudomonas*-Stämmen mittels Objektträger Agglutination. *Zbl. Bakt. I. Abt. Orig.*, **170**, 570–583.

Kleinmaier, H. & Müller, H. (1958). Vergleichende Prüfung der Präzipitation und Agglutination als Methode zur Bestimmung der O-Antigene von *Pseudomonas aeruginosa*. *Zbl. Bakt., I. Abt. Orig.*, **172**, 54–65.

Kleinmaier, H. & Quincke, G. (1959). Über das vorkommen der Serotypen von *Pseudomonas aeruginosa*. *Arch. Hyg.* (*Berl.*), **143**, 125–134.

Kleinmaier, H., Schreiner, E. & Graeff, H. (1958). Untersuchungen über die serodiagnostischen Differenzierungsmöglichkeiten mit thermolabilen Antigenen von *Pseudomonas aeruginosa*. *Z. Immun.-Forsch.*, **115**, 492–508.

Klyhn, K. M. & Gorrill, R. H. (1967). Studies on the virulence of hospital strains of *Pseudomonas aeruginosa*. *J. gen. Microbiol.*, **47**, 227–235.

Knights, H. T., France, D. R. & Harding, S. (1968). *Pseudomonas aeruginosa* cross infection in a neonatal unit. *N.Z. med. J.*, **67**, 617–620.

Kobayashi, F. (1971a). Experimental infection with *Pseudomonas aeruginosa* in mice. I. The virulence of *Pseudomonas aeruginosa* for mice. *Jap. J. Microbiol.*, **15**, 295–300.

Kobayashi, F. (1971b). Experimental infection with *Pseudomonas aeruginosa* in mice. II. The fate of highly and low virulent strains in the peritoneal cavity and organs of mice. *Jap. J. Microbiol.*, **15**, 301–307.

Köhler, W. (1957). Zur Serologie der *Pseudomonas aeruginosa*. *Z. Immun.-Forsch.*, **144**, 282–302.

Kominos, S. D., Copeland, C. E. & Grosiak, B. (1972a). Mode of transmission of *Pseudomonas aeruginosa* in a burn unit and an intensive care unit in a general hospital. *Appl. Microbiol.*, **23**, 309–312.

Kominos, S. D., Copeland, C. E., Grosiak, B. & Postic, B. (1972b). Introduction of *Pseudomonas aeruginosa* into a hospital via vegetables. *Appl. Microbiol.*, **24**, 567–570.

Kozaczek, W., Bergan, T., Lachowic, T. & Szczepański, K. (1973). Wyhrywanie źródel i dróg zakażenia paleczka ropy blekitnej w oddziale urologicznym. *Przeg. Epid.* (*Warsaw*), **27**, 37–44.

Lantos, J., Kiss, M., Lányi, B. & Völgyesi, J. (1969). Serological and phage typing of *Pseudomonas aeruginosa* invading a municipal water supply. *Acad. microbiol. Acad. Sci. hung.*, **16**, 333–336.

Lányi, B. (1966/67). Serological properties of *Pseudomonas aeruginosa*. I. Group-specific somatic antigens. *Acta. microbiol. Acad. Sci. hung.*, **13**, 295–318.

Lányi, B. (1968). Biochemical and cultural characters of serologically grouped *Pseudomonas aeruginosa* strains. *Acta. microbiol. Acad. Sci. hung.*, **15**, 337–355.

Lányi, B. (1969). Amino acid utilization by serologically grouped *Pseudomonas aeruginosa* strains. *Acta microbiol. Acad. Sci. hung.*, **16**, 357–361.

Lányi, B. (1970). Serological properties of *Pseudomonas aeruginosa*. II. Type-specific thermolabile (flagellar) antigens. *Acta microbiol. Acad. Sci. hung.*, **17**, 35–48.

Lányi, B., Gregács, M. & Ádám, M. M. (1966/67). Incidence of *Pseudomonas aeruginosa* serogroups in water and human faeces. *Acta microbiol. Acad. Sci. hung.*, **13**, 319–326.

Lewis, M. S. (1967). Another method of pyocine typing. *J. clin. Path.*, **20**, p. 103.

Liljedahl, S.-O., Malmborg, A.-S., Nystrøm, B. & Sjöberg, L. (1972). Spread of *Pseudomonas aeruginosa* in a burns unit. *J. med. Microbiol.,* **5**, 473–481.

Lindberg, R. B., Latta, R. L., Brame, R. & Moncrief, J. A. (1963a). Bacteriophage typing of *Pseudomonas aeruginosa*: epidemiological observations based on type distribution. Progress Report. U.S. Army Surgical Research Unit. Brooke Army Medical Center, Fort Sam, Houston, Texas, pp. 1–19. Unpublished.

Lindberg, R. B., Brame, R., Latta, R. L., Mason, A. D. & Moncrief, J. A. (1963b). Relationship between phage type and antigenic structure of *Pseudomonas aeruginosa* strains from infected burns. *Fed. Proc., Abstract, no. 276.*

Lindberg, R. B., Latta, R., Brame, R. & Moncrief, J. A. (1963c). Bacteriophage typing of *Pseudomonas aeruginosa*: epidemiologic observations based on type distribution. *Bact. Proc.,* p. 72.

Lindberg, R. B., Latta, R. L., Brame, R. E. & Moncrief, J. A. (1964). Definitive bacteriophage typing system for *Pseudomonas aeruginosa. Bact. Proc.,* p. 81.

Lindberg, R. B., Latta, R. L., Brame, R. E. & Moncrief, J. A. (1966). Alterations in *Pseudomonas aeruginosa* flora and phage type with topical Sulfamylon treatment of severe burns. *Bact. Proc.,* p. 65.

Lindberg, R. B., Curreri, P. W. & Pruitt, B. A. (1970). Microbiology of burns treated with carbenicillin: experimental and clinical observations. *J. infect. Dis.,* **122**, S34–S39.

Liu, P. V. (1969). Changes on somatic antigens of *Pseudomonas aeruginosa* induced by bacteriophages. *J. infect. Dis.,* **119**, 237–246.

Losonczy, G., Tóth, L., Petrás, G., Bognár, S., Lányi, B. & Csekes, J. (1971). *Pseudomonas aeruginosa* infections in an artificial respiratory ward. *Acta microbiol. Acad. Sci. hung.,* **18**, 261–269.

Lowbury, E. J. L. (1974). Medical aspects of *Pseudomonas aeruginosa.* In *Genetics and Biochemistry of* Pseudomonas, (Eds. P. H. Clark & M. H. Richmond), John Wiley, London.

Lowbury, E. J. L. & Fox, J. (1954). The epidemiology of infection with *Pseudomonas pyocyanea* in a burns unit. *J. Hyg.,* **52**, 403–416.

Lowbury, E. J. L., Thom, B. T., Lilly, H. A., Babb, J. R. & Whittall, K. (1970). Sources of infection with *Pseudomonas aeruginosa* in patients with tracheostomy. *J. med. Microbiol.,* **3**, 39–56.

MacPherson, J. N. & Gillies, R. R. (1969). A note on bacteriocine typing techniques. *J. med. Microbiol.,* **2**, 161–165.

Malmborg, A.-S., Liljedahl, S.-O., Nyström, B., Seim, S. & Sjöberg, L. (1969). Infections with *Pseudomonas* in a burns unit. *Acta path. microbiol. scand.,* **76**, 329–336.

Martin, D. R. (1973). Mucoid variation in *Pseudomonas aeruginosa* induced by the action of phage. *J. med. Microbiol.,* **6**, 111–118.

Maruyama, S., Takimoto, M., Suehiro, T., Kawamura, S., Iwata, T., Ono, H., Murayama, T. & Yoshioka, H. (1971). Faecal carriage of *Pseudomonas aeruginosa* among newborns in a hospital nursery. Incidence and epidemiological consideration by serological typing. *Acta neonat. Jap.,* **7**, 146–150.

Matsumoto, H. & Tazaki, T. (1969). Relationships of O antigens of *Pseudomonas aeruginosa* between Hungarian types of Lányi and Habs' type or Verder and Evans' types. *Jap. J. Microbiol.,* **13**, 209–211.

Matsumoto, H., Tazaki, T. & Kato, T. (1968). Serological and pyocine types of *Pseudomonas aeruginosa* from various sources. *Jap. J. Microbiol.,* **12**, 111–119.

Mayr-Harting, A. (1948). The serology of *Pseudomonas pyocyanea. J. gen. Microbiol.,* **2**, 31–39.

Mead, T. H. & van den Ende, M. (1953). Bacteriophage inhibition by extracts from phage-insensitive bacteria of the genus *Pseudomonas. J. Hyg.,* **51**, 108–124.

Meitert, E. (1965). Schéma de lysotypie pour *Pseudomonas aeruginosa*. *Arch. roum. Path. exp.*, **24**, 439–458.

Meitert, T. (1964). Contribution à l'étude de la structure antigénique des *B. pyocyaniques*. (*Pseudomonas aeruginosa*). II. Individualisation des groupes sérologiques au moyen des antigenes 'O'. *Arch. roum. Path. exp.*, **23**,679–688.

Meitert, E., Meitert, T., Rusu, R. & Zaharia, I. (1967). Considérations sur l'incidence du bacille pyocyanique (*Pseudomonas aeruginosa*) dans un service de bronchopneumologie. *Arch. roum. Path. exp.*, **26**, 787–796.

Meitert, E. & Meitert, T. (1973). *Pseudomonas aeruginosa*. In *Lysotypie und andere spezielle epidemiologische Laboratoriumsmethoden.*, VEB Gustav Fischer Verlag, Jena.

Meitert, T. & Meitert, E. (1960). Contribution à l'étude de la structure antigénique des *P. pyocyaniques* (*Pseudomonas aeruginosa*). I. Emploi des réactions d'agglutination pour l'étude de 181 souches. *Arch. roum. Path. exp.*, **19**, 623–634.

Meitert, T. & Meitert, E. (1961). Über die Lysogenie und Lysosensibilität bei *Pseudomonas aeruginosa*. Lysotypieversuche. *Arch. roum. path. exp.*, **20**, 277–285.

Meitert, T. & Meitert, E. (1966). Utilisation combinée du sérotypage et de la lysotypie des souches de *Pseudomonas aeruginosa* en vue d'approfondir les investigations épidémiologiques. *Arch. roum. Path. exp.*, **25**, 427–434.

Meitert, T. & Meitert, E. (1971). Virulence pour la souris blanche de quelques souches de *Pseudomonas aeruginosa* provenant de cas sporadiques et d'infections nosocomiales. *Arch. roum. Path. exp.*, **30**, 37–44.

Meitert, E., Meitert, T., Cazacu, E. & Moscuna, M. (1967). Elucidarea mechanismilu de contaminare cu *Pseudomonas aeruginosa* a unor unituri dentare prin utilizarea combinată a lizotipiei și serotipajuliu. *Microbiologia, parazitol., Epidemiol.*, **12**, 329–338.

Merrikin, D. J. & Terry, C. S. (1972). Variability of pyocine type and pyocine sensitivity in some strains of *Pseudomonas aeruginosa*. *J. appl. Bact.*, 35, 667–672.

Mikkelsen, O. S. (1968). Serotyping of *Pseudomonas aeruginosa*. 1. Studies on the production of anti O sera. *Acta. path microbiol. scand.*, **73**, 373–390.

Mikkelsen, O. S. (1970). Serotyping of *Pseudomonas aeruginosa*. 2. Results of an O group classification. *Acta path microbiol. scand.*, **78B**, 163–175.

Minamishima, Y., Takeya, K., Ohnishi, Y., & Amako, K. (1968). Physicochemical and biological properties of fibrous *Pseudomonas* bacteriophages, *J. Virol.*, **2**, 208–213.

Moody, M. R., Young, V. M., Kenton, D. M. & Vermeulen, G. D. (1972). *Pseudomonas aeruginosa* in a center for cancer research. I. Distribution of intraspecies types from human and environmental sources. *J. infect. Dis.*, **125**, 95–101.

Muraschi, T. F., Miller, J. K., Bolles, D. M. & Hedberg, M. (1966a). *Pseudomonas aeruginosa* serotypes encountered in hospitals in Albany, New York. *N. Y. St. J. Med.*, **66**, 3033–3035.

Muraschi, T. F., Bolles, D. M., Moczulski, C. & Lindsay, M. (1966b). Serologic types of *Pseudomonas aeruginosa* based on heat-stable O antigens: correlation of Habs' (European) and Verder and Evans' (North American) classifications. *J. infect. Dis.*, **116**, 84–88.

Mushin, R. & Ziv, G. (1973a). An epidemiological study of *Pseudomonas aeroginosa* in cattle and other animals by pyocine typing. *J. Hyg.*, **71**, 113–122.

Mushin, R. & Ziv, G. (1973b). Epidemiological aspects of *Pseudomonas aeruginosa* in man, animals and the environment. *Israel J. med. Sci.*, **9**, 155–161.

Naito, T., Koura, M. & Iwanaga, Y. (1972). Studies on pyocine typing of *Pseudomonas aeruginosa*. IV. Comparison of media, pyocine production and sensitivity to pyocine by different colonial types under parallel use of two typing methods. *Trop. Med. (Nagasaki)*, **14**, 71–85.

Naito, T., Koura, M. & Iwanaga, Y. (1973). Studies on pyocine typing of *Pseudomonas aeruginosa*. V. The first application and comparison of pyocines produced by different colonial types using isolates under parallel use of two typing methods. *Trop. Med. (Nagasaki)*, **15**, 46–55.

Neussel, H. (1971). Die Bedeutung der Pyocin-Typisierung bei Kontrollen des Verlaufes von Harnweginfektionen mit *Pseudomonas aeruginosa*. *Arzneimittel-Forsch.*, **21**, 333–335.

Nishimura, T., Takagi, M. & Kotani, Y. (1973). The identification and serological typing of *Pseudomonas aeruginosa* by fluorescent antibody technique. *Jap. J. exp Med.*, **43**, 43–45.

Nord, C.-E., Sjöberg, L. & Wadström, T. (1972). *Pseudomonas aeruginosa* in oral infections. *Acta odont. scand.*, **30**, 371–381.

O'Callaghan, R. J., O'Mara, W. & Grogan, J. B. (1969). Physical stability and biological and physicochemical properties of twelve *Pseudomonas aeruginosa* bacteriophages. *Virology.* **37**, 642–648.

Oeding, P. & Williams, R. E. O. (1958). The type classification of *Staphylococcus aureus*: a comparison of phage-typing with serological typing. *J. Hyg.*, **56**, 445–454.

Olsen, R. H., Metcalf, E. S. & Todd, J. K. (1968). Characteristics of bacteriophages attacking psychrophilic and mesophilic *Pseudomonas*. *J. Virol.*, **2**, 357–364.

Osman, M. A. M. (1965). Pyocine typing of *Pseudomonas aeruginosa*. *J. clin. Path.*, **18**, 200–202.

Papavassiliou, J. (1961). Actions antibiotiques reciproques chez *Pseudomonas aeruginosa*. *Arch. Inst. Pasteur Tunis.*, **38**, 57–63.

Paterson, A. C. (1965). Bacteriocinogeny and lysogeny in the genus *Pseudomonas. J. gen. Microbiol.*, **39**, 295–303.

Pavlatou, M. P. & Kaklamani, E. H. (1961). Recherches en vue d'une lysotypie des bacilles pyocyaniques. *Ann. Inst. Pasteur*, **101**, 914–927.

Pavlatou, M. & Kaklamani, E. (1962). Stabilité des lysotypes de *Pseudomonas pyocyanea in vivo* et *in vitro*. *Ann. Inst. Pasteur*, **102**, 300–308.

Phillips, I. (1966). Postoperative respiratory-tract infection with *Pseudomonas aeruginosa* due to contaminated lignocaine jelly. *Lancet*, **i**, 903–904.

Piguet, J. D. & Kékessy, D. A. (1972). Repartition de l'activité de phages de *Pseudomonas aeruginosa* sur des souches de différentes origines. *Progr. immunobiol. Standard*, **5**, 406–409.

Plehn, M. & Trommsdorff, R. (1916). *Bacterium salmonicida* und *Bacterium fluorescens*, zwei wohldifferenzierte Bakterienarten. *Zbl. Bakt., I. Abt. Orig.*, **78**, 142–157.

Postic, B. & Finland, M. (1961). Observations on bacteriophage typing of *Pseudomonas aeruginosa*. *J. clin. Invest.*, **40**, 2064–2075.

Potel, J. (1957). Versuche einer Lysotypie bei *Pseudomonas aeruginosa*. *Naturwissenschaften*, **44**, 332–333.

Rabin, E. R., Graber, C. D., Vogel, E. H., Finkelstein, R. A. & Tumbusch, W. A. (1961). Fatal *Pseudomonas* infection in burned patients—a clinical, bacteriologic and anatomic study. *New Engl. J. Med.*, **265**, 1225–1231.

Rose, H. D., Babock, J. B. & Heckman, M. G. (1971). Subtyping of pyocin type 1 *Pseudomonas aeruginosa*: one year of experience. *Appl. Microbiol.,*, **22**, p. 475.

Rouques, R., Vieu, J.-F., Mignon, F. & Leroux-Robert, C. (1969). Épidémiologie des infections a bacille pyocyanique (*Pseudomonas aeruginosa*) dans un centre de traitement de l'insuffisance rénale. *Presse med.*, **77**, 509–511.

Rubbo, S. D., Gardner, J. F. & Franklin, J. C. (1966). Source of *Pseudomonas aeruginosa* infection in premature infants. *J. Hyg.*, **64**, 121–128.

Sandvik, O. (1960a). The serology of *Pseudomonas aeruginosa* from bovine udder infections. *Acta vet. scand.*, **1**, 221–228.

Sandvik, O. (1960b). Serological comparison between strains of *Pseudomonas aeruginosa* from human and animal strains. *Acta. path. microbiol. scand.*, **48**, 56–60.

Shionoya, H., Goto, S., Tsukamoto, M. & Homma, J. Y. (1967). Relationship between pyocine and temperate phage of *Pseudomonas aeruginosa*. I. Isolation of temperate phages from strain. P1–III and their characteristics. *Jap. J. exp. Med.*, **37**, 359–372.
Shionoya, H. & Homma, J. Y. (1968). Dissociation in *Pseudomonas aeruginosa*. *Jap. J. exp. Med.*, **38**, 81–94.
Shooter, R. A. (1971). Changes of the infectious pool in the hospital with regard to *Pseudomonas aeruginosa* and *Escherichia coli*. In *Bacterial Infections. Changes in their Causative Agents. Trends and Possible Basis*, (Eds. M. Finland, W. Marget & K. Bartmann), Springer Verlag. Stuttgart, pp. 125–130.
Shooter, R. A. (1973). The hospital epidemiology of *Pseudomonas aeruginosa* and *Escherichia coli*. In *Brit. Encycl. med. Pract. Medical Progress*, Butterworths, London, pp. 47–53.
Shooter, R. A., Walker, K. A., Williams, V. R., Horgan, G. M., Parker, M. T., Asheshov, E. H. & Bullimore, J. F. (1966). Faecal carriage of *Pseudomonas aeruginosa* in hospital patients. Possible spread from patient to patient. *Lancet*, **ii**, 1331–1334.
Shooter, R. A., Faiers, M. C., Cooke, E. M., Breaden, A. L., O'Farrell, S. M. (1971). Isolation of *Escherichia coli*, *Pseudomonas aeruginosa*, and *Klebsiella* from food in hospitals, canteens, and schools. *Lancet*, **ii**, 390–392.
Sjöberg, L. & Lindberg, A. A. (1967). Phage and pyocine typing of *Pseudomonas aeruginosa*. *Acta path. microbiol. scand.*, **70**, 639–640.
Sjöberg, L. & Lindberg, A. A. (1968). Phage typing of *Pseudomonas aeruginosa*. *Acta path. microbiol. scand.*, **74**, 61–68.
Smith, H. W. (1948). Investigations on the typing of staphylococci by means of bacteriophage. II. The significance of lysogenic strains in staphylococcal type designation. *J. Hyg.*, **46**, 82–89.
Southern, P. M., Mays, B. B., Pierce, A. K. & Sanford, J. P. (1970). Pulmonary clearance of *Pseudomonas aeruginosa*. *J. Lab. clin. Med.*, **76**, 548–559.
Stewart, D. J. & Young, H. (1971). Factors affecting the adsorption of a pyocin by cells of *Pseudomonas aeruginosa*. *Microbios*, **3**, 15–22.
Stoodley, B. J. & Thom, B. T. (1970). Observations on the intestinal carriage of *Pseudomonas aeruginosa*. *J. med. Microbiol.*, **3**, 367–375.
Sutter, V. L. & Hurst, V. (1966). Sources of *Pseudomonas aeruginosa* infection in burns: study of wound and rectal cultures with phage typing. *Ann. Surg.*, **163**, 597–602.
Sutter, V. L., Hurst, V. & Fennell, J. (1965). A standardized system for phage typing *Pseudomonas aeruginosa*. *Hlth Lab. Sci.*, **2**, 7–16.
Sutter, V. L., Hurst, V., Grossman, M. & Calonje, R. (1966). Source and significance of *Pseudomonas aeruginosa* in sputum. Patients requiring tracheal suction. *J. Amer. med. Ass.*, **197**, 854–858.
Tagg, J. R. & Mushin, R. (1971). Epidemiology of *Pseudomonas aeruginosa* infection in hospitals. 1. Pyocin typing of *Pseudomonas aeruginosa*. *Med. J. Aust.*, **i**, 847–852.
Takeya, K., Mori, R., Ueda, S. & Toda, T. (1959). Bacteriophage of *Pseudomonas aeruginosa* with unfamiliar head morphology. *J. Bact.*, **78**, 332–335.
Terry, C. S.: PHD Thesis. University of Glasgow. 1972.
Thörne, H. & Kyrkjebø, A. (1966). Serological group differentiation of *Pseudomonas aeruginosa* from various sources. *Acta vet. scand.*, **7**, 289–295.
Verder, E. & Evans, J. (1961). A proposed antigenic schema for the identification of strains of *Pseudomonas aeruginosa*. *J. infect. Dis.*, **109**, 183–193.
Véron, M. (1961). Sur l'agglutination de *Pseudomonas aeruginosa*: subdivision des groupes antigéniques O:2 et O:5. *Ann. Inst. Pasteur*, **101**, 456–460.
Vieu, J.-F. (1969). La lysotypie et la pyocinotypie de *Pseudomonas aeruginosa*. Leur role dans l'épidémiologie des infections hospitalières. *Bull. Inst. Pasteur*, **67**, 1231–1249.
Wahba, A. H. (1963). The production and inactivation of pyocines. *J. Hyg.*, **61**, 431–441.

Wahba, A. H. (1965a). Pyocine typing of *Pseudomonas pyocyanea* and its relation to serological typing. *Zbl. Bakt., I. Abt. Orig.,* **196**, 389–394.

Wahba, A. H. (1965b). Hospital infection with *Pseudomonas pyocyanea*: an investigation by a combined pyocine and serological typing method. *Brit. med. J.,* **I**, 86–89.

Warner, P. T. J. C. P. (1950). The isolation of the bacteriophages of *Ps. pyocyanea. Brit. J. exp. Path.,* **31**, 112–129.

Whitby, J. L. & Rampling, A. (1972). *Pseudomonas aeruginosa* contamination in domestic and hospital environments. *Lancet,* **i**, 15–17.

Williams, R. J. & Govan, J. R. W. (1973). Pyocine typing of mucoid strains of *Pseudomonas aeruginosa* isolated from children with cystic fibrosis. *J. med. Microbiol.,* **6**, 409–412.

Williams, R. E. O. & Rippon, J. E. (1952). Bacteriophage typing of *Staphylococcus aureus. J. Hyg.,* **50**, 320–353.

Wokatsch, R. (1964). Serologische Untersuchungen an *Pseudomonas aeruginosa (Bact. pyocyaneum)* aus verschiedenen Tierarten. *Zbl. Bakt., I. Abt. Orig.,* **192**, 468–476.

Wretlind, B., Hedén, L., Sjöberg, L. & Wadström, T. (1973). Production of enzymes and toxins by hospital strains of *Pseudomonas aeruginosa* in relation to serotype and phage-typing pattern. *J. med. Microbiol.,* **6**, 91–100.

Yabuuchi, E., Miyajima, N., Hotta, H. & Furu, Y. (1971). Serological typing of 31 achromogenic and 40 melanogenic *Pseudomonas aeruginosa* strains. *Appl. Microbiol.,* **22**, 530–533.

Yamada, K. (1960). Studies on *Pseudomonas* phage (Phage typing for pseudomonas). *Mie. med. J.,* **10**, 359–365.

Yoshioka, H., Takimoto, M., Maruyama, S., Furuyama, M. & Murayama, T. (1970). Serotypes and antibiotic susceptibility of *Pseudomonas aeruginosa* isolated from clinical materials in the Hokkaido University Hospital 1967. *J. Jap. Ass. infect. Dis.,* **44**, 340–344.

Young, H. & Stewart, D. J. (1971). A turbidimetric method for the assay of pyocin activity. *J. gen. Microbiol.,* **68**, 227–230.

Zabransky, R. J. & Day, F. E. (1967). Pyocine typing of clinical strains of *Pseudomonas aeruginosa. Bact. Proc.,* p. 97.

Zabransky, R. J. & Day, F. E. (1969). Pyocine typing of clinical strains of *Pseudomonas aeruginosa. Appl. Microbiol.,* **17**, 293–296.

Zanen, H. C. & van den Berge, M. (1963). Een epidemie van *Pseudomonas aeruginosa*-infecties, opgehelderd met behulp van faagtypering. *Nederl. T. Geneesk.,* **107**, 1700–1703.

Zierdt, C. H. & Schmidt, P. J. (1964). Dissociation in *Pseudomonas aeruginosa. J. Bact.,* **87**, 1003–1010.

Ziv, G., Mushin, R. & Tagg, J. R. (1971). Pyocine typing as an epidemiological marker in *Pseudomonas aeruginosa* mastitis in cattle. *J. Hyg.,* **69**, 171–177.

CHAPTER 7

Treatment and Prophylaxis for *Pseudomonas* Infections

E. J. L. LOWBURY and R. J. JONES

INTRODUCTION

Chemotherapy for pseudomonas infection presents a number of difficulties which arise both from the nature of infection with this organism and from limitations of the antibiotics. *Pseudomonas aeruginosa* has little or no pathogenic activity against healthy adults or tissues with good antimicrobial resistance. In persons or tissues with poor resistance, however, it can play the part of an 'opportunist' pathogen, causing severe and potentially fatal sepsis (Lowbury, 1975); under these circumstances, antibiotics used for treatment of invasive infections are poorly supported, or completely unsupported, by the humoral and cellular host defences which complement therapeutic action in

237

patients whose defences are normal. Moreover, the organisms tend to colonize dead or devitalized tissue (e.g. the slough of burns) in which the access of circulating antibiotic to the site of infection is prevented, or at least restricted. As regards the availability of effective antibiotics, only three—polymyxin, gentamicin and carbenicillin, including near homologues—have clinically relevant activity against most strains of *P. aeruginosa*, and in each case there are factors which limit the effectiveness of the antibiotic in therapy. The narrow range and limited value of chemotherapy for *P. aeruginosa* have been major factors in determining the emergence of this species as an opportunist pathogen, especially in hospitals where the use of antibiotics exerts a selection-pressure favouring the resistant flora.

Because of these limitations of chemotherapy it is important that the clinician should have alternative methods for controlling infection with the organism. Prevention, when possible, is preferable to cure, and in the case of some pseudomonas infections it is also more likely to succeed. The factors which limit the usefulness of chemotherapy also limit the potential value of chemoprophylaxis, but a number of other prophylactic measures are available, including asepsis, protective isolation, topical chemoprophylaxis and the use of immunological methods; topical application of antimicrobial agents and injection of specific immunoglobulins or antisera may also have a role in the treatment of established infection.

This chapter is concerned with the treatment and prophylaxis of pseudomonas infection and, in particular, with the problems arising out of antibiotic resistance. We consider the ways in which antibiotics active *in vitro* against *P. aeruginosa* may fail to achieve therapeutic effects, the emergence of resistant variants, the ways in which the emergence of such variants may be prevented, and how a reversion to sensitivity among strains colonizing patients in a ward can sometimes be obtained. We also discuss the avoidance of antibiotics and preservation of their sensitivity by use of other measures of treatment and prophylaxis, in particular the use of immunological methods for the control of pseudomonas infection.

TREATMENT

Chemotherapy

Sensitivity of P. aeruginosa *to Antibiotics*

In vitro sensitivity tests are designed to show the probable effectiveness or ineffectiveness of antibiotics in the treatment of infected patients. In practice, a strain is considered sensitive to an antibiotic if the minimal inhibitory concentration (M.I.C.), as shown by a tube or plate *dilution test*, is exceeded by the concentration of the antibiotic in the serum of a patient under treatment for and appreciable part of the interval between doses. This is an approximation, because the level of antibiotic in tissue fluid is normally lower than that in the blood (Chisholm *et al.*, 1973), and some tissues, especially the central nervous system, may receive very little of the circulating antibiotic; the kidney, by contrast, excretes many of the antibiotics (including polymyxin, gentamicin and carbenicillin) at higher concentration in the urine than the concentration present in the blood. If local chemotherapy is used, still higher concentrations may be brought in contact with infecting bacteria, and strains may be sensitive to an antibiotic administered locally though resistant to the same antibiotic given by the systemic route. The definitive knowledge about sensitivity or resistance, in a clinical sense, comes from assessment of the results of therapy against infection with strains of known *in vitro* sensitivity, by which the *in vitro* test criteria can be confirmed or adjusted.

The usual way of assessing sensitivity of bacteria in a clinical microbiology laboratory is by a *diffusion test*, in which zones of inhibition of growth on agar plates around discs containing a measured quantity of the antibiotic are compared with those obtained with a 'control' strain of known sensitivity (M.I.C.). By the use of a calibration curve a presumptive M.I.C. can be calculated from the zone of inhibition, provided standard conditions are used for the test (Ericsson & Sherris, 1971); it is more usual, however, for a less quantitative type of diffusion test to be used. For reasons discussed below, the direct measurement of M.I.C. from dilution tests is advantageous in assessments of the sensitivity of *P. aeruginosa* to the three main antibiotics active against this organism. Assessments of bactericidal action are desirable before selecting a drug for treatment of septicaemia or endocarditis; this can be roughly assessed by subculture from the tubes in a tube dilution test, or more accurately by Chabbert's cellophane transfer technique (see Garrod *et al.*, 1973). Since polymyxin, gentamicin and carbenicillin are predominantly bactericidal in action, the minimal inhibitory concentration gives a useful presumptive index of bactericidal activity.

All strains of *P. aeruginosa* are resistant *in vitro* to benzyl penicillin, ampicillin, methicillin and cloxacillin, the cephalosporins, the macrolides, lincomycin and clindamycin, novobiocin, vancomycin and fusidic acid, and usually also to chloramphenicol, the sulphonamides, trimethoprim, nitrofurantoin and nalidixic acid. Some strains are moderately sensitive to streptomycin, kanamycin (also neomycin) and tetracycline, but the M.I.C. is usually too high for effective therapy except, sometimes, in urinary tract infection. The polymyxins (including colistin), gentamicin and tobramycin, and carbenicillin are usually active enough to have potential value in therapy of *P. aeruginosa* infection, as judged by the M.I.C. of *P. aeruginosa* and the blood levels of the antibiotics which can normally be obtained under systemic therapy. If a single antibiotic is used, the last three are the only agents from which useful results may often be expected, but combinations of other agents may have some value, and the combination of gentamicin with carbenicillin is probably the most effective chemotherapy available for pseudomonas infections.

The Polymyxins

General. These antibiotics were first obtained from aerobic sporing bacilli (*Bacillus polymyxa*) by three independent groups of workers in the same year

(Ainsworth, Brown & Brownlee, 1947; Benedict & Langlykke, 1947; Stansly, Shepherd & White, 1947). They have been identified as basic deca-peptides containing a seven-membered ring with an α-connected side chain ending in a fatty acid (Vogler & Studer, 1966). Five fractions (A, B, C, D and E) are described; fractions A, C and D are too toxic for use in chemotherapy, but fractions B and E have been extensively used. Colistin ('Colomycin'), which was described in Japan by Koyama and others (1950), was subsequently found to be identical with polymyxin E (Suzuki *et al.*, 1964).

The polymyxins are 'narrow-spectrum' antibiotics, with predominantly bactericidal action against a wide range of Gram-negative bacilli, but inactive against the Proteus group; Gram-positive bacteria and fungi are also resistant. All strains of *P. aeruginosa* are sensitive or relatively sensitive by *in vitro* tests, with M.I.C.s commonly in the range of 0.1 to 3.0 μg (1 to 30 units) per ml, and less than 10 μg per ml (Jawetz, 1956; Florey, 1960; Adler & Finland, 1971). The antibiotic causes disruption of bacterial cells with loss of nuclear material and of cytoplasmic granularity (Chapman, 1962), associated with injury to the cell membrane (Newton, 1956).

As polymyxins are not absorbed from the intestine, the drug must be injected for systemic use. Polymyxin B or E may be injected by the intramuscular route either as the sulphate or as the sulphomethyl compound, the latter being less toxic but also less active than the sulphate (Nord & Hoeprich, 1964; O'Grady & Pennington, 1967). The most serious toxic effect is damage to the renal tubular epithelium, which can be prevented by avoidance of overdosage and control of dose in relation to creatinine clearance in treatment of patients who already have impaired renal function (Atuk *et al.*, 1964). Minor neurotoxic effects may occur, especially tingling around the mouth and dizziness. The sulphomethyl polymyxins dissociate in the body into more active antimicrobial compounds (Beveridge & Martin, 1967). In both mouse and dog, sulphomethyl colistin (colistin sulphomethate) is shown to be the least toxic of the polymyxin products (Vinnicombe & Stamey, 1969; Nord & Hoeprich, 1964); on intramuscular injections at a dosage of 4 mg per kg body weight, it gives a peak serum level of 17–25 μg per ml in a human adult: i.e. appreciably higher than the M.I.C. range for *P. aeruginosa*.

Clinical use. In spite of their promising *in vitro* activity and the attainment of effective blood levels after intramuscular injection, treatment of severe *P. aeruginosa* infection with polymyxins has been disappointing. This is especially true in the case of septicaemic infections. For example, Forkner *et al.* (1958) reported 22 out of 23 cases of pseudomonas septicaemia which had a fatal outcome in spite of treatment with polymyxin. Markley *et al.* (1957) and Tumbusch *et al.* (1961) also reported failure in treatment of pseudomonas septicaemia in patients with burns. Jones, Jackson & Lowbury (1966) had better results in a series of 10 patients with pseudomonas septicaemia; 4 of these patients survived, all having received colistin sulphomethate (1 gram per day), while only one of the 6 patients who died had been treated with the drug. Fekety, Norman & Cluff (1962) have also reported successful treatment with colistin sulphomethate for pseudomonas septicaemia. In the series of Jones *et al.* (1966), a patient died in spite of the clearance of *P. aeruginosa* from the blood and the burns while under treatment with colistin sulphomethate. At autopsy, meningitis was found, but very few bacteria were isolated from the meningeal lesions; it seemed likely that the patient had already suffered irreparable damage at the time when septicaemia was diagnosed and chemotherapy started. Tumbusch *et al.* (1961) have suggested that successful chemotherapy may, in fact, precipitate an exacerbation of symptoms by the release of endotoxin from the killed organisms into the circulation, causing a local and general Schwartzman reaction.

In other types of infection with *P. aeruginosa* treatment with polymyxin has been found to have some value. Manoukian (1953) has reported successful treatment of a case of pseudomonas osteomyelitis with local and systemic polymyxin. Meningitis has been successfully treated with combined intramuscular and intrathecal administration of polymyxin (Hayes & Yow, 1950; Jawetz, 1952; Trapnell, 1954). Successful treatment has also been recorded in urinary tract infection; e.g. Pulaski & Rosenberg (1949) reported successful clearance, by polymyxin in intramuscular dosage of 2·0 to 5·6 mg per kg per day, of *P. aeruginosa* from the urine in 10 out of 10 patients who had urinary tract infections with pure cultures of the organism; 8 of the patients had clinical recovery. Good results are also reported by Rodger, Nixon and Tonning (1965) and Brumfitt, Black & Williams (1966). In chronic urinary tract infections recurrences must be expected. Chest infections have usually responded poorly to polymyxin therapy, probably because there was some functional or structural abnormality of the respiratory tract (Kagan *et al.*, 1951; Jawetz, 1956). Pines and others (1970) used a large dosage of colistin (4–6 million units per day by intramuscular injection and 2–4 million units per day by aerosol inhalation) in 13 patients with chronic purulent bronchial infections; treatment failed in all the patients, and bronchial inhalation was not well tolerated. Local treatment with a polymyxin cream has been found in a controlled trial to have some value in treatment of infected burns (Jackson, Lowbury & Topley, 1951); it has also been reported to have therapeutic value in infected surgical wounds (Jawetz, 1956), pleural cavities and joints (Jawetz, 1952). Corneal ulcers infected with *P. aeruginosa* have been successfully treated with subconjunctional injection of polymyxin B, 20–25 mg per day (Ainslie, 1953; Fraser, 1953). Pseudomonas infections of the external ear have been effectively treated with a solution containing 10% polymyxin B sulphate in propylene glycol, acidified with acetic acid (Farrar, 1954).

The use of polymyxin in combination with other antimicrobial agents is discussed below.

Resistance. By gradual habituation to polymyxin *in vitro, P. aeruginosa* can acquire high degrees of resistance; e.g. Jawetz & Coleman (1949) showed that 14 daily transfers of large inocula in subinhibitory concentrations of polymyxin B led to a thousandfold increase in resistance; Hirsch, McCarthy & Finland (1960) have shown *in vitro* habituation to polymyxin B and colistin, with complete cross-resistance to these antibiotics. Brown, Fenton & Watkins (1972) obtained increases in M.I.C. of polymyxin from 10 to 20,000 units per ml, with cross-resistance to carbenicillin, gentamicin and several membrane-active agents; the polymyxin-resistant variants were found to have an increased sensitivity to tetracycline, chloramphenicol and erythromycin. Brown & Melling (1969) have shown that high degrees of resistance to polymyxin can be obtained by growing *P. aeruginosa* in a magnesium-deficient medium; on subculture to a standard culture medium these strains reverted to sensitivity (see also Chapter 3).

Resistance to polymyxin acquired *in vitro* probably has no relevance to the clinical situation, in which strains of *P. aeruginosa* have retained their sensitivity in hospital environments where the antibiotic has been much used. For example, Jackson *et al.* (1951) found no emergence of more resistant strains during two years at the Birmingham Accident Hospital while polymyxin was used on many patients. In the same hospital eighteen years later, Lowbury and others (1969) found no increase in polymyxin resistance of strains isolated from burns over a period of three years, the mean M.I.Cs being in the same range as those of strains isolated in the 1950s. There was a small reduction in the mean M.I.C. between 1966 and 1969, probably due to the displacement of polymyxin by carbenicillin and gentamicin for treatment of most pseudomonas infections.

Though resistance of *P. aeruginosa* to the polymyxins, as shown by raised M.I.C., has not emerged in hospital patients, there is a degree of 'therapeutic resistance', as shown by the failure of these drugs to achieve effective therapy of severe infections even when the infecting organisms were judged sensitive by *in vitro* tests. Mouse protection tests, in which mice were challenged by inoculation of *P. aeruginosa* on to experimental burns, showed that colistin sulphomethate, unlike gentamicin and carbenicillin, did not prevent invasive infection and death (Jones & Lowbury, 1967). Therapeutic resistance may be caused, in part, by poor penetration to sites of infection by the large polymyxin molecule; partly, also, to the appreciable inhibition of polymyxin by serum, and to the fact that rapid invasion, causing irreparable damage to the patient, is likely to have occurred at the time when treatment is started—a difficulty which would apply to any antibiotic. Another factor of possibly greater importance is the inactivation of polymyxin by the tissues, because the antibiotic is bound to the phospholipids of tissue cell membranes, as it is to phospholipids of bacterial cells (Kunin & Bugg, 1971).

Combined action of polymyxin with other antibiotics. Polymyxin has often been used topically in combination with neomycin and bacitracin or with tetracycline to obtain a wider range of activity against the bacteria of mixed infections in wounds, in the intestine or in the urinary tract. Potentiation of the bactericidal activity of colistin by sulphamethoxazole has been demonstrated by Simmons (1969) in 19 out of 20 strains of *P. aeruginosa*: neither carbenicillin nor gentamicin showed synergy with these sulphonamides. Trimethoprim, which has poor activity against *P. aeruginosa*, shows synergy with sulphamethoxazole, and the combination was apparently effective in the treatment of a patient with pseudomonas infection of the urinary tract (Grüneberg & Kolbe, 1969). Cox & Harrison (1971) compared a mixture of polymyxin and kanamycin with gentamicin alone in the treatment of pseudomonas bacteraemia; the former caused eradication of the infection in 4/5, the latter in 15/15 cases. Potentiation of polymyxin by other compounds, e.g. the non-ionic surface-active compound polysorbate (Brown & Winsley, 1971) and ethylenediaminetetraacetic acid (EDTA) (Brown & Richards, 1965), suggests directions in which chemotherapy with polymyxin might be developed.

Gentamicin

General. Between 1947 and 1963 polymyxin was the sole antibiotic of choice for the treatment of pseudomonas infections. In 1963 gentamicin, an antibiotic highly active against *P. aeruginosa*, was introduced (Weinstein *et al.*, 1963); tobramycin, a closely related compound with slightly greater activity against *P. aeruginosa*, was introduced some years later (Meyer, Young & Armstrong, 1971).

Gentamicin is a member of the aminoglycoside group of antibiotics, produced by a strain of *Micromonospora purpurea*. It has a broad spectrum of activity against Gram-positive and Gram-negative organisms, in many ways similar to that of kanamycin and neomycin, but differing in various respects: e.g. in the absence of cross-resistance to gentamicin of naturally occurring neomycin or kanamycin-resistant staphylococci (though cross-resistance does occur when strains are habituated *in vitro* to gentamicin: Klein, Eickhoff and Finland, 1964). Gentamicin is active against a wider range of Gram-negative bacilli than any of the other antibiotics. It is 5 to 10 times more active than kanamycin against most strains of *P. aeruginosa*, the M.I.C. usually being in the range of $0 \cdot 1$ to $2 \cdot 0$ μg per ml. (Klein *et al.*, 1964; Barber & Waterworth, 1966; Jones & Lowbury, 1967); the M.I.C. varies with the magnesium content of the medium (Garrod & Waterworth, 1969) and the wide range of reported sensitivities of *P. aeruginosa* strains to gentamicin reflects the varied magnesium content of media used for the tests. Sensitivity tests should be done in a medium with a magnesium content similar to that of blood or tissue fluids, i.e. about 2 mg per 100 ml. Gentamicin has bactericidal activity at two to three times the minimal inhibitory concentration.

Like the other aminoglycosides, gentamicin is not absorbed from the intestine and must therefore be given parenterally (usually by intramuscular injection) for systemic treatment. If the dosage is raised above a critical level, giving a serum level of 10 μg per ml or more, gentamicin is likely to have ototoxic effects, the main damage being to the vestibular branch of the eighth cranial nerve, though minor degrees of deafness, especially to higher frequencies, may also occur. An adult dosage of 80 mg eight-hourly is found to give therapeutic blood levels consistent with safety (Gingell & Waterworth, 1968). With this dosage, bacteristatic blood levels can usually be maintained over a period of 4–6 hr, with an average peak concentration of 7 μg per ml at about

1 hr after injection; the peak level is independent of renal function, but if renal function is impaired, the fall in serum level is delayed. It is important that blood levels should be measured in patients who have renal failure, so that dosage can be adjusted to active but safe levels; to achieve such conditions, the individual dose injected should be the same as in patients with normally functioning kidneys, but with a longer interval between doses. Gingell & Waterworth (1968) have proposed a dosage schedule by reference to blood urea and creatinine clearance; e.g. with blood urea over 200 mg per 100 ml and creatinine clearance less than 3 ml per min, it is suggested that 80 mg of gentamicin should be given every 40 hr. A rapid assay method (e.g. Noone, Pattison & Samson, 1971) is useful.

Chisholm and others (1968) have shown, in experimental animals, that gentamicin is distributed rapidly and uniformly throughout the blood and lymph, but is concentrated in the urine. Over 80% of the gentamicin injected can be recovered within 24 hr from the urine, in which a concentration of about 200 μg per ml may be present 1 hr after a dose of 0·8 mg per Kg body weight (Black *et al.*, 1963); lower levels occur in some patients (Bulger, Sidell & Kirby, 1963). Barber & Waterworth (1966) have shown that gentamicin is sixteen times more active in alkaline than in acid or neutral urine.

Clinical use.   Stone *et al.* (1965b) report the survival of 10 out of 13 patients with severe burns and pseudomonas septicaemia following treatment with gentamicin: the antibiotic was given systemically for 14 to 16 days and applied locally in an ointment containing gentamicin at a concentration of 0·1%. Good results in the treatment of pseudomonas infection of burns with topical and systemic gentamicin are also reported by Müller (1967). Cox & Harrison (1971) report 15 out of 15 successful eradications by gentamicin of *P. aeruginosa* in patients with bacteraemia. The findings of Jackson (1967) in the treatment of *P. aeruginosa* bacteraemia were less satisfactory; he reported 1 out of 8 cases in which there was a cure, in contrast with 8 out of 9 cures of bacteraemia caused by *E. coli*.

Urinary tract infections with *P. aeruginosa* have been successfully treated with gentamicin, sometimes when other antibiotics have failed. For example, Bulger *et al.* (1963) report 18 out of 23 patients successfully treated for such infections, several of which were severe and complicated. Klein *et al.* (1964), Brayton & Louria (1964) and Jao & Jackson (1964) also report successful therapy for pseudomonas infection of the urinary tract. A proportion of failures occurred where the underlying condition hindered chemotherapy.

Other severe pseudomonas infections have also been successfully treated with gentamicin. Klein *et al.* (1964) reported the cure of pseudomonas meningitis in an infant after the failure of treatment with polymyxin. Suppurative bronchitis was reported by Brun, Perrin-Fayelle & Sedaillan (1967) to have been successfully treated with gentamicin after the failure of other antibiotics: however, Pines and co-workers (1970) obtained only marginal improvement in a series of 28 patients with severe pseudomonas infections of the bronchi treated with gentamicin by systemic administration and by aerosol;

better results were obtained by these workers with carbenicillin alone or combined with gentamicin (see below). Local treatment for pseudomonas infection of wounds and burns has been favourably reported (Stone, Martin & Kolb, 1965).

Resistance. Resistance of *P. aeruginosa* to gentamicin has been obtained with some difficulty on habituation *in vitro*. Different strains have shown different results; e.g. Barber & Waterworth (1966) passaged four strains daily on a ditch plate containing gentamicin; two showed an eightfold and two a thirty-twofold increase in resistance after 20 transfers. Graber *et al.* (1963) tested 8 strains of different phage type; after ten transfers on nutrient agar containing subinhibitory concentrations of gentamicin, seven strains showed no increase in resistance and one showed a two-fold increase. Jones & Lowbury (1967) found that resistant strains obtained on habituation *in vitro* were small colony variants with diminished virulence for mice challenged by inoculation of experimental burns.

The clinical importance of resistance obtained by habituation *in vitro* is uncertain. Because toxic effects are likely to occur when the blood level of gentamicin exceeds about $10 \mu g$ per ml, strains with a minimal inhibitory concentration of $10 \mu g$ per ml or more must be considered resistant, and an M.I.C. of $5 \mu g$ per ml would indicate marginal sensitivity. Strains described in early reports on the antibiotic include some which, by these criteria, were marginally sensitive or even resistant (Weinstein *et al.*, 1963; Graber *et al.*, 1963). Out of 135 isolates of *P. aeruginosa*, Jackson (1967) reported five with M.I.Cs of $40 \mu g$ per ml. Stone (1971) reports the emergence and subsequent predominance of gentamicin-resistant *P. aeruginosa* in the flora of many burns late in the course of treatment. A small proportion of gentamicin-resistant *P. aeruginosa* has been found by the authors in the Burns Unit of the Birmingham Accident Hospital; the M.I.C. of these strains has been in the range of 16 to 32 μg per ml gentamicin (the most sensitive strains were found to have an M.I.C. of $1 \mu g$ per ml).

Witchitz & Chabbert (1972) have described 26 strains of Gram-negative bacilli, isolated from patients in an intensive care unit in Paris, which were resistant to gentamicin at concentrations ranging from 16 to 256 μg per ml; the resistance to gentamicin and associated resistance to ampicillin, chloramphenicol and sulphonamides were transferable from those bacteria, which included *P. aeruginosa*, by conjugation to a sensitive recipient strain of *E. coli* K12 and by transduction from *E. coli* K12 to suitable recipients; among the organisms which received the R-factor determining this resistance were *E. coli, Proteus mirabilis* and Providencia. Gentamicin-resistant strains of *P. aeruginosa* isolated at Birmingham Accident Hospital have failed to transfer resistance to a sensitive *E. coli* K12.

Tobramycin, an antibiotic closely related to gentamicin, is reported by Meyer, Young & Armstrong (1971) and Traub & Raymond (1972) to have about twice the activity of gentamicin against *P. aeruginosa*; it was found to be slightly less active than gentamicin against *Serratia marcescens*. Brzezinska *et al.* (1972) describe strains of *P. aeruginosa* which are resistant to gentamicin but sensitive to tobramycin; the difference between the antibiotics in this respect is associated with inactivation of gentamicin, but not of tobramycin, by an enzyme which causes acetylation of the 3-amino group in the 2-deoxy-streptamine moiety of the antibiotic. Combined use of gentamicin with other antibiotics is discussed below.

Carbenicillin

General. This antibiotic, disodium–carboxybenzyl penicillin, is a semi-synthetic, broad-spectrum penicillin, sensitive to penicillinase, and unique among the penicillins in its activity against *P. aeruginosa* (Knudsen, Rolinson & Sutherland, 1967). Carbenicillin is acid-sensitive and must be given by parenteral routes (especially intravenous infusion, because of the large dosages required); an acid-stable derivative, indanyl carbenicillin, which is suitable for treatment of urinary tract infections, has been developed (English, Retsema, Ray & Lynch, 1972).

Though a small proportion of strains of *P. aeruginosa* are highly sensitive to carbenicillin, the great majority are only moderately sensitive, the M.I.C. at the time when the antibiotic was introduced being usually in the range of 25 to 50 μg per ml. (Brumfitt *et al.*, 1967; Jones & Lowbury, 1967). Like all penicillins, this antibiotic is bactericidal. Though in some later reports (e.g. Smith & Finland, 1968) most strains continued to show a similar sensitivity range, other workers report a higher incidence of insensitive strains; e.g. Bodey & Terrell (1968) found that only 4% of their isolates were inhibited by 50 μg per ml carbenicillin, and referred to strains with M.I.Cs of 200 and 400 μg per ml. Other Gram-negative bacilli, e.g. *Escherichia* and *Proteus* spp., are usually more sensitive to carbenicillin than *P. aeruginosa*, but Klebsiella is commonly resistant or relatively resistant.

Like other penicillins, carbenicillin is remarkably free from toxic effects, apart from sensitization reactions which it shares with the related antibiotics. It is therefore usually safe to treat patients with very large doses of carbenicillin, so that blood levels active against *P. aeruginosa* may be reached. A dosage of 20 to 30 grams (or 500–750 mg per kg body weight) per day, given intermittently in an intravenous infusion, produces blood levels of 200 to 400 μg per ml, which can be enhanced by simultaneous treatment with probenecid to reduce renal excretion of the drug. Several patients receiving such large dosages have been found to develop temporary bleeding disorders, with epistaxis, petechiae, a prolonged bleeding time and reduced platelet adhesiveness and aggregation (McLure *et al.*, 1970); in general, however, large dosage of carbenicillin by intravenous infusion is well tolerated. The antibiotic is stable and more active in acid than alkaline pH. It is excreted by the kidneys, and high urine concentrations are obtained when relatively small doses (e.g. 4 to 8 grams per day) are given by intramuscular injection. Ticarcillin (AB2288) is an antibiotic closely related to carbenicillin with slightly greater activity (Lynn, 1973).

Clinical use.   Though carbenicillin is active against a wide range of bacteria, it has been used mainly for the treatment of infection with *P. aeruginosa*. Brumfitt *et al.* (1967) reported successful treatment for *E. coli* and Proteus infections of the urinary tract with a relatively small dosage of carbenicillin, but only 2 out of 7 patients with *P. aeruginosa* infection responded to such treatment. Van Rooyen *et al.* (1967) found that a large dosage of carbenicillin was successful in the treatment of 4 patients with extensive burns infected with *P. aeruginosa*. Jones & Lowbury (1967) found that carbenicillin and gentamicin, unlike colistin, protected mice against invasion by *P. aeruginosa* from experimental burns: they also obtained evidence that systemic use of carbenicillin with probenecid could remove *P. aeruginosa* from burns in some patients; an effect which may have been helped by simultaneous topical chemoprophylaxis with silver nitrate and other agents. Eickhoff & Marks (1970) report two cures in a series of 6 cases of pseudomonas septicaemia; results of treatment for lower respiratory infections were disappointing. Pines *et al.* (1970) report successful treatment of chronic pseudomonas infection of the bronchi with carbenicillin; gentamicin, by contrast, gave poor results in such patients.

Since Brumfitt *et al.* (1967), Smith *et al.* (1969) and Sonne & Jawetz (1969) showed synergy of carbenicillin with gentamicin, this combination has been widely used and found effective in the treatment of severe pseudomonas infections. Cooper, Rice & Penfold (1969) reported successful treatment with this combination for pseudomonas infections, including two with septicaemia. Good results are also reported by Smith *et al.* (1970) and Eickhoff & Marks (1970). McLaughlin and Reeves (1971) have reported that the antimicrobial activity of gentamicin was antagonized by carbenicillin *in vitro*, and possibly also *in vivo*, when large doses of carbenicillin were given with gentamicin to patients with normal renal function, or when moderate doses were given to patients with renal failure; if the infecting organism of a patient under treatment is sensitive to gentamicin only, treatment might, in these circumstances, fail. But since the inactivation of gentamicin by carbenicillin is slow, it is unlikely to occur *in vivo* during therapy, or to interfere with synergy of the two drugs. Riff & Jackson (1971) have pointed out that, with normal kidney function, the renal elimination of gentamicin given intravenously is considerably faster than the inactivation of gentamicin by carbenicillin at 37 °C. What must be avoided is continuous infusion of mixed carbenicillin and gentamicin (see Eykyn, Phillips & Ridley, 1971; Noone & Pattison, 1971). Combined therapy, though not proven to be superior to the use of gentamicin or carbenicillin alone, is rational, and may be valuable not only because of synergy, but also by covering a wider range of organisms and, possibly, by preventing the emergence of mutants resistant to one of the agents (see Lowbury & Ayliffe, 1974).

Resistance. With few exceptions, normal strains of *P. aeruginosa* are no more than moderately sensitive to carbenicillin; the range of M.I.Cs is much above the blood levels which could be safely allowed with most antibiotics, notably gentamicin and the other aminoglycosides. A slight increase in resistance of a strain with an M.I.C. of 50 μg per ml would render it clinically resistant, because blood levels much above 200 μg per ml cannot be obtained with the largest practicable dosage.

Resistant variants of *P. aeruginosa* have been obtained by 'training' *in vitro*, but these were small colony variants with reduced virulence for burned mice (Jones & Lowbury, 1967; Van Rooyen *et al.*, 1967). Jones & Lowbury also found evidence of the emergence of some strains with increased carbenicillin resistance during treatment of patients with pseudomonas infection of burns; though the increases were small, they might have been clinically significant.

Increases in the proportion of strains with higher M.I.Cs of carbenicillin were reported from several centres in the years following the introduction of carbenicillin. Bodey & Terrell's (1968) findings reported above showed a majority of *P. aeruginosa* strains to be resistant in clinical terms. Resistant strains which retained their mouse virulence were obtained on habituation *in vitro* by Bell & Smith in 1969. In the same year there were several reports on the isolation of highly carbenicillin-resistant *P. aeruginosa* from patients (Darrell & Waterworth, 1969; Lowbury *et al.*, 1969; Black & Girdwood, 1969; Newsom, 1969).

The strains isolated by Lowbury *et al.* (1969) in the Burns Unit of the Birmingham Accident Hospital were highly resistant to carbenicillin (M.I.C. 4000 μg per ml) and produced a carbenicillin-inactivating enzyme ('carbenicillinase'). They first appeared in March 1969, after three years during which many patients had been treated with the antibiotic and all isolates of *P. aeruginosa* had been tested for sensitivity to carbenicillin. The first highly resistant strains were of two different phage and serotypes, and these were found at almost the same time in burns previously colonized with carbenicillin-sensitive *P. aeruginosa* of the same types (see Table 1). For this reason it seemed likely that the high-level carbenicillin resistance was determined by an R-factor, a view supported by the instability of resistance of these strains on subculture, especially in the presence of an acridine dye.

Table 1. Emergence of carbenicillin-resistant *P. aeruginosa* carrying R-factor RP$_1$ in a burns unit

	P. aeruginosa in burns			
Patient	Carbenicillin-sensitive		Carbenicillin-resistant with (RP$_1$)	
	Date	Phage type	Date	Phage type
A	4 Feb. 1969	44/F8/109/119X/1214	3 March 1969	44/F8/109/119X/1214
B	28 Feb. 1969	7/21/68/119X	4 March 1969	7/21/119X

The first isolates of carbenicillin-resistant *P. aeruginosa* carrying the R-factor RP$_1$ were from patients A and B, each being of a different phage type. Carbenicillin sensitive *P. aeruginosa* of the same phage type had previously been isolated from these burns.

Transfer of carbenicillin resistance from these strains to *E. coli* K12 was demonstrated by Sykes & Richmond (1970) and by Fullbrook, Elson & Slocombe (1970). Resistance determined by the R-factor (RP₁) present in these bacteria was associated with a β-lactamase substrate profile of a type (R_{TEM}) found among Enterobacteria and different from that of the enzymes commonly produced by *P. aeruginosa*. R_{TEM} enzyme and 'carbenicillinase' activity were also found in the strains isolated by Black & Girdwood (1969). Two other highly resistant strains, one reported by Newsom (1969) and Newsom, Sykes & Richmond (1970), the other by Jephcott, Lowbury & Richmond (1973), showed enzyme substrate profiles which were different from those of *E. coli* R_{TEM} and did not transfer carbenicillin resistance to *E. coli.*

The clinical role of the R-factor RP₁ was shown by experience in the Birmingham Burns Unit, where carbenicillin-sensitive strains of *P. aeruginosa* were largely replaced by highly resistant strains within a few weeks of their first appearance (see Figure 1). A linked resistance to tetracycline, kanamycin, carbenicillin, ampicillin and cephaloridine (resistance pattern TKCACe) was transferred by the R-factor from *P. aeruginosa*/R to *E. coli* K12/S, from *E. coli* K12/R to *P. aeruginosa*/S and from various Enterobacteria (including Proteus spp. & Klebsiella spp.) present in burns to sensitive *E. coli* K12 or *P. aeruginosa*: such transfers could be demonstrated in experimental mouse burns (Roe, Jones & Lowbury, 1971). A large proportion of the Enterobacteria isolated from burns carried the R-factor, and an unusually large proportion of the Proteus spp and *E. coli* were found to be resistant to kanamycin and ampicillin (Roe & Lowbury, 1972). Though organisms carrying the R-factor RP₁ spread vigorously in the Burns Unit, they were not found in other wards of the same Hospital; a study on Klebsiella and Proteus spp and *P. aeruginosa* from 11 other hospitals in England, Scotland and Wales showed only one centre, a burns unit in Scotland, where an R-factor determining the resistance pattern TKCACe was present; it was present in both Proteus and Pseudomonas (Ayliffe, Lowbury & Roe, 1972).

Attempts to clear the Birmingham Burns Unit of *P. aeruginosa* carrying the R-factor by stopping the use of carbenicillin were apparently successful, but Enterobacteria carrying the R-factor continued to be prevalent, selected by the use of antibiotics other than carbenicillin in the pattern TKCACe, to which they were commonly sensitive; these other antibiotics were usually inactive against *P. aeruginosa*, so their use exerted no selection pressure in favour of this organism. On two occasions carbenicillin treatment for sensitive pseudomonas infection led to the prompt appearance in the same burns of highly resistant *P. aeruginosa* of the same phage type, apparently through the emergence, by selection, of *P. aeruginosa* which had received the R-factor RP₁ from Enterobacteria (Klebsiella or Proteus) colonizing the same burns (Lowbury, Babb & Roe, 1972; Ingram *et al.*, 1973). The clearance of Enterobacteria, as well as *P. aeruginosa*, carrying the R-factor was clearly essential if carbenicillin was to be effectively used in treatment, and this could be achieved only by banning or severely restricting the use of tetracycline, kanamycin, ampicillin

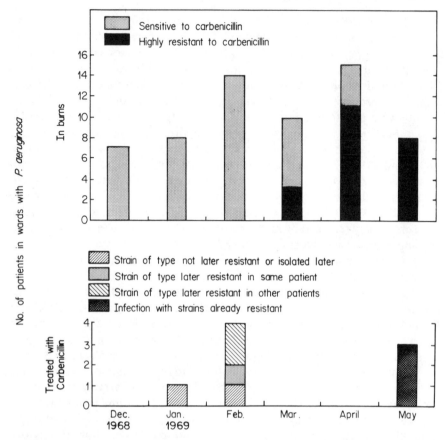

Figure 1. The upper histogram shows the numbers of patients in each month (December, 1968 to May, 1969) from whose burns *P. aeruginosa* was isolated; the black columns show the numbers of carbenicillin-resistant strains. The lower histogram shows the number of patients in the same period who were being treated with carbenicillin and the types of *P. aeruginosa* for which they were having treatment. Reproduced with permission from *Lancet*, **ii**, 448 (1969)

and cephalosporins, as well as carbenicillin; the result of adopting such restrictions was successful (Lowbury *et al.*, 1972) (see Figure 2).

Other methods of preventing transfer of R-factors to *P. aeruginosa* have been tried in experimental animals. Roe & Jones (1972) found that the transfer of linked antibiotic resistance by RP₁ from *K. aerogenes* to *P. aeruginosa* on a mouse burn could be prevented by application of a cream containing nalidixic acid to the burn; nalidixic acid stops DNA synthesis in the male cell, thereby preventing conjugation between Gram-negative bacilli (Hane, 1971). For clinical use another agent which acts in the same way would be required, because nalidixic acid is a valuable chemotherapeutic agent for urinary tract infections, and resistance emerges readily in Gram-negative bacilli exposed to this compound.

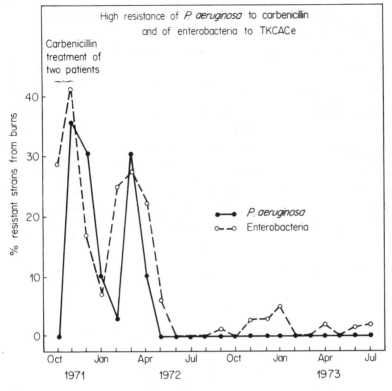

Figure 2. Effects of using carbenicillin in November 1971 and, from summer of 1972, of restricting use of antibiotics TKCACe in Burns Unit

Comments on Antibiotic Resistance of P. aeruginosa and its Prevention

The prospects for successful treatment of pseudomonas infection have been greatly improved since gentamicin and carbenicillin, as well as polymyxin, have been available, but each of these antibiotics has shortcomings. Polymyxin, to which *P. aeruginosa* does not acquire resistance *in vivo*, has relatively poor therapeutic activity, especially against systemic infections. Gentamicin has too great a potential toxicity to be used at dosages high enough to raise the blood level much above the M.I.C. Carbenicillin can be given in high dosage, but the margin between the M.I.C. and the highest practicable blood level is also narrow. A small increase in M.I.C. can convert a sensitive strain into one which is resistant. Accurate sensitivity tests are therefore necessary, and it is wise to use a plate-dilution or tube-dilution technique, which gives the result in terms of M.I.C., rather than a disc diffusion method in which discrepancies are likely to occur; e.g. Traub & Raymond (1972) have shown that wide zones of inhibition were given in tobramycin and gentamicin disc diffusion tests, with 10 μg discs, on cultures of rather resistant organisms. Diffusion tests are not suitable for polymyxin, because large differences in M.I.C. of this antibiotic are associated with very small differences in the zone of inhibition; dilution tests should therefore also be used for polymyxin (Ericsson & Sherris, 1971).

To preserve antibiotics for continuing use, it is essential that they should be used with special care to avoid the emergence and spread of resistant variants. This involves (i) restrictions in the use of antibiotics, especially in hospitals, with a policy by which certain antibiotics are more freely available than others, while some are used only when absolutely necessary: (ii) precautions to avoid cross-infection, by which resistant strains emerging in one patient may spread to others in the ward and (iii) combined therapy with two or more antibiotics (e.g. gentamicin and carbenicillin), so that mutants, which very rarely show simultaneous emergence of resistance to more than one antibiotic, may be destroyed by the antibiotic to which resistance has not emerged. Combined therapy is obviously of no use in preventing the acquisition of resistance by transfer of an R-factor determining resistance to both of the antibiotics used; this does not apply in the case of RP_1, which does not determine resistance to gentamicin.

Since *P. aeruginosa* may, with little increase in M.I.C., become resistant to carbenicillin and to gentamicin, these antibiotics should be reserved for use in severe infections and should not be used for prophylaxis of uninfected patients or in topical applications for minor infection. Polymyxin, which is free from resistance hazards, is more suitable for these purposes. Other antibiotics and antibiotic combinations have sometimes been used against *P. aeruginosa*; e.g. streptomycin and tetracycline, which are moderately active against some strains, and combinations of colistin with carbenicillin and sulphonamides (Dalton & Meyers, 1971). Neomycin has been reported effective in treatment of a case of pseudomonas endocarditis (Kenoyar, Stone & Levine, 1952). The use of erythromycin with alkali was reported by Zinner *et al.* (1971) to be effective in the treatment of a series of urinary tract infections, including one in which *P. aeruginosa* was the pathogen. None of these agents, however, is as likely to succeed in the treatment of pseudomonas infection as gentamicin, carbenicillin and polymyxin.

Immunotherapy

Immunological methods of prophylaxis against *P. aeruginosa* have received considerable attention in recent years and will be considered in a later section (see page 256). Therapy of established infection with vaccines and immune sera has also been studied and some successes have been reported. In an early report, Groves (1909) described the successful treatment of a case of pseudomonas septicaemia with a specific vaccine. Since some time is required for the development of active immunity, passive immunization is much more likely to be effective in the treatment of established infection, and there are several reports of successful therapeutic use of antiserum. Feingold and Oski (1965), for example, reported a remission in a case of pseudomonas septicaemia when convalescent serum from another case of pseudomonas infection was injected. Bocanegra *et al.* (1966) reported some clinical improvement in children with pseudomonas septicaemia when they were given hyperimmune serum. Jones, Alexander & Fisher (1970), using hyperimmune globulin from human volunteers immunized with a heptavalent pseudomonas vaccine, describe the successful treatment of *P. aeruginosa* septicaemia in patients with severe burns, cystic fibrosis and organ transplants. According to Spiers, Selwyn & Nicholson (1963), γ globulin probably helped to prevent recurrences of pseudomonas septicaemia in a case of congenital hypo-gammaglobulinaemia. However, Stone *et al.* (1965a) found γ globulin ineffective in the treatment of pseudomonas infections of burns, and Bodey, Molberg & Friedreich (1964) report a similar disappointment in the treatment of leukaemic patients. Unless it contains protective antibodies against *P. aeruginosa*, γ globulin cannot be expected to have useful therapeutic (or prophylactic) effects.

The value of hyperimmune serum or immunoglobulin, though strongly suggested by the evidence of some studies in human patients, is hard to evaluate for a number of reasons, in particular the complexity of the pathological processes, the variety of treatment and the absence of controls in many of the studies. Experiments in animals have shown clearly that pseudomonas infection can be arrested by passive immunotherapy, provided that it is given early enough (Jones & Lowbury, 1966). Millican & Rust (1960) showed that hyperimmune serum prevented invasive infection in mice which had 3 hours previously been given an intraperitoneal challenge which was lethal in unprotected animals. In an earlier study, the spread of pseudomonas keratitis was arrested by a hyperimmune serum (Jackson & Hartman, 1927). Rabbits challenged intravenously with live *P. aeruginosa* survived when given passive protection with a hyperimmune serum provided that this was not delayed for more than 12 hr (Feller *et al.*, 1964). Jones & Lowbury (1966) reported a similar finding in mice, in which the longest interval between challenge by inoculation of *P. aeruginosa* on to experimental burns and successful passive immunotherapy was 24 hr; presumably the time required for the pseudomonas to multiply in the burn to a lethal invasive dose was longer than this. In these studies serum from unvaccinated rabbits had no therapeutic effect.

PROPHYLAXIS

The incidence of antibiotic-resistant bacteria in hospital is commonly proportional to the amount of antibiotic used in the treatment of infection. Prevention of infection, by removing the need for therapy, is therefore a rational way of reducing the emergence of resistant species or variants. Several methods of prophylaxis have been found useful in preventing infection with *P. aeruginosa*.

Prophylactic methods can be classified under two headings: (i) methods of preventing contamination of the patient and his tissues by micro-organisms (the 'first line of defence'), and (ii) methods of preventing the invasion of tissues and blood stream from lesions (e.g. burns) already contaminated or colonized by the bacteria (the 'second line of defence'). In hospital practice both first and second lines of defence are used; e.g. the aseptic and antiseptic methods used in the operating theatre and in the ward help to protect the patient's wound or other susceptible areas against contamination, while the careful handling of wounds to preserve the viability of tissues, the removal of slough, prophylactic chemotherapy in some patients, and immunization (e.g. against tetanus) are methods used to prevent invasion or general effects of infection.

Defences Against Contamination: Asepsis and Antisepsis

Because *P. aeruginosa* is able to survive in water with minimal nutrient additives, special importance is given, in the control of pseudomonas infection, to sterilization and the maintenance of sterility of fluids (e.g. eyedrops and antiseptic-solutions), and to the avoidance or elimination of moist reservoirs of contamination in hospital equipment (e.g. respiratory ventilators, nebulizers) and in the environment. Some of the environmental reservoirs, e.g. standing water in sinks and gulleys, are probably of little importance as sources of infection, but they may play a role in some circumstances; it is desirable to prevent, by all practical measures, the contamination of nurses' hands from environmental sources, and of objects handled by patients, including food sent from kitchens, in wards where 'high-risk' patients are under treatment.

Urinary tract infection after instrumentation, which is sometimes caused by *P. aeruginosa* (Gould, 1968), has been greatly reduced by closed drainage, urethral disinfection, improved disinfection and sterilization of equipment and other methods of blocking the access of bacteria from external sources to the bladder via the urethra (Gillespie *et al.*, 1960; Miller *et al.*, 1960).

Another situation in which a potential site of infection has been successfully protected by topical prophylaxis against bacteria coming from an external source is in the treatment of burns, where *P. aeruginosa* is a particularly dangerous pathogen. In an early controlled trial of topical chemoprophylaxis (antisepsis), Jackson *et al.* (1951) found a significantly lower incidence of infection with *P. aeruginosa* (11/160, 7%) in burns treated prophylactically with a cream containing polymyxin E (1 mg per gram) than in a comparable series treated with a cream containing no polymyxin (50/207, 24%); no polymyxin-resistant strains of *P. aeruginosa* emerged during the trial. More recent developments have been the introduction of 0·5% silver nitrate solution (Moyer *et al.*, 1965), of 11% mafenide ('sulfamylon') cream (Lindberg *et al.*, 1965) and silver sulphadiazine cream (Fox, 1968), each of which was reported to be successful in preventing infection with *P. aeruginosa*. Controlled trials of silver nitrate (Cason *et al.*, 1966), mafenide cream and silver sulphadiazine cream (Lowbury *et al.*, 1971), have confirmed the prophylactic value of these topical applications. In a trial on severely burned patients, the proportion of burns infected with *P. aeruginosa* was 12/64 (18·8%) in the series treated with 0·5% silver nitrate compresses, but 33/41 (80·5%) in the control series treated with a cream containing no agent active against *P. aeruginosa*; the prophylactic effect of silver nitrate was greater against *P. aeruginosa* than against *Staph. aureus* and there was no apparent effect against miscellaneous Enterobacteria. Significant clinical effects of topical chemoprophylaxis were shown in the lower mean temperature and respiration rates of patients treated with silver nitrate or an alternative topical chemoprophylaxis. Bull (1971) and Mason *et al.* (1970) report reduced mortality associated with a reduction in pseudomonas infection after the introduction of more effective topical chemoprophylaxis. Good results have also been described with the use of topical gentamicin cream (Stone, Martin & Kolb, 1965; Lowbury & Jackson, 1968), but the emergence of gentamicin-resistant *P. aeruginosa* in some hospitals where the antibiotic has been used shows this to be an inadvisable form of topical prophylaxis for general use.

Physical (aseptic) measures include primary excision and grafting for deep burns of relatively small extent and, for patients with more extensive burns, segregation in protective isolation rooms or isolators. In a burns unit, isolation of patients in one- or two-bedded rooms did not, by itself, give sufficient protection to reduce the acquisition of *P. aeruginosa* (Cason *et al.*, 1966). However, a plastic isolator was found, in a controlled trial, to give significant protection against *P. aeruginosa* in patients with burns of moderate extent; 4/37 (10·8%) of the patients treated in isolators acquired *P. aeruginosa*, compared with an acqusition rate of 11/17 (64·7%) in patients concurrently treated in the open ward (Lowbury, Babb & Ford, 1971). Protection against other bacteria was much less satisfactory, and the isolator gave no protection against intestinal coliform bacilli. A more rigorous application of the technique combined with other prophylactic measures, including topical chemo-prophylaxis, appears to have greater effectiveness; for example, Burke (1971) has described the virtual elimination of infection in a burns unit where isolators with laminar flow ventilators were used in conjunction with silver-nitrate compresses and other prophylactic measures; it is impossible, however, to say how much, if anything, is contributed by a single component of a system of multiple barriers against infection.

In leukaemic patients who are receiving treatment with cytotoxic drugs invasive infection with *P. aeruginosa* is a potential cause of death. When patients are treated in 'ultraclean' units or protective isolators with sterile supplies (including food), exogenous infection is either eliminated or reduced to very small proportion, but infection with *P. aeruginosa* may still occur in patients who carry the organism in their intestinal flora (Jameson *et al.*, 1971). It has been suggested by some authors that a mixture of non-absorbed antibiotics (e.g. neomycin and polymyxin) should be given by mouth to disinfect the colonic contents in such patients.

Defences Against Invasion: Chemoprophylaxis and Immunoprophylaxis

The second line of defence consists of immunological, chemotherapeutic and general supportive measures. Among the general methods which can be expected to contribute to the natural antimicrobial defences is maintenance of physiological conditions: e.g. control of diabetes, haemoglobin, electrolyte and water balance. Systemic prophylaxis with polymyxin in patients with burns has been found to cause no reduction in the colonization of burns with *P. aeruginosa* (Cason & Lowbury, 1960; Jones, Jackson & Lowbury, 1966); although patients who received such prophylaxis in a controlled trial showed a lower incidence of septicaemia than patients in the control series the numbers were too small for assessments of statistical significance. Systemic chemo-prophylaxis with gentamicin or carbenicillin against *P. aeruginosa* is likely to select resistant mutants and should be avoided except in patients who are judged, on clinical and bacteriological grounds, to be developing invasive infection with the organism; this is, in effect, early chemotherapy, which has already been discussed (see page 238). The difficulties experienced with chemotherapy and topical chemoprophylaxis, especially microbial resistance and toxicity to the patient, may, perhaps, be avoided in the future by the use of active and passive immunoprophylaxis. A considerable amount of laboratory work and some clinical study has in recent years been devoted to these methods of treatment, which are discussed in the next section.

Immunoprophylaxis

Resistance to *P. aeruginosa* can be enhanced either by active immunization with an antigenic preparation ('vaccine'), or by passive immunization with serum antibody from an actively immunized person or animal. The protection conferred by active immunization persists but takes some time to develop; passive immunization, by contrast, gives immediate protection which only lasts for a short time.

Immunization depends, for its success, on production of an adequate amount of protective antibody, and on effective phagocytic and bactericidal functioning of leucocytes. It is important also for the patient requiring immunoprophylaxis to receive the treatment as early as possible, because the effects of immuniza-tion in established infection are relatively poor and only apparent in the early stages (see above, p. 252).

Active Immunization

The injection of vaccines prepared from *P. aeruginosa* and from its extracell-ular products into man or animals has been repeatedly shown to stimulate the production of antibodies and of immunity. For example, control of local sepsis at the site where living pseudomonas suspension had been injected intradermally into immunized rabbits was reported by Fox & Lowbury (1953). Many workers have demonstrated protection against potentially fatal sep-ticaemia after active immunization, and some of the studies are discussed below.

Vaccines for immunization against *P. aeruginosa* have been made in a number of different ways: as live bacterial suspensions (Charrin, 1889; Walker, Mason & Raulston, 1964); as suspensions of bacteria killed by heat (Groves,

1909; Jackson & Hartman, 1927; Feller *et al.*, 1964; Millican, Evans & Markley, 1966), formaldehyde (Fox & Lowbury, 1953; Sachs, 1970), or phenol (Fajardo & Laborde, 1968), phenol and heat (Pierson & Feller, 1970); extracts of cell walls (Alexander *et al.*, 1966; Homma, 1971; Vidal & Mynard, 1972; Milerova, 1974); bacterial slime (Liu, Abe & Bates, 1961; Alms & Bass, 1967); and culture filtrates (Charrin, 1889; Markley & Smallman, 1968; Jones, 1968; Liu & Hsieh, 1973).

The most effective vaccines make use of antigens present on the surface of the bacteria (Alexander *et al.*, 1969; Jones & Roe, 1975). Such antigens arc highly immunogenic, are easily extracted from the bacteria (Alms & Bass, 1967; Jones, 1968) and can be refined and detoxified (Jones, 1969). Vaccines made from surface antigens of a single strain have the capacity to cross-protect against a wide range of strains of different serotype (Fisher, Devlin & Gnabasik, 1969; Jones, 1972).

As most patients for whom immuniziation against *P. aeruginosa* is desirable require such protection at the earliest possible time (e.g. in burns soon after the injury), it is necessary to rely on the early immunity which appears within about 2 days of the first injection of vaccine (Markley & Smallman, 1968; Jones, 1971); such immunity which is associated with the IgM fraction of immunoglobulin (Jones, Hall & Ricketts, 1972) has been shown to protect burned mice against challenge from infected burns (Jones & Lowbury, 1972).

Development of Multivalent Vaccines

In 1969 Fisher *et al.* published a scheme by which strains of *P. aeruginosa* could be 'immuno-typed' by reference to the presence or absence of fatal infection in mice actively immunized with a set of antigenically distinct pseudomonas vaccines (bacterial suspensions). Each vaccine gave cross-protection against a number of strains of different serotype, seven type-strains being sufficient to cover 98% of a range of isolates tested at that time. By ethanol precipitation of extracts of cell 'pastes' from a strain of each of the seven representative serotypes, stable, soluble vaccines of low toxicity were developed (Alexander *et al.*, 1969; Hanessian *et al.*, 1971). During the trial of a heptavalent vaccine containing each of these seven components, Alexander & Fisher (1970) found that about 87% of the strains of *P. aeruginosa* isolated from patients in the Burns Unit showed serological reactions with one of the seven immunotypes.

A trivalent vaccine was prepared by Jones (1972) from culture filtrates of three strains of *P. aeruginosa*; mice immunized with this vaccine were protected against challenge by strains representing 14 different serotypes (i.e. agglutination types) of *P. aeruginosa*. Better protection, however, was obtained by the use of new vaccines prepared from surface antigens; (Jones & Lowbury, 1971; Milerova, 1974). These vaccines, which are still being developed, have been prepared from representative strains of each of the 13 available serotypes, including the 12 types described by Habs (1957). Protection of mice against 10 out of 10 strains of each representative serotype was given by 11 out of 13 of these vaccines, while the two other vaccines protected mice against 9 out of 10 strains. As well as homologous protection, these vaccines gave cross-protection against some other serotypes; but such cross-protection, unlike homologous-type protection, was obtained with some strains but not with others of the heterologous type. For this reason it was considered necessary to prepare a multivalent vaccine with components from each of the 13 serotypes rather than trying to cover the whole range by the use of a vaccine made from a small range of types, which would depend partly on cross-protective properties (Jones & Roe, 1975). No mutual interference has been found to occur between components of a multivalent vaccine (Alexander *et al.*, 1969; Jones, 1972). The 13-fold multivalent vaccine was found to give satisfactory protection against each of the three most virulent strains of each of the 13 serotypes.

Clinical Trials of Vaccines

Multivalent vaccine.   Trials of the heptavalent vaccine (Parke-Davis & Co.) in patients with burns have shown a reduced incidence of septicaemia and a lower death rate, as compared with previous levels (Alexander *et al.*, 1969; Alexander & Fisher, 1970); these authors refer to treatment by this method of over 100 patients with severe burns. The response to immunization was shown to depend on the dose of vaccine; in patients given large doses (25 μg per kg per day, by intradermal injection) no deaths from sepsis were recorded, but malaise, fever, and local tenderness and induration occurred, apparently caused by the treatment. Approximately twice as much vaccine could be given without side-effects to patients with burns as to healthy volunteers (Alexander & Fisher, 1970). The best protective results and antibody titres were found when immunization was started immediately after injury; with increasing intervals between burning and first injection of vaccine there was a decrease in response to immunization (Alexander, 1971). This could be partly overcome by giving a larger initial dose of vaccine. There was a good correlation between increased antibody titre and reduced sepsis rate (Nance *et al.*, 1970); serum from vaccinated patients showed haemagglutinin titres with vaccine-coated erythrocytes of <1/4 to 1/128, the majority being in the range of 1/16 to 1/64. Passive protection of mice with serum from vaccinated burned patients was obtained when the haemagglutinin titre in the IgG fraction of the serum was 1/10 or higher. With the use of the vaccine, only 3 out of 96 patients with burns of more than 20% of body surface died with *P. aeruginosa* as a primary or contributory cause; by contrast, 14 out of 75 patients not given the vaccine during the period before vaccination was introduced died with pseudomonas infection.

Young, Meyer & Armstrong (1973) have reported a controlled trial of the heptavalent vaccine in the treatment of patients with malignant tumours. Fatal pseudomonas infection occurred in 31/176 unvaccinated patients in the control series, but in only 13/185 patients who had received the vaccine (P < 0·001). Recovery from *P. aeruginosa* infection in the vaccinated was associated with high serum titres of opsonizing antibody to the infecting strain (Young & Armstrong, 1972). Although the heptavalent vaccine had significant protective value, toxic side-effects occurred in a number of the vaccinated patients.

Sachs (1970) reported on the use of formolized vaccine containing six strains, of different serotype, of *P. aeruginosa*, combined with staphylococcal suspensions and toxoid. Serum titres of agglutinin to *P. aeruginosa* were increased after 3 doses of vaccine; though vaccination did not cause a fall in infection rate, it appeared to prolong the survival of patients who eventually died.

Monovalent vaccine. Feller (1966) and Pierson & Feller (1970) have reported the use of heat-killed suspension prepared from a single strain of *P. aeruginosa* isolated in a burns unit. This vaccine was used for the preparation of hyperimmune serum in healthy volunteers, to be given as a passive immunizing agent to patients with burns: the vaccine was also used for active immunization of burned patients. After a skin sensitivity test on arrival, patients who gave no reaction were injected subcutaneously with 0·5 ml of the vaccine, and further doses of 0·5 ml were given at weekly intervals until discharge of the patient. In a later series, patients received the vaccine and also daily injections of 250 ml of plasma with a titre of 1/512 of agglutinin to the immunizing strain of *P. aeruginosa*, until the patient was judged capable of resisting infections. Deaths from pseudomonas septicaemia fell after the introduction of the vaccine, and fell to a still lower incidence after the introduction of combined active and passive immunization.

Passive Immunization

It has been shown by many workers that injection of serum from actively immunized animals protects susceptible animals against the immunizing organism or related strains; similar findings on passive immunization of human subjects have been reported. An early study (Jackson & Hartman, 1927) showed beneficial effect of serum from an immunized rabbit in preventing extension of *P. aeruginosa* infection of the eye. Protection by antiserum against fatal septicaemic invasion in mice has been reported by Millican & Rust (1960); Jones, Jackson & Lowbury (1966), Crowder *et al.* (1972) and others. Immunoglobulin fractions of immune serum have been shown by Jones, Alexander & Fisher (1970) and Jones, Hall & Ricketts (1972) to cause passive protection of mice. Evidence that human subjects with burns can be protected by passive immunization with the plasma of immunized human volunteers has been reported by Feller (1966), Bocanegra *et al.* (1970) and Alexander (1973). Experiments in animals have shown that immune serum protects not only healthy animals but also animals which have been burned (Jones *et al.*, 1966; Markley & Smallman, 1968) or treated with an immunosuppressive drug (Rosenthal, Millican & Rust, 1957).

Patients with severe burns are particularly susceptible to invasive infection during the first few days after injury, and passive immunization must be considered potentially more useful than active immunization against this hazard, even though active immunity can appear at an early stage. In patients whose natural antibacterial defences, including antibody forming powers are reduced by disease or immunosuppressive treatment, passive rather than active prophylaxis is the appropriate method of immunological protection.

Antibodies in the Serum

Jones & Lowbury (1965) and Bass & McCoy (1971) have shown that agglutinin levels in sera correlated well with passive protective effects. Alexander & Fisher (1970) showed a rise in the level of haemagglutinin after vaccination which was associated with protection of patients against *P. aeruginosa*. Protective activity appears in the serum of immunized mice before agglutinins are detected (Jones, 1971; Liu & Hsieh, 1973), but passive haemagglutinins are usually present at the stage when the serum first shows passive immunizing properties: e.g. 3 to 4 days after a single vaccinating dose. This early immunity is associated with the IgM fraction; agglutinins, which are associated with the IgG fraction, first appear on about the seventh day after vaccination (Jones *et al.*, 1972). In man, pseudomonas antibodies also appear first in the IgM and later in the IgG fraction (Alexander & Fisher, 1970). Absorption of antibodies from the serum with vaccine-coated erythrocytes removes its protective property (Roe & Jones, 1975). Both of the serum immunoglobulin fractions appear to play a role in protection. IgG persists longer than IgM in the blood after immunization and, being of smaller molecular size, penetrates more effectively into extravascular spaces; it is therefore of greater potential value in passive protection.

Antibodies to *P. aeruginosa* are commonly assessed by agglutination tests (e.g. Fox & Lowbury, 1953; Walker *et al.*, 1964; Pierson & Feller, 1970; Bass & McCoy, 1971) and by the passive haemagglutinin test (Gaines & Landy, 1955; Graber *et al.*, 1961; Kefalides *et al.*, 1964; Alexander *et al.*, 1969); immuno-diffusion tests have also been used (Young, Yu & Armstrong, 1970; Crowder *et al.*, 1972). The protective activity of antisera is evaluated by animal protection tests and, indirectly, by tests of phagocytic and bactericidal activity of leucocytes exposed to the sera (Alexander & Fisher, 1970; Jones & Dyster, 1973).

Most normal human subjects have antibodies to *P. aeruginosa* in their sera (e.g. Gaines & Landy, 1955; Graber *et al.*, 1961; Jones & Lowbury, 1965), possibly due to immunizing effects of previous exposure to *P. aeruginosa* or to bacteria which produce antigens similar to those of the pseudomonas, e.g. *Klebsiella aerogenes* (Jones *et al.*, 1971) or *Enterobacter cloacae* (Homma, Abe & Hirao, 1973).

It is uncertain how important the naturally occurring antibodies are in protection against *P. aeruginosa*; Björnson & Michael (1972) found that natural IgG had poor complement fixing properties as compared with immune IgG. Alexander (1971) and Young *et al.* (1973) have found that antibody has little protective value unless the supporting defence mechanisms of reticulo-endothelial cells, leucocytes and complement are functioning effectively (Lowbury, 1975).

COMMENTS

Though *P. aeruginosa* infections can sometimes be effectively treated with appropriate antibiotics, such treatment is indicated only when there is evidence or likelihood of severe clinical effects: e.g. in septicaemia, or when the organism colonizes tissues, such as the urinary tract or the anterior chamber of the eye, which are normally sterile. In minor wounds and in burns of small or moderate extent there is rarely any need to give systemic or even local chemotherapy, as such infections will normally respond to the natural defences. Topical prophylaxis, however, is rational in a burns unit (e.g. by application of suitable antimicrobial agents active against all strains) both for the protection of the patient on whom it is used and to prevent the accumulation of a continuing source or reservoir of endemic infection.

Successful methods for controlling the spread of *P. aeruginosa* have led in the last few years to a reduced incidence of clinical infection with the organism in many hospitals; in these environments the antibiotics with particular value against *P. aeruginosa* are less used, and resistant variants are less likely to emerge. In burns, topical chemoprophylaxis has, by itself, proved sufficiently effective in some centres to make immunoprophylaxis unnecessary; a high standard of asepsis and nursing care may have similar effect in hospitals with good facilities and a small number of patients (Birke *et al.*, 1964). But where such methods cannot be effectively used (e.g. in developing countries, or in situations where long delays in the admission of patients to hospital are inevitable), there is a rational place for immunological prophylaxis and therapy.

REFERENCES

Adler, J. L. & Finland, M. (1971). Susceptibility of recent isolates of *Pseudomonas aeruginosa* to gentamicin, polymyxin and 5 penicillins with observations on the pyocin and immunotypes of the strains. *Applied Microbiology*, **22**, 870–875.

Ainslie, D. (1953). Treatment of corneal infection with *Pseudomonas pyocyanea* by subconjuctival injection of polymyxin. *British Journal of Ophthalmology*, **37**, 336–342.

Ainsworth, G. C., Brown, A. M. & Brownleee, G. (1947). 'Aerosporin', an antibiotic produced by *Bacillus aerosporus* Greer. *Nature*, **160**, 263.

Alexander, J. W. (1971). Immunological considerations and the role of vaccination in burn management. In *Contemporary Burn Management*, (Eds. H. Polk & H. H. Stone), Little Brown, Boston, p. 265.

Alexander, J. W. (1973). Personal communication

Alexander, J. W., Brown, W., Walker, H. C., Mason, A. D. & Moncrief, J. A. (1966). Studies on the isolation of infective-protective antigens from pseudomonas. *Surgery, Gynaecology and Obstetrics*, 123, 965.

Alexander, J. W., Fisher, M. W., Macmillan, B. G. and Altemeier, W. A. (1969). Prevention of invasive pseudomonas infection in burns with a new vaccine. *Archives of Surgery*, **99**, 249–256.

Alexander, J. W. & Fisher, M. W. (1970). Immunological control of pseudomonas infections in burn patients: A clinical evaluation. *Archives of Surgery*, **102**, 31–35.

Alms, T. H. & Bass, J. A. (1967). Immunisation against *Pseudomonas aeruginosa* 1. Induction of protection by an alcohol precipitated fraction of slime layer. *Journal of Infectious Diseases*, **117**, 249–256.

Atuk, N. O., Mosca, A. & Kunin, C. (1964). The use of potentially nephrotoxic antibiotics in the treatment of Gram-negative infections in uraemic patients. *Annals of internal medicine*, **60**, 28–38.

Ayliffe, G. A. J., Lowbury, E. J. L. & Roe, E. (1972). Transferable carbenicillin resistance in *Pseudomonas aeruginosa*. *Nature (New Biology)*, **235**, 141–143.

Barber, M. & Waterworth, P. M. (1966). Activity of gentamicin against pseudomonas and hospital staphylococci. *British Medical Journal*, **i**, 203–205.

Bass, J. A. & McCoy, J. C. (1971). Passive immunisation against experimental pseudomonas infection. 'Correlation of Protection to Verder and Evans 'O' Serotypes'. *Infection and Immunity*, **3/1**, 51.

Bell, S. M. & Smith, D. D. (1969). Resistance of *Pseudomonas aeruginosa* to carbenicillin. *Lancet*, **i**, 753–755.

Benedict, R. G. & Langlykke, A. F. (1947). Antibiotic activity of *Bacillus polymyxa*. *Journal of Bacteriology*, **54**, 24.

Beveridge, E. G. & Martin, A. J. (1967). Sodium sulphomethyl derivatives of polymyxin. *British Journal of Pharmacology and Chemotherapy*, **29**, 125–135.

Birke, G., Liljedahl, S. O., Backdahl, M. & Nylen, B. (1964). Studies on burns. VIII Analysis of mortality and length of hospital care for 603 burned patients referred for primary treatment. *Acta chirugica Scandinavia*, **128**, Supplement 337, p. 3–100.

Bjornson, A. B. & Michael, J. G. (1972). Contribution of humoral and cellular factors to the resistance to experimental infection by *Pseudomonas aeruginosa* in mice. *Infection and Immunity*, **5/5**, 775–782.

Black, J., Calesnick, B., Williams, D. & Weinstein, M. J. (1963). Pharmacology of gentamicin, a new broad spectrum antibiotic. *Antimicrobial agents and chemotherapy*, 138–147.

Black, W. A. & Girdwood, R. W. A. (1969). Carbenicillin resistance in *Pseudomonas aeruginosa*. *British medical Journal*, **iv**, 234.

Bocanegra, M., Minostroza, F., Bazan, A., Verlarde, N., Yoza, V. & Rosenthal, S. M. (1966). Convalescent burn plasma for severely burned children. *Annals of Surgery*, **163**, 461.

Bodey, G. P., Molberg, N. R. & Friedreich, E. J. (1964). Use of gamma globulin in infections in leukaemia. *Journal of the American Medical Association*, **190**, No. 13, 1099.

Bodey, G. P. & Terrell, L. M. (1968). *In vitro* activity of carbenicillin against Gram-negative bacilli. *Journal of Bacteriology*, **95**, 1587–1590.

Brayton, R. G. & Louria, D. B. (1964). Gentamicin in Gram-negative urinary and pulmonary infections. *Archives of Internal Medicine*, **114**, 205–212.

Brown, M. R. W., Fenton, E. M. & Watkins, W. M. (1972). Tetracycline-sensitive polymyxin resistant *Pseudomonas aeruginosa*. *Lancet*, **ii**, 86.

Brown, M. R. W. & Melling, J. (1969). Role of divalent cations in the action of polymyxin B and EDTA on *Pseudomonas aeruginosa*. *Journal of General Microbiology*, **59**, 263–273.

Brown, M. R. W. & Richards, R. M. E. (1965). Effect of ethylenediamine tetracetate on the resistance of *Ps. aeruginosa* to antibacterial agents. *Nature*, **207** (ii), 1391–1393.

Brown, M. R. W. & Winsley, B. E. (1971). Synergism between polymyxin and polysorbate 80 against *Pseudomonas aeruginosa*. *Journal of General Microbiology*, **68**, 367–373.

Brumfitt, W., Black, M. & Williams, J. D. (1966). Colistin in *Pseudomonas pyocyanea* infection and its effect on renal function. *British Journal of Urology*, **38**, 495–500.

Brumfitt, W., Percival, A. & Leigh, D. A. (1967). Clinical and laboratory studies with carbenicillin. A new pencillin active against *Ps. pyocyanea*. *Lancet*, **i**, 1289–1293.

Brun, J., Perrin-Fayelle, M. & Sedaillan, A. (1967). In *Gentamicin First International Symposium*, Schwabe, Basel, p. 129.

Brzesinska, M., Benveniste, R., Davies, J., Daniels, P. J. L. & Weinstein, J. (1972). Gentamicin resistance in strains of *Pseudomonas aeruginosa* mediated by enzymatic *N*-acetylation of the deoxystreptomine moiety. *Biochemistry*, **ii**, 761–765.

Bulger, R. J., Sidell, S. & Kirby, W. M. M. (1963). Laboratory and clinical studies of gentamicin. A new broad spectrum antibiotic. *Annals of Internal Medicine*, **59**, 593–604.

Bull, J. P. (1971). Revised analysis of mortality due to burns. *Lancet*, **ii**, 1133–1134.

Burke, J. F. (1971). Isolation techniques and their effectiveness. In *Contemporary Burn Management*, (Eds. H. S. Polk & H. H. Stone), Little Brown, Boston, pp. 141–150.

Cason, J. S., Jackson, D. M., Lowbury, E. J. L. & Ricketts, C. R. (1966). Antiseptic and aseptic prophylaxis for burns: Use of silver nitrate and of isolators. *British Medical Journal*, **ii**, 1288–1294.

Cason, J. S. & Lowbury, E. J. L. (1960). Prophylactic chemotherapy for burns. Studies on the local and systemic use of combined therapy. *Lancet*, **ii**, 501–507.

Chapman, G. B. (1962). Cytological aspects of antimicrobial antibiosis. 11. Cytological changes associated with the exposure of *Pseudomonas aeruginosa* and *Bacillus megaterium* to colistin sulphate. *Journal of Bacteriology*, **84**, 180–185.

Charrin, A. (1889). *La maladie pyocyanique*, (Ed. G. Steinheil), G. Steinheil, 2 Rue Casimir, Delavigne 2, Paris.

Chisholm, G. D. Calnan, J. J., Waterworth, P. M. & Reiss, N. D. (1968). Distribution of gentamicin in body fluids. *British Medical Journal*, **ii**, 22–24.

Chisholm, G. D. Waterworth, P. M. & Reiss, N. D. (1973). Concentration of antibacterial agents in interstitial tissue fluid. *British Medical Journal*, **ii**, 569–573.

Cox, C. E. & Harrison, L. H. (1971). Comparison of gentamicin, polymyxin B and kanamycin in therapy of bacteremia due to Gram-negative bacilli. *Journal of Infectious Diseases*, **124**, s156–s163.

Crowder, J. G., Fisher, M. W. & White, A. (1972). Type specific immunity in pseudomonas disease. *Journal of Laboratory and Clinical Medicine*, **i**, 47.

Cooper, R. G., Rice, J. C. & Penfold, J. L. (1969). Pseudomonas infection treated with carbenicillin and gentamicin. *Medical Journal of Australia*, **i**, 517–519.

Dalton, A. C. & Meyers, S. D. (1971). Sensitivity of *Pseudomonas aeruginosa* to sulphamethoxazole. *American Journal of Clinical Pathology*, **56**, 371–374.

Darrell, J. H. & Waterworth, P. M. (1969). Carbenicillin resistance in *Pseudomonas aeruginosa* from clinical material. *British Medical Journal*, **iii**, 141–143.

Eickhoff, T. C. & Marks, M. I. (1970). Carbenicillin in therapy of systemic infection due to pseudomonas. *Journal of Infectious Diseases*, **122**, Supplement s84–s90.

English, A. R., Retsema, J. A., Ray, V. A. & Lynch, J. E. (1972). Carbenicillin indanyl sodium, an orally active derivative of carbenicillin. *Antimicrobial Agents and Chemotherapy*, **i**, 185–191.

Ericsson, H. M. & Sherris, J. C. (1971). Antibiotic Sensitivity Testing: Report of an International Collaborative Study. *Acta Pathologica Microbiologica Scandanavica*, Section B, Supplement 217.

Eykyn, S., Phillips, I. & Ridley, M. (1971). Gentamicin plus carbenicillin. *Lancet*, **i**, 545–546.

Fajardo, C. L. & Laborde, H. F. (1968). Pseudomonas vaccine. *Journal of Bacteriology*, **95**, 1968.

Farrar, D. A. R. (1954). Use of polymyxin B in the external ear. *British Medical Journal*, **ii**, 629.

Feingold, D. S. & Oski, D. (1965). Pseudomonas infection. *Archives of Internal Medicine*, **116**, 326.

Fekety, F. R., Norman, P. S. & Cluff, L. E. (1962). The treatment of Gram-negative bacillary infections with colistin. The toxicity and efficacy in 48 patients. *Annals of Internal Medicine*, **57**, 214–229.

Feller, I. (1966). The use of pseudomonas vaccine and hyperimmune plasma in the treatment of seriously burned patients. Research in Burns, (Eds. A. B. Wallace & A. W. Wilkinson), Livingstone, Edinburgh and London, pp. 470–480.

Feller, I., Burgess, V., Callahan, W. & Waldyke, J. (1964). Use of vaccine and hyperimmune serum for protection against Pseudomonas septicaemia. *Journal of Trauma*, **4**, 451.

Fisher, M. W., Devlin, H. B. & Gnabasik, F. J. (1969). New immunotype schema for *Pseudomonas aeruginosa* based on protective antigens. *Journal of Bacteriology*, **98**, 835–836.

Florey, M. E. (1960). *The Clinical Application of Antibiotics*, Volume iv, Oxford University Press, London.

Fox, C. L. (1968). Silver sulphadiazine—a new topical therapy for pseudomonas in burns. *Archives of Surgery, Chicago*, **96**, 184.

Fox, J. E., & Lowbury, E. J. L. (1953). Immunity and antibody to *Pseudomonas pyocyanea* in rabbits. *Journal of Pathology and Bacteriology*, **65**, 533–542.

Fraser, H. (1953). Subconjunctival injection of polymyxin B. *British Journal of Ophthalmology*, **37**, 369–373.

Forkner, C. E., Frei, E., Edgcombe, J. H. & Utz, J. P. (1958). Pseudomonas septicaemia: Observations on 23 cases. *American Journal of Medicine*, **25**, 877–889.

Fullbrook, P. D. S., Elson, S. W. & Slocombe, B. (1970). R-factor mediated β-lactamase in *Pseudomonas aeruginosa*. *Nature (London)*, **226**, 1054.

Gaines, S. & Landy, M. (1955). Prevalence of antibody to Pseudomonas in normal human sera. *Journal of Bacteriology*, **69**, 628.

Garrod, L. P. & Waterworth, P. M. (1969). Effect of medium composition on the apparent sensitivity of *Pseudomonas aeruginosa* to gentamicin. *Journal of Clinical Pathology*, **22**, 534–538.

Garrod, L. P., Lambert, H. P., O'Grady, F. & Waterworth, P. M. (1973). *Antibiotic and Chemotherapy*. Churchill, Livingstone, Edinburgh and London.

Gillespie, W. A., Linton, K. B., Miller, A. & Slade, N. (1960). The diagnosis, epidemiology and control of urinary infections in urology and gynaecology. *Journal of Clinical Pathology*, **13**, 187–194.

Gingell, J. L. & Waterworth, P. M. (1968). Dose of gentamicin in patients with normal renal function and renal impairment. *British Medical Journal*, **ii**, 19–22.

Gould, J. C. (1968). *Urinary Tract Infection*, (Eds. F. O'Grady and W. Brumfitt), Oxford University Press, Oxford, p. 43.

Graber, C. D. Cummings, D., Vogel, E. H. & Tumbusch, W. T. (1961). Measurement of the protective effect of antibody in burned and unburned patients' sera for *Ps. aeruginosa* infected mice. *Texas Reports of Biology and Medicine*, **19**, 268–276.

Graber, C. D., Stone, H. H., Kolb, L. & Martin, J. D. (1963). *In vitro* sensitivity of bacterial flora from burned patients to gentamicin sulphate. *Antimicrobial agents and Chemotherapy*, 161–163.

Groves, E. H. (1909). Case of *Bacillus pyocyaneus* pyaemia successfully treated by vaccine. *British Medical Journal*, **i**, 1169.

Grüneberg, R. H. & Kolbe, R, (1969). Trimethoprim in the treatment of urinary infections in hospital. *British Medical Journal*, **i**, 545–547.

Habs, I. (1957). Untersuchungen uber die O-antigene von *Ps. aeruginosa. Zeitschrift fur Hygiene und Infectionskrankheiten*, **144**, 218–228.

Hane, M. (1971). Some effects of nalidixic acid on conjugation on *E. coli* K12. *Journal of Bacteriology*, **105**, 46.

Hanessian, S., Regan, W., Watson, D. & Haskell, T. H. (1971). Isolation and characterization of antigenic components of a new heptavalent Pseudomonas vaccine. *Nature (New Biology)*, **229**, 209–210.

Hayes, E. R. & Yow, E. (1950). Meningitis due to *Pseudomonas aeruginosa* treated with polymyxin B. *American Journal of Medical Science*, **220**, 633–637.

Hirsch, H. A., McCarthy, C. G. & Finland, M. (1960). *Proceedings of the Society of Experimental Biology (New York)*, **103**, 338.

Homma, J. Y. (1971). Recent investigations on *Pseudomonas aeruginosa*. *Japanese Journal of Experimental Medicine*, **41/5**, 387–400.

Homma, J. Y., Abe, C. & Hirao, I. (1973). Common protective antigen of *Pseudomonas aeruginosa*. *Journal of the Japanese Association for Infectious Diseases*, **47**, 169.

Ingram, L., Richmond, M. H. & Sykes, R. B. (1973). Molecular characterisation of the R-factors implicated in the carbenicillin resistance of a sequence of *Pseudomonas aeruginosa* strains isolated from burns. *Antimicrobial Agents and Chemotherapy*, **3**, 279–288.

Jackson, D. M., Lowbury, E. J. L. & Topley, E. (1951). *Pseudomonas pyocyanea* in burns. Its role as a pathogen and the value of local polymyxin therapy. *Lancet*, **ii**, 137–165.

Jackson, E. & Hartman, F. W. (1927). Experimental Bacillus pyocyaneus keratitis. *Journal of Laboratory and Clinical Medicine*, **12**, 442–450.

Jackson, G. G. (1967). *The Practitioner*, **198**, 855.

Jameson, B., Gamble, D. R., Lynch, J. & Kay, H. E. M. (1971). Five-year analysis of protective isolation. *Lancet*, **i**, 1034–1040.

Jao, R. L. & Jackson, G. G. (1964). Gentamicin sulphate, a new antibiotic against Gram-negative bacilli. Laboratory, Pharmacological and clinical evaluation. *Journal of the American Medical Association*, **189**, 817–822.

Jawetz, E. (1952). Infections with *Pseudomonas aeruginosa* treated with polymycin B. *Archives of Internal Medicine*, **89**, 90–98.

Jawetz, E. (1956). Polymyxin, Neomycin, Bacitracin, Medical Encyclopaedia Inc., New York.

Jawetz, E. & Coleman, V. R. (1949). Laboratory and clinical observations on aerosporin (polymyxin B). *Journal of Laboratory and Clinical Medicine*, **34**, 751–760.

Jephcott, A. E., Lowbury, E. J. L. & Richmond, M. H. (1973). Non-transferable carbenicillin resistance of *Pseudomonas aeruginosa* from a burn. *Lancet*, **i**, 272.

Jones, C. E., Alexander, J. W. & Fisher, M. W. (1970). Clinical evaluation of pseudomonas hyperimmune globulin and plasma. *Surgical Forum*, **21**, 238.

Jones, R. J. (1968). Protection against *Pseudomonas aeruginosa* infection by immunisation with fractions of culture filtrates of *Ps. aeruginosa*. *British Journal of Experimental Pathology*, **49**, 411–420.

Jones, R. J. (1969). Detoxification of an immunogenic fraction from a culture filtrate of *Pseudomonas aeruginosa*. *Journal of Hygiene, Cambridge*, **67**, 241–247.

Jones, R. J. (1970). Passive immunisation against Gram-negative bacilli in burns. *British Journal of Experimental Pathology*, **51**, 53–58.

Jones, R. J. (1971). Early protection by vaccines in burns. *British Journal of Experimental Pathology*, **52**, 100–109.

Jones, R. J. (1972). Specificity of early protective responses induced by pseudomonas vaccines. *Journal of Hygiene, Cambridge*, **70**, 343–351.

Jones, R. J. & Dyster, R. E. (1973). The role of polymorphonuclear leucocytes in protecting mice vaccinated against *Pseudomonas aeruginosa* infections. *British Journal of Experimental Pathology*, **54**, 416–421.

Jones, R. J., Hall, M. & Ricketts, C. R. (1972). Passive protective properties of serum fractions from mice inoculated with an antipseudomonas vaccine. *Immunology*, **23**, 889–895.

Jones, R. J., Jackson, D. M. & Lowbury, E. J. L. (1966). Antisera and antibiotics in the prophylaxis of burns against *Pseudomonas aeruginosa*. *British Journal of Plastic Surgery*, **5**, 43–57.

Jones, R. J., Lilly, H. A. & Lowbury, E. J. L. (1971). Passive protection of mice against *Pseudomonas aeruginosa* by serum from recently vaccinated mice. *British Journal of Experimental Pathology*. **52**, 264–270.

Jones, R. J. & Lowbury, E. J. L. (1966). Antiserum and antibiotic in the prophylaxis against *Pseudomonas aeruginosa*. *Research in Burns* (Eds. A. B. Wallace & A. W. Wilkinson), Livingstone, Edinburgh and London, pp. 474–485.

Jones, R. J. & Lowbury, E. J. L. (1967). Prophylaxis and therapy for *Pseudomonas aeruginosa* infection with carbenicillin and with gentamicin. *British Medical Journal*, **iii**, 79–82.

Jones, R. J. & Lowbury, E. J. L. (1972). Early protection by vaccine against *Pseudomonas aeruginosa* colonising burns. *British Journal of Experimental Pathology*, **53**, 659–664.

Jones, R. J. & Roe, E. (1975). Vaccination against different serotypes of *Pseudomonas aeruginosa*. Unpublished.

Jones, R. J. & Roe, E. A. (1975). Protective properties and haemaglutins in serum from humans and in serum from mice injected with a new polyvalent *Pseudomonas* vaccine. *British Journal of Experimental Pathology*, **56**, 34–44.

Kagan, B. M., Krevsky, D., Milzer, A. & Locke, M. (1951). Polymyxin B and Polymyxin E. Clinical and laboratory studies. *Journal of Laboratory and Clinical Medicine*, **37**, 402.

Kefalides, N. A., Arana, J. A. Bazan, A., Verlarde, N. & Rosenthal, S. M. (1964). Evaluation of antibiotic prophylaxis and gamma globulins, plasma, albumin and saline solution therapy in severe burns. *Annals of Surgery*, **159**, 496.

Kenoyar, W. L., Stone, C. T. & Levine, W. C. (1952). Bacterial endocarditis due to *Pseudomonas aeruginosa*. *American Journal of Medicine*, **13**, 108.

Klein, J. O., Eickhoff, T. C. & Finland, M. (1964). Gentamicin. Activity *in vitro* and observations in 26 patients. *American Journal of Medical Science*, **248**, 528–543.

Koyama, Y., Kurosasa, A., Tsuchiya, A., Takakuta, K. (1950). *Journal of Antibiotics (Tokyo)*, **3**, 457.

Knudsen, E. T., Rolinson, G. N. & Sutherland, R. (1967). Carbenicillin: A new semisynthetic penicillin active against *Pseudomonas pyocyaneas*. *British Medical Journal*, **iii**, 75–78.

Kunin, C. M. & Bugg, A. (1971). Binding of polymyxin antibiotics to tissues: The major determinant of distribution and persistence in the body. *Journal of Infectious Diseases*, **124**, 394–400.

Lindberg, R. B., Moncrief, J. A., Switzer, W. E., Order, S. E. & Mills, W. (1965). The successful control of burn wound sepsis. *Journal of Trauma*, **5**, 601.

Liu, P. V., Abe, Y. & Bates, J. L. (1961). The role of various fractions of *Pseudomonas aeruginosa* in its pathogenesis. *Journal of Infectious Diseases*, **108**, 218.

Liu, P. V. & Hsieh, H. (1973). Exotoxins of *Pseudomonas aeruginosa* 111. Characteristics of antitoxin A. *Journal of Infectious Diseases*, **128/4**, 520.

Lowbury, E. J. L. (1975). Ecological importance of *P. aeruginosa*: medical aspects. In *The Biochemistry and Genetics of Pseudomonas*, (Ed. P. H. Clarke & M. H. Richmond), John Wiley, London.

Lowbury, E. J. L. & Ayliffe, G. A. (1974). In *Drug Resistance in Antimicrobial Therapy*, Charles C. Thomas, Springfield, Illinois.

Lowbury, E. J. L., Babb, J. R. & Ford, P. M. (1971). Protective isolation in a burns unit: the use of plastic isolators and air curtains. *Journal of Hygiene, Cambridge*, **69**, 529–546.

Lowbury, E. J. L., Babb, J. R. & Roe, E. (1972). Clearance from a hospital of Gram-negative bacilli that transfer carbenicillin-resistance to *Pseudomonas aeruginosa*. *Lancet*, **ii**, 941–945.

Lowbury, E. J. L. & Jackson, D. M. (1968). Local chemoprophylaxis for burns with gentamicin and other agents. *Lancet*, **i**, 654–657.

Lowbury, E. J. L., Jackson, D. M., Lilly, H. A., Bull, J. P., Cason, J. S., Davies, J. W. L. & Ford, P. M. (1971). Alternative forms of local treatment for burns. *Lancet*, **ii**, 1105–1111.

Lowbury, E. J. L., Kidson, A., Lilly, H. A., Ayliffe, G. A. J. & Jones, R. J. (1969). Sensitivity of *Pseudomonas aeruginosa* to antibiotics: emergence of strains highly resistant to carbenicillin. *Lancet*, **ii**, 448–452.

Lynn, B. (1973). Administration of carbenicillin and ticarcillin: pharmaceutical aspects. *European Journal of Cancer*, **9**, 425–433.

Manoukian, M. (1953). Osteomyelitis pubis due to *Pseudomonas aeruginosa* treated with polymyxin B sulphate. *Archives of Surgery*, **67**, 937–938.

Markley, K., Gurmendi, G., Chavez, P. M. & Bazan, A. (1957). Fatal pseudomonas septicaemia in burned patients. *Annals of Surgery*, **145**, 175.

Markley, K. & Smallman, E. (1968). Protection by vaccination against Pseudomonas infection after thermal injury. *Journal of Bacteriology*, **96/4**, 867.

Mason, A. D., Pruitt, B. A., Lindberg, R. B., Moncrief, J. A. & Foley, F. D. (1970). Topical sulfamylon chemotherapy in the treatment of patients with extensive thermal burns. *Research in Burns*, (Eds. P. Matter, T. L. Barclay and Z. Koničková), Hans Huber, Berne, pp. 120–123.

Meyer, R. D., Young, L. S. & Armstrong, D. (1971). Tobramycin (Nebramycin factor 6): *In Vitro* activity against *Ps. aeruginosa*. *Applied Microbiology*, **22**, 1147–1151.

McClure, P. D., Casserby, J. G., Monier, C. & Grozier, D. (1970). Carbenicillin-induced bleeding disorder. *Lancet*, **ii**, 1307–1308.

McLaughlin, J. E. & Reeves, D. S. (1971). Clinical and laboratory evidence for inactivation of gentamicin by carbenicillin. *Lancet*, **i**, 261–264.

Milerova, L. (1974). Personal communication.

Miller, A., Linton, K. B., Gillespie, W. A., Slade, N. & Mitchell, J. P. (1960). Catheter drainage and infection in acute retention of urine. *Lancet*, **i**, 310–312.

Millican, R. C., Evans, G. & Markley, K. (1966). Susceptibility of burned mice to *Pseudomonas aeruginosa* and protection by vaccination. *Annals of Surgery*, **163**, 603–610.

Millican, R. C. & Rust, J. D. (1960). Efficacy of rabbit pseudomonas antiserum in experimental *Pseudomonas aeruginosa* infections. *Journal of Infectious Diseases*, **107**, 389.

Moyer, C. A., Brentano, L., Gravens, D. L., Margraf, H. W. & Monafo, W. W. (1965). Treatment of large burns with 0·5% silver nitrate solution. *Archives of Surgery*, **90**, 812.

Müller, F. E. (1967). Gentamicin in the treatment of pseudomonas infections complicating burns. (First International Symposium on Gentamicin), Schwabe, Basel, p. 148.

Murdoch, J. M. C. (1964). Proceedings of Third International Congress of Chemotherapy, Stuttgart, p. 319.

Nance, F. C., Hines, J. L., Fulton, R. E. & Bornside, G. H. (1970). Treatment of experimental burn wound sepsis by postburn immunisation with polyvalent pseudomonas antigen. *Surgery*, **68**, 248.

Newsom, S. W. B. (1969). Carbenicillin-resistant pseudomonas. *Lancet*, **ii**, 1140.

Newsom, S. W. B., Sykes, R. B. & Richmond, M. H. (1970). Detection of a β-lactamase markedly active against carbenicillin in a strain of *Pseudomonas aeruginosa*. *Journal of Bacteriology*, **101**, 1079–1080.

Newton, B. A. (1956). The properties and mode of action of the polymyxins. *Bacteriological Reviews*, **20**, 14–27.

Noone, P. & Pattison, J. R. (1971). Therapeutic implications of interaction of gentamicin and pencillin. *Lancet*, **ii**, 575–578.

Noone, P., Pattison, J. R. & Samson, D. (1971). Simple rapid method for assay of aminoglycoside antibiotics. *Lancet*, **ii**, 16–22.

Nord, N. M. & Hoeprich, P. D. (1964). Polymyxin B and Colistin: a critical comparison. *New England Journal of Medicine*, **270**, 1030–1035.

O'Grady, F. & Pennington, J. H. (1967). Screening of antibacterial agents for *in vivo* activity against pseudomonas infections. *Postgraduate Medical Journal*, (Supplement), **43**, 72–73.

Pierson, C. & Feller, I. (1970). A reduction of pseudomonas septicaemia in burned patients by the immune processes. *Surgical Clinics of North America,* **50,** 1377.

Pines, A., Raafat, H., Siddiqui, E. & Greenfield, J. S. B. (1970). Treatment of severe pseudomonas infections of the bronchii. *British Medical Journal,* **i,** 663–665.

Pulaski, E. J. & Rosenberg, M. L. (1949). Use of polymyxin in Gram-negative urinary tract infections. *Journal of Urology (Baltimore),* **62,** 564–573.

Riff, L. & Jackson, G. G. (1971). Gentamicin plus carbenicillin. *Lancet,* **i,** 592.

Rodger, K. C., Nixon, M. & Tonning, H. O. (1965). Treatment of infections with colistimethate sodium (Coly-mycin). *Canadian Medical Association Journal,* **93,** 143–146.

Roe, E. & Jones, R. J. (1972). Effects of topical chemoprophylaxis on transferable antibiotic resistance in burns. *Lancet,* **ii,** 109–111.

Roe, E., Jones, R. J. & Lowbury, E. J. L. (1971). Transfer of antibiotic resistance between *Pseudomonas aeruginosa, Escherichia coli* and other Gram-negative bacilli in burns. *Lancet,* **i,** 149–152.

Roe, E. & Lowbury, E. J. L. (1972). Changes in antibiotic sensitivity patterns of Gram-negative bacilli in burns. *Journal of Clinical Pathology,* **25,** 176–178.

Rosenthal, S. M. (1966). Convalescent burn plasma therapy for severaly burned children. Control study of 81 cases and tests for Pseudomonas antibodies. *Annals of Surgery,* **163,** 461–469.

Rosenthal, S. M., Millican, R. C. & Rust, J. (1957). A factor in human gamma globulin preparations active against *Pseudomonas aeruginosa* infections. *Proceedings of the Society of Experimental Biology and Medicine,* **94,** 214–217.

Sachs, A. (1970). Active immunoprophylaxis in burns with a new multivalent vaccine. *Lancet,* **ii,**(93), 959.

Simmons, N. (1969). Potentiation of inhibitory activity of colistin on *Pseudomonas aeruginosa* by sulphamethoxazole and sulphamethiazole. *British Medical Journal,* **iii,** 693–696.

Smith, C. B., Dans, P. E., Wilfort, J. N. & Finland, M. (1969). Use of gentamicin in combinations with other antibiotics. *Journal of Infectious Diseases,* **119,** 370–377.

Smith, C. B. & Finland, M. (1968). Carbenicillin activity *in vitro* and absorption and excretion in normal young men. *Applied Microbiology,* **16,** 1753–1760.

Smith, C. B., Wilfort, J. N., Dans, P. E., Kurrus, T. A. & Finland, M. (1970). *In vitro* activity of carbenicillin and results of treatment of infections due to pseudomonas with carbenicillin singly and in combination with gentamicin. *Journal of Infectious Diseases,* **122,** Supplement, p. 14.

Sonne, M. & Jawetz, E. (1969). Combined action of carbenicillin and gentamicin on *Pseudomonas aeruginosa in vitro. Applied Microbiology,* **17,** 893–896.

Spiers, C. F., Selwyn, S. & Nicholson, D. N. (1963). Hypogammaglobulinaemia presenting as pseudomonas septicaemia. *Lancet,* **ii,** 710.

Stansly, P. G., Shepherd, R. G. & White, H. J. (1947). Polymyxin: A new chemotherapeutic agent. *Bulletins of the Johns Hopkins Hospital,* **81,** 43.

Stone, H. (1971). Wound care with topical gentamicin. *Contemporary Burn Management,* Little Brown, Boston, pp. 203–216.

Stone, H. H., Graber, C. D., Martin, J. D. & Kolb, L. (1965a). Evaluation of γ-globulins for prophylaxis against burn sepsis. *Surgery,* **58,** 810.

Stone, H. H., Martin, J. P. & Kolb, L. (1965). Experiences in the use of gentamicin sulphate ointment. *Antimicrobial agents and Chemotherapy,* 156–159.

Stone, H. H., Martin, J. P., Huger, W. E. & Kolb, L. (1965b). Gentamicin sulphate in the treatment of pseudomonas sepsis in burns. *Surgery, Gynaecology and Obstetrics,* **120,** 351–352.

Suzuki, T., Hayashi, K., Fujkawa, K. & Tsutamoto, K. (1964). *Journal of Biochemistry,* **56,** 535.

Sykes, R. B. & Richmond, M. H. (1970). Intergeneric transfer of a β-lactamase gene between *Pseudomonas aeruginosa* and *Escherichia coli*. *Nature (London)*, **226**, 951.
Trapnell, D. H. (1954). Pseudomonas pyocyanea meningitis successfully treated with polymixin. *Lancet*, **i**, 759–761.
Traub, U. P. & Penn, W. P. (1964). Third International Congress of Chemotherapy, Volume 1, Stuttgart 284.
Traub, W. H. & Raymond, E. A. (1972). Evaluation of the *in vitro* activity of tobramycin as compared with that of gentamicin sulphate. *Applied Microbiology*, **23**, 4–7.
Tumbusch, W. J., Vogel, E. H., Butkiewicz, C. D., Graber, C. D., Larson, D. L. & Mitchell, E. T. (1961). The rising incidence of pseudomonas septicaemia following burn injury. *Research in Burns*, (eds. Artz), Philadelphia, pp. 235–241.
Van Rooyen, C. E., Ross, J. F., Bethune, G. W. & MacDonald, A. C. (1967). Bacteriological observations on carbenicillin in the control of *Pseudomonas aeruginosa* infection in burns. *Canadian Medical Association Journal*, **97**, 1227–1229.
Vidal, G. & Mynard, M. C. (1972). Infection experimentale pars des sérotypes homolgues et heterologues de '*Pseudomonas aeruginosa*' chez la souris immunisée. *Annales de l'Institut Pasteur*, **122**, 1129–1135.
Vinnicombe, J. & Stamey, T. A. (1969). *Investigations in Urology*, **6**, 503.
Vogler, K. & Studer, R. O. (1966). The chemistry of the polymyxin antibiotics. *Experientia*, **22**, 345–416.
Waisbren, B. A. & Hastings, E. V. (1953). Bacterial endocarditis due to *Pseudomonas aeruginosa*. *Archives of Pathology*, **55**, 218–222.
Walker, H. C., Mason, A. D. & Raulston, G. L. (1964). Surface infection with *Pseudomonas aeruginosa*. *Annals of Surgery*, **160**, 297.
Weinstein, M. J., Luedemann, G. M., Oden, E. M. & Wagman, G. H. (1963). Gentamicin, a new broad-spectrum antibiotic complex. *Antimicrobial Agents and Chemotherapy*, **1**.
Witchitz, J. L. & Chabbert, Y. A. (1972). Résistance transférable à la gentamicine. II Tranmissions et liasons du charactère de résistance. *Annales de l'Institut Pasteur*, **122**, 367–378.
Young, L. S., Yu, B. H. & Armstrong, D. (1970). Agar gel precipitating antibody in *Ps. aeruginosa* infections. *Infection and Immunity*, **2**, 495.
Young, L. S. & Armstrong, D. (1972). Human immunity to pseudomonas 1. *In vitro* interaction of bacteria, polymorphonuclear leucocytes, and serum factors. *Journal of Infectious Diseases*, **126**, 257.
Young, L. S., Meyer, R. D. & Armstrong, D. (1973). *Pseudomonas aeruginosa* vaccine in cancer patients. *Annals of Internal Medicine*, **79**, 518–527.
Zinner, S. H., Sabath, L. D., Casey, J. I. & Finland, M. (1971). Erythromycin and alkalinisation of the urine in the treatment of urinary tract infections due to Gram-negative bacilli. *Lancet*, **i**, 1267–1271.

CHAPTER 8

In vitro Eradication of Pseudomonas aeruginosa

R. M. E. RICHARDS

STATING THE PROBLEM

The Fact of Contamination

The first workers to implicate the contamination of a pharmaceutical with *Pseudomonas aeruginosa* appear to have been Garretson & Cosgrove (1927) who suspected a 4% boric acid solution, used in a factory first-aid unit, to be the source of a series of *P. aeruginosa* eye infections. Wilson (1929) mentioned the contamination of a cocaine solution with this organism and Shrewsbury (1934) reported the development of *P. aeruginosa* meningitis after the intrathecal injection of a nupercaine solution. Eight years later Lepard (1942) and Cooper (1942) each reported cases of corneal ulcers resulting from the use of fluorescein eye drops contaminated with *P. aeruginosa*. McCulloch (1943) investigated the origin and pathogenicity of *P. aeruginosa* in the conjunctival sac and found that several solutions were occasionally contaminated. These were pontocaine hydrochloride, pilocarpine hydrochloride, ethyl morphine hydrochloride, scopolamine hydrobromide and atropine sulphate. Other solutions were always contaminated; physostigmine salicylate 0·5 and 1·0% and fluorescein 2%. Pharmacy stocks of the latter three solutions yielded positive cultures. From about that time onwards pharmacists and ophthalmologists were made increasingly aware of the problem of the contamination of ophthalmic solutions (Theodore, 1951; Theodore & Feinstein, 1952; Allen, 1952; Vaughan, 1955; Crompton, 1961, 1963a,b). These publications showed that contamination of ophthalmic solutions with *P. aeruginosa* was occurring over a wide geographical area and at far too great a rate for preparations which should have been sterile. The range of products contaminated was also wide and included fluorescein solutions (Theodore & Feinstein, 1952; Vaughan, 1955; Crompton, 1961, 1963a), physostigmine solutions (Theodore & Feinstein, 1952), silver proteinate solutions (Soet, 1952), saline solutions (Ayliffe, Barry, Lowbury, Roper-Hall & Walker, 1966), sulphonamide solutions (Theodore, 1951; Theodore & Feinstein, 1952; Allen, 1952; Vaughan, 1955) and cortisone suspensions (Theodore, 1951; Theodore & Feinstein, 1952). In addition, penicillin solutions were implicated as being contaminated with *P. aeruginosa* (Bignell, 1951).

Ophthalmic solutions, however, are by no means the only class of preparation to be contaminated by this organism (Brown, 1971). Kallings, Ringertz, Silverstolpe & Ernerfeldt (1966) reported eight cases of eye infection caused by *P. aeruginosa* which occurred in 1964. All the patients concerned had been treated with an imported hydrocortisone–neomycin–amphomycin ophthalmic ointment after having foreign bodies removed from the cornea. *P. aeruginosa* having identical characteristics and antibiotic sensitivity patterns were isolated from the infected eyes, from the used ointment and from unopened ointment tubes of the same batch. Six of fifteen further batches of the same manufacturer's ointment were also contaminated with this organism.

P. aeruginosa has been reported as a contaminant of a steroid cream (Noble & Savin, 1966), hand creams (Ayliffe, Lowbury, Hamilton, Small, Asheshov & Parker, 1965) and detergent solutions (Victorin, 1967; Cooke, Shooter, O'Farrell & Martin, 1970). Contamination of cosmetics with *P. aeruginosa* is also well substantiated. Baker (1959) cited three cases where serious production problems had been caused by *P. aeruginosa* contamination. Two cases involved shampoos and the third case involved a facial lotion which had 10^7 *P. aeruginosa*/ml in the marketed product. It seems that *Pseudomonads* are especially well equipped for multiplying in shampoos (Yasufuku, Hashimoto,

Hamai & Uesugi, 1968). Dunnigan (1968) reported that the Food and Drugs Administration had 25 recalls of cosmetic products due to microbiological contamination during 1966, 1967 and part of 1968. Fifteen manufacturers were involved in these recalls which included 16 lots of lotion, six of eye solutions and three of carmine red. *P. aeruginosa* was the contaminant in 14 of 16 lotions. The six eye solutions contained unidentified bacteria. Wilson, Kuehne, Hall & Ahearn (1971) investigated microbial contamination in partially used ocular cosmetics (mascara, eyeliner and eye shadow). All six of 428 samples which were contaminated with *P. aeruginosa* were from eyeliners which had been diluted with tap water as directed by the manufacturers. The same organism was also present in at least one eye of each of the six users of the contaminated eyeliners. One sample had approximately $2 \cdot 10^6$ organisms/ml.

The contamination of non-sterile preparations was investigated in England by the Public Health Laboratory Service Working Party (Report, 1971). As the result of this survey Hooper (1971) stated 'It became abundantly clear that aqueous medicines containing no preservative were very favourable breeding grounds for water-borne gram-negative bacteria including *Pseudomonas/ Alcaligenes/Achromobacter* groups. Mixtures such as magnesium trisilicate, aluminium hydroxide, ammonia and ipecacuanha, kaolin, magnesium carbonate, magnesium sulphate and magnesium hydroxide were often found to contain enormous numbers of organisms and counts of 10^6 ml^{-1} were commonplace'. *P. aeruginosa* was found in 3·2% (33 of 995) of preparations made in hospital pharmacies and 15 of 33 samples of peppermint water from a number of different hospitals were found to be contaminated with this organism (Report, 1971). Peppermint water has been found to be virtually a selective medium for *P. aeruginosa* (Shooter, Cooke, Gaya, Kumar, Patel, Parker, Thom & France, 1969; Brown, W. R. L., 1971).

Disinfectants are not exempt from contamination by *P. aeruginosa* (Brown, 1971). Quaternary ammonium compounds were implicated by Lowbury (1951) and Allen (1959). A phenolic was shown to be contaminated by Jellard & Churcher (1967) and chloroxylenol by Ayliffe *et al.* (1965). Maurer (1969) quoted a personal communication which reported contamination in 40 of 46 bottles of a diluted phenolic disinfectant which was investigated microbiologically before use. Other species of *Pseudomonas*, however, have been isolated from disinfectant solutions more often than *P. aeruginosa* (Burdon & Whitby, 1967; Bassett, Stokes & Thomas, 1970; Mitchell & Hayward, 1966; Hardy Ederer & Matsen, 1970; Phillips, Eykyn, Curtis & Snell, 1971; Speller, Stephens & Viant, 1971; Phillips, Eykyn & Laker, 1972).

Only one instance of the contamination of medicinal powders with *P. aeruginosa* appears to have been reported in the literature and that is in the report of Kallings *et al.* (1966). It is not clear whether the powders contaminated were baby powders or wound powders or one of each.

It can readily be seen from the foregoing that the contamination of pharmaceuticals and cosmetics with *P. aeruginosa* is a very real possibility unless conditions are deliberately designed to prevent the access of the organism to the products during preparation and to ensure as far as possible the death of any organism which subsequently gains access to the products.

THE SOURCE OF CONTAMINATION

1. *Raw Materials*

Raw materials, particularly those from natural sources such as dried plants, tragacanth, talc, kaolin, chalk, pancreatin, thyroid and rice starch are obvious sources of microbial contamination. Schiller, Kuntscher, Wolff & Nekola, (1968) found *Pseudomonadaceae* contaminating jaborandi and senna leaves but these organisms disappeared completely during the extraction processes. These authors concluded that synthetic or semi-synthetic substances can be considered free from micro-organisms but that care is to be observed with extracts of animal organs. Robinson (1971) suspected that magnesium hydroxide prepared from sea water and used in antacid preparations may have been responsible for contamination of the final preparations with this organism. No *P. aeruginosa* was found by Kallings *et al.* (1966) in the various components of the hydrocortisone–neomycin–amphomycin ointment. Refined oils, fats and waxes are not usually a source of serious contamination (Herbold, 1943).

2. *Manufacturing Plant*

The need for clean operating conditions and for carefully designed manufacturing plant for the production of pharmaceuticals and cosmetics has been stressed on many occasions (Davis, 1960; Deeley, 1962; Wedderburn, 1964, 1965; Kallings *et al.*, 1966; Monograph, 1970). Manufacturing plant having inaccessible stagnation areas must be avoided and routine testing of the manufacturing plant should include microbiological investigations.

Investigations at the manufacturer's plant by Kallings *et al.* (1966) showed that *P. aeruginosa* contaminating the hydrocortisone–antibiotic ointment was present in the production area in a runway, on towels and on the shoes, gloves and hands of personnel engaged in the manufacturing and bulk packaging of the ointment. Part of the manufacturing process consisted of pouring molten ointment into bulk containers. As this ointment cooled to the solid state a film of water condensed on its surface. The contaminating *P. aeruginosa* was shown to be multiplying in the aqueous film and the cells growing in this environment were resistant to both the neomycin and the amphomycin contained in the ointment. Many of the eye ointment tubes which had been packed with the bulk ointment prepared in this way contained more than 2000 *P. aeruginosa* cells/gram.

3. *Water*

The literature on the contamination of pharmaceuticals and cosmetics with *P. aeruginosa* does not often give details of how a particular product became contaminated. Nevertheless it appears that the preparation is frequently contaminated through some association with contaminated water. *P. aeruginosa* has very simple growth requirements and certain strains have been shown to be capable of growth in filter-sterilized distilled water (Favero, Bond, Peterson & Carsen, 1970). Brown (1968) found that aqueous vehicles supported the viability of large populations of *P. aeruginosa* for periods of a year or more. Inocula maintained viability to about the same extent in 2% fluorescein solution, tris buffer and water.

Water used to suspend, dissolve or emulsify the active components of the medicines manufactured in hospital pharmacies was cited by Hooper (1971) as the major source of contamination of the medicines with Gram-negative organisms. Twenty-one percent of the Gram-negative contamination was in fact *P. aeruginosa*.

Report No. 71 (1970) on public health and medical subjects entitled *The Bacteriological Examination of Water Supplies* is the basis on which bacteriological purity of water is usually judged. Potability is assessed on the presumptive and faecal coli tests and colony counts at 22 °C and 37 °C. The presence of *P. aeruginosa* in public water supply would not therefore render the water non-potable from a public health point of view. This does not mean, however, that potable water is *ipso facto* suitable for using in the preparation of pharmaceuticals and cosmetics. The conditions of manufacture and storage may be such that any *P. aeruginosa* originally present may be subjected to conditions which are suitable and even selective for the multiplication of this organism. The peppermint water contamination cited by Brown W. R. L. (1971) provides an example of how the medicament could selectively encourage the multiplication of small numbers of *P. aeruginosa* present in the water used in making up the final preparation. In addition to certain solutions providing selective conditions for *P. aeruginosa* the storage of water in tanks and passage through pipelines, pumps, filters and softeners often provides conditions for further contamination and multiplication. The resin beds of ion-exchangers are often responsible for contamination (Chambers & Clarke, 1966) which under warm storage conditions can result in 10^6 bacteria/ml (Olson, 1967).

The following two examples give ample illustration of the necessity for strict microbiological control on the water sources. Davis (1972) described how water contaminated with *P. aeruginosa* had been used to wash the udders of a valuable dairy herd and had caused severe cases of mastitis. The source of contamination was traced to a dead rat in the water tank! The second example is given by Phillips *et al.* (1972) who reported on the contamination of autoclaved fluids. The organism responsible was a *Pseudomonad* which apparently had not been described before and was given the name *Pseudomonas thomasii*. Figure 1 shows diagramatically the distribution of the contamination of the hospital pharmacy water supply system. The result was that contaminated water was widely distributed throughout the hospital.

4. People

Wilson *et al.* (1971) found that samples from unused ocular cosmetics were 'essentially free' of microbial contamination and considered that the user was the main source of bacterial contamination. This included *P. aeruginosa*.

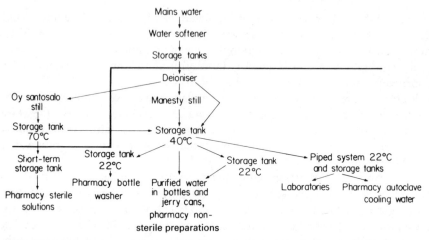

Figure 1. Pharmacy system for producing softened, deionised and distilled water. All sites below the line were contaminated with *P. thomasii.* Reproduced with permission from Phillips, I., Eykyn, S., and Laker, M., *Lancet,* **i**, 1258–1260 (1972)

P. aeruginosa can very occasionally be cultivated from normal human skin (Lilley & Bearup, 1928; Wilson & Miles, 1964) from sinuses (Wilson & Miles, 1964) and from a small percentage of human stools (Ringen & Drake, 1952; Wilson & Miles, 1964). Sutter, Hurst & Landucci (1966) found that about 5% of normal healthy people carried this organism in the saliva. Hospital staff and patients show a very variable but often greater than normal carriage rate of *P. aeruginosa* in the stools (Gould, 1963; Lowbury & Fox, 1954; Ayliffe *et al.,* 1965, 1966; Shooter, Walker, Williams, Horgan, Parker, Asheshov & Bullimore 1966; Jellard & Churcher, 1967; Noble & White, 1969; White, 1971), in urine (McLeod, 1958; Gould, 1963), in sputum (Phillips & Spencer, 1965; Tinne, Gordon, Bain & Mackay, 1967) and on the skin (Lowbury & Fox, 1954; Gould, 1963).

The human body is therefore a potential source of *P. aeruginosa* contamination for pharmaceuticals and cosmetics. Actual contamination by a given individual is nevertheless very difficult to demonstrate. The findings of Falcao, Mendonca, Scrassolo, De Almeida, Hart, Farmer & Farmer (1972) in a closely related field are therefore very interesting. A sensitive pyocine typing technique was used to determine the precise epidemiological relations between 36 isolates of *P. aeruginosa* in a nursery outbreak of severe diarrhoea. A nursery worker was shown to be carrying in her intestine a strain of *P. aeruginosa* which was also found contaminating an oxygen bubbler. Three children were infected by the oxygen bubbler and it was thought that the sequence of contamination had been the nursery worker, the oxygen bubbler and then the children.

5. *Hospital Environment*

Whitby & Rampling (1972) compared the domestic and hospital environments for contamination with *P. aeruginosa.* It was found that certain objects such as sink traps, floor cloths, dish cloths and mops were much more frequently contaminated in the hospital environment. There is a danger that these reservoirs of infection could become a source of *P. aeruginosa* contamination in cosmetics and pharmaceuticals used in hospitals. Pharaoh's ants (Monomorium pharaohnis) could be one means of transporting *P. aeruginosa* from the reservoir of infection to the medicament. It is known from the findings of Beatson (1972) that, owing to the predilection of these ants for visiting drains and sluices, they can be involved in the transport of infection including *Pseudomonas* species. Rupp & Forni (1972) reported observing an ant in a solution of glucose which was being administered to a patient. Presumably formulations high in carbohydrate are likely to be a particular attraction for ants and special care should be taken to prevent contamination of these solutions from such a source. Beatson (1972) recommended that expert advice should be taken to ensure removal of all ants from the hospital environment.

Kominos, Copeland, Grosiak & Postic (1972) showed that *P. aeruginosa* could be introduced into the hospital environment via vegetables. *P. aeruginosa* was isolated from tomatoes, radishes, celery, carrots, endive, cabbage, cucumbers, onions and lettuce obtained from the kitchen of a general hospital. Tomatoes yielded both the highest frequencies of isolation and the highest counts. It was estimated that a patient consuming an average portion of tomato salad might injest as many as $5 \cdot 10^3$ colony-forming units of *P. aeruginosa*. Pyocine types of *P. aeruginosa* isolated from clinical specimens were frequently identical to those recovered from vegetables, thus implicating tomatoes and other vegetables as an important source and vehicle by which *P. aeruginosa* colonizes the intestinal tract of patients.

Samish & Etinger-Tulcyzynska (1963) suggest that *P. aeruginosa* is an epiphyte which colonizes tomatoes. It is found mostly in the stem scar and underlying cores of healthy tomatoes. The stem depression was shown to be the point of entry of the *P. aeruginosa* into the tomato.

The Significance of Contamination

1. *Resistance*

It is the general ability of strains of *P. aeruginosa* to survive contact with concentrations of chemical antibacterials which other species of bacteria do not survive that has made this organism so infamous. Curtin, Petersdorf & Bennet (1961) stated that '*Pseudomonas aeruginosa* is so notoriously resistant that it occupies an almost unique position'. Gould (1963) described the situation very well: '*Pseudomonas pyocyanea* is an organism well adapted to survive an environment selective because of antibiotics. Biologically active to an extreme degree, it can live on simple substrates, survive for long periods under a wide range of environmental conditions apart from severe dehydration, and adapt to the presence of high concentrations of most antibiotics and antibacterial substances.'

Evidence will be given later in the chapter of the resistance of *P. aeruginosa* to a wide range of antibacterials. In contrast to the vast majority of reports however, there have been a few which would indicate that *P. aeruginosa* does not possess exceptional resistance to chemical agents (Hess & Speiser, 1959a,b; Bean & Farrell, 1967). Brown (1971) attempts to set this in context by clarifying the meaning of the term 'resistance' with special reference to *P. aeruginosa*.

Despite having high resistance to chemical antibacterials, *P. aeruginosa* is sensitive to both heat treatment (Burdon & Whitby, 1967; Tenenbaum, 1971; Dallos & Hughes, 1972; Drewett, Payne, Tuke & Verdon, 1972) and radiation (Niven, 1958; Darmady, Hughes, Burt, Freemand & Powell, 1961; Thornley, 1963).

2. *Pathogenicity*

P. aeruginosa is considered to have very little invasive power of its own except under exceptional circumstances (Jawetz, 1952; Editorial, 1966a) and is considered by many to penetrate the body's defences as the result of some other predisposing factor providing suitable conditions for *P. aeruginosa* to set up an infection. Parker (1972) refers to *P. aeruginosa* (along with certain other Gram-negative bacteria) as a 'conditional pathogen'. That is to say, it is harmless to completely healthy adults unless free access is gained to areas of the body which are normally sterile, such as the bladder, but may cause serious disease in the very young and those debilitated because of illness. Rogers (1960) named *P. aeruginosa* as being the most dangerous cross-infecting pathogen in a large children's hospital.

The significance of the contamination of a given product with *P. aeruginosa* therefore largely depends on the route of administration and the level of contamination of the product, together with the state of health of the recipient. The concurrent administration of an antibiotic may also be a significant factor in whether or not an infection is established (Buck & Cooke, 1969).

Perry & Nichols (1956) instilled *P. aeruginosa* into the ears of volunteers without giving rise to clinical infection and Buck & Cooke (1969) administered *P. aeruginosa* in milk to three normal volunteers without causing clinical symptoms. Intact corneal epithelium also appears to be highly resistant to *P. aeruginosa* (Vaughan, 1955) but, as Vaughan points out, this is the situation where *P. aeruginosa* is best able to show its opportunist powers. When the organism gains effective entrance through an injury to the corneal epithelium it can be totally destructive to the eye and will almost certainly cause rapid, severe and permanent damage. Even minute abrasions such as those due to the improper use of contact lenses can result in *P. aeruginosa* infection. (Gerke & Magliocco, 1971). Allen (1959) stated that *P. aeruginosa* was the most lethal in its effect on the eye of all bacteria found contaminating aqueous solutions. 50–100 cells injected intraocularly were able to establish an infection in the rabbit and cause panophthalmitis (Riegelman, Vaughan & Okumoto, 1956; Crompton, Anderson & Kennare, 1962).

Fisher & Allen (1958) showed that the method of corneal destruction caused by this organism is due to the production of an enzyme. This enzyme will actively degrade casein, haemoglobin, tendon collagen and two different corneal fractions, one of which is related to corneal collagen. This enzyme caused corneal damage when injected intracorneally into the eyes of rabbits. Recent work (Marzulli, Evans & Yoder, 1972) has also shown the elaboration of a cologenolytic enzyme by *P. aeruginosa*.

Although ingestion of *P. aeruginosa* in liquid medicines may not cause intestinal disease (Buck & Cooke, 1969) it is nevertheless undesirable and could result in auto-infections with bacteria from the patient's own bowel (Darrell & Wahba, 1964; Shooter *et al.*, 1966).

It may be concluded that *P. aeruginosa* is a very significant contaminant of pharmaceuticals and cosmetics and its presence in such products must be eliminated.

SOLVING THE PROBLEM

Disinfectants in Hospital Practice

A practical and effective hospital disinfectant policy would seem to be a prerequisite for an adequate control of hospital infection. It was not until 1961, however, that a rational approach was begun to be made to the use of disinfectants in British hospitals as a whole. This was done by the setting up of a committee by the Public Health Laboratory Service to study the situation. This committee's preliminary findings (Report, 1965) emphasized the confused situation existing in many hospitals. For example, a wide range of disinfectants was being used by different hospitals for a similar purpose and many of the disinfectants so used were ineffective in that situation. Disinfectant usage was often irrational, wasteful and even dangerous. This meant that disinfection was ineffective and large sums of money were being wasted. There were a few hospitals which were notable exceptions to this general position and where a more intelligent approach was being made to the disinfection problem. The report emphasized that chemical antimicrobial agents cannot be relied upon to kill viruses and spores quickly and efficiently and that heat and ionizing irradiation should be used wherever applicable. An interesting illustration of this point is provided by the investigations of Drewett *et al.* (1972) who traced the source of a recurring *P. aeruginosa* infection in a nursery, over a period of two years, to contaminated resuscitation apparatus in the delivery room. The adaptability of the organism to grow in the presence of antibacterials is demonstrated by this report. The authors found that subatmospheric steam sterilizers (80 °C for six min) gave a quick and reliable method of disinfecting the resuscitation apparatus. It was also apparent from the Report (1965) that *P. aeruginosa*, particularly in the presence of organic matter, was likely to survive contact with several of the commonly used disinfectants such as chloroxylenol, chlorhexidine and quaternary ammonium compounds. Davis (1960) warned that disinfectants could be highly specific in their action and that in choosing a disinfectant consideration must always be given to this fact. The findings of Ayliffe, Brightwell, Collins & Lowbury (1969) confirmed that *P. aeruginosa* often survived disinfection processes. The statement of Cook (1960) that lysol has a wide bactericidal spectrum including activity against *P. aeruginosa* is therefore very relevant to the hospital situation.

The Report (1965) suggested that three categories of disinfectant were needed in hospital practice. These were general disinfectants, surface disinfectants and disinfectants for use on skin and mucous membranes. The first category should have a wide spectrum of activity in the presence of organic matter and would be used for such purposes as washing down premises, steeping linen, transporting contaminated instruments, storing mops, neutralizing spilt discharges and for discarding contaminated laboratory materials. A black or white fluid to British Standard Specifications 2462:1961 or a clear soluble fluid of the lysol type were recommended as being suitable general disinfectants. Soaking linen in a chemical disinfectant, however, is not now recommended as a routine practice because bed linen, towels, gowns, uniforms, curtains and tea towels can all be laundered at a temperature sufficiently high for disinfection (Kelsey & Wagg, 1969).

The surface disinfectants should have a wide spectrum of activity and rapid action and would be used for disinfecting clean surfaces such as trolley tops, kitchen tables and clinical thermometers. Certain alcohols and hypochlorites are suitable for this function and general disinfectants could also be used in certain situations. The recommendations for skin disinfections were those of Lowbury & Lilly (1960) and Lowbury, Lilly & Bull (1960; 1963; 1964a,b).

Kelsey & Maurer (1967) recommend use-dilutions appropriate to hospital usage for a range of disinfectants which were available in the United Kingdom at that time. A further substance is included in the list of Kelsey & Sykes (1969) and a list of the commoner type of disinfectants together with notes about each is given by Kelsey & Maurer (1972).

The survey of Ayliffe *et al.* (1969) on the varieties of aseptic practice in hospital wards indicated, however, that the problem of hospital disinfection was by no means solved. Fourteen hospitals, which were all in one region, were included in the survey. Most of these hospitals had a disinfectant policy but the choice of disinfectants for similar purposes in the different hospitals varied considerably. More disturbing still was the comment that strict observance of the policies was rare, either as regards the type of disinfectant or the concentration used. Contamination of equipment seemed to relate more to the use of inadequate concentrations of disinfectant, or a failure to change solutions, than to the type of disinfectant used. Mops, whether sponge or string, rarely had adequate disinfection after use and 47% of both types of mop were found to be contaminated. *P. aeruginosa* was amongst the most frequently isolated organisms. Locker-top cleaning cloths, bath mops and brushes, nailbrushes, shaving brushes and toilet brushes were frequently contaminated with Gram-negative bacteria including *P. aeruginosa*. Kelsey & Maurer (1972) recommend that nailbrushes be discarded from wards and autoclaved for use in theatres.

As the result of their survey, Ayliffe *et al.* (1969) considered that 'codes of practice' for the use of disinfectants should be formulated where changes of technique seem to be desirable. Many hospitals do have well-established hospital disinfection policies and examples are given by Kelsey & Maurer (1972). Useful information is also contained in the Northern Ireland Hospitals Authority Code of Practice (Gibson, 1971). Those people involved in planning a hospital disinfection policy (a microbiologist, a nurse and a pharmacist would form the basis of such a group) would do well to adapt from these existing 'in use' but continually evolving policies. The work of Ayliffe *et al.* (1969), however, shows that in addition to having a hospital disinfection policy, staff training in the implementation of the policy is needed. All hospital staff having contact with patients at any time should be fully acquainted with the day-to-day functioning of the policy. It is interesting to note that Farrand & Williams (1973) have shown the feasibility of basing a hospital disinfection policy on the use of single-use packs of disinfectants and this apparently made compliance with the disinfection policy much easier.

Hospital pharmaceutical aspects involve the production of sterile 'in use' concentrations of disinfectants. Returned disinfectant dregs should be discarded, the bottles and caps thoroughly washed and all traces of detergent rinsed away. Thermostable disinfectants may be autoclaved in the final containers but the activity of the finished preparation needs to be checked. Meyers (1972) reported that a 40% loss of chlorhexidine could occur on autoclaving in new soft glass bottles when the pH went from $6 \cdot 0$ to $9 \cdot 5$.

Disinfectant Evaluation with Particular Reference to Hospital Use

1. *Phenol coefficient tests*

Surprisingly few advances were made in the evaluation of disinfectants between the publication of the Report (1909) on the standardization of disinfectants and the publication of the Report (1965) on the use of disinfectants in hospitals. It had been concluded in 1909 that the Rideal–Walker (1903) test for disinfectant activity gave accurate information under well-defined and strictly limited conditions but that it afforded little information on the activity of the disinfectants under practical conditions. Much work was anticipated in order to determine the effects of (i) the presence of foreign substances in the material to be disinfected; (ii) the temperature at which the disinfecting process is carried on; (iii) the fluid with which the disinfectant is diluted: hard water, soft water, sea water etc.; (iv) the type of micro-organism that has to be destroyed in the process of disinfection; (v) the nature of the substance and the character of the surface of the material to be disinfected and (vi) the duration of the disinfecting process.

The Report (1965) pointed to the need for further work to be done in the area of disinfectant evaluation to attempt to produce tests which were both realistic and reproducible. At that time the Rideal–Walker and Chick–Martin tests were still the best known and most widely used for phenolic disinfectants.

In these tests the performance of the unknown disinfectant against a standard organism is compared with that of a solution of phenol. The Chick–Martin test is performed in the presence of a 5% yeast suspension in an attempt to simulate in-use conditions where organic matter would be present. It has often been pointed out that use-dilutions derived from phenol coefficients are only applicable when the active ingredients of the disinfectants concerned are closely related to phenol, as in black or white fluids, or the lysols (Berry, 1951; Sykes, 1962; Kelsey, Beeby & Whitehouse, 1965). Use-dilutions of other disinfectants cannot be determined by phenol coefficient tests because these other agents vary from phenol in respect to such things as pH, temperature, organic matter, spectrum of activity and dilution.

2. *Surface film tests*

This type of test dates from the experiments of Kronig & Paul (1897). Stuart, Ortenzio & Friedl (1955) described a use-dilution test in which comparison with a standard disinfectant was dispensed with. Ten stainless steel cylinders were dipped in a broth culture of either *Salmonella choleraesuis* or *Staphylococcus aureus* and after drying were dipped in the test disinfectants for a fixed time before transferring to culture medium and incubating. The disinfectant passes the test if no cylinder causes growth. Statistical treatment of the results is given by Ortenzio & Stuart (1961). The test has been criticized because it does not distinguish between disinfection and detergency and the choice of organism is not very realistic (Kelsey *et al.*, 1965).

Hare *et al.* (1963) described a similar method in which overnight cultures of a number of organisms, including *P. aeruginosa*, were dried onto the outer surfaces of the base of glass tablet tubes and immersed in the test substance for a specified time. The antibacterial was then removed by holding the tube in a rapid stream of tap water. Survivors were detected by placing the base of the tubes on to the surface of a suitable solid culture medium. Some of the rather unusual results obtained, particularly the rapid sterilization times obtained against *P. aeruginosa*, might have been the result of the tap-water wash. It is now known that *P. aeruginosa* is particularly sensitive to this type of treatment (Brown, 1968). This test procedure is also open to the criticism of not distinguishing between disinfection and detergency.

3. *Capacity Tests*

Cantor & Shelanski (1951) proposed a capacity test for evaluating halogen disinfectants. Basically the test consists of adding the suspension of test organisms in a series of increments, at one min. intervals, to the disinfectant test dilution. A sample is removed from the mixture and tested for sterility immediately before each addition of organism. The results are expressed as the number of additions before a positive culture is obtained. *Salmonella typhi* and *S. aureus* are the test organisms used.

The International Dairy Federation (1963) adopted a similar test procedure and Kelsey *et al.* (1965) further modified the procedure for their capacity use-dilution test for disinfectants. In the introduction to another paper (Kelsey & Maurer, 1966), the procedure of Kelsey *et al.* (1965) was described as 'not being particularly easy to perform and interpret' and being unduly stringent in its use of 5% yeast. Nevertheless, the selection of *P. aeruginosa* NCTC 6749 by Kelsey *et al.* (1965) adds realism to the test and is to be commended. The test organism was chosen because it proved to be the most resistant of many possible test organisms when evaluated against the test disinfectants. Kelsey & Maurer (1966) indicate that the capacity use-dilution test described above had been modified to include only three successive additions of test organism and only 1% yeast for simulating 'dirty' conditions. The end point was 'that initial dilution of disinfectant which after the second incremental addition gives only a defined small number of survivors.' (Kelsey & Sykes, 1969).

Kelsey & Sykes (1969) combined their wide experience in disinfectant evaluation to propose a new test for the assessment of disinfectants with particular reference to their use in hospitals. While Kelsey had been developing test methods with various colleagues, Sykes had been evolving a test structure in collaboration with the British Disinfectant Manufacturers Association. The result of collaboration by Kelsey & Sykes was the further modification of the Kelsey tests to produce the Kelsey–Sykes test which is a test of major importance for the assessment of disinfectants intended for use in the hospital situation. Four test organisms are used; *S. aureus* NCTC 4163; *Escherichia coli* NCTC 8196; *P. aeruginosa* NCTC 6749 and *Proteus vulgaris* NCTC 4635. Twenty-four-hr broth cultures incubated at 30–32 °C and containing 10^8–10^9 organisms/ml form the sources of inocula. The inocula are added in three increments of 1 ml at ten min intervals to an initial 3 ml of disinfectant dilution freshly prepared in standard hard water (300 p.p.m. hardness). The concentration of yeast to simulate 'dirty' conditions is 2% (dry weight). Eight min after each addition a sample of mixture is removed with a '50 dropper' pipette and one drop transferred to each of five tubes of the liquid recovery medium. The initial test is carried out at 20–22 °C and all subcultures are incubated at about 32 °C for 48 hr. A starting dilution is considered to pass the test if, after the second increment, not more than three tubes show growth. Alternatively, five drops may be placed separately on a nutrient agar plate. Here the accepted dilution is that which gives not more than five colonies from the five drops subcultured (presumably after the second increment). It is stated that it must not be presumed that a reliable result can be obtained from a single test but that the test should be repeated several times on different occasions and the mean response calculated.

Bergan & Lystad (1971) evaluated ten disinfectants by a capacity use-dilution test similar to that of Kelsey & Sykes (1969) and considered that the test realistically simulated practical conditions and gave reasonable results. Gardner (1972) was in favour of adopting the Kelsey–Sykes (1969) test as the primary test for the evaluation and estimation of use-dilutions of disinfectants for hospital use.

4. *In-use test*

In addition to the disinfectant use-dilution tests which have evolved as outlined above it has been found necessary to introduce two further tests for the effective evaluation of disinfectants in hospital use. The first of these is the in-use test described by Kelsey & Maurer (1966). This test checks the survival of organisms in the liquid phase of the disinfectant in practical situations. Disinfectant samples are taken from in-use situations and diluted 1:10 in ¼ strength Ringer's solution or, for non-phenolics, in a suitable inactivator. Ten drops of this dilution are then plated out on an overdried agar plate and incubated for 72 hr at 37 °C. Failure is defined as any growth on more than five drops out of ten. This was said to correspond to about 1000 recoverable organisms/ml of liquid sampled and a use-dilution was thought to be satisfactory when only an occasional sample failed. When used and interpreted with care the in-use test can provide useful information on whether a selected disinfectant, at the use-dilution indicated by the capacity test, is effective under the conditions of use. The in-use test also provides a check as to whether procedural techniques such as correctness of dilution, frequency of changing solutions, frequency of cleaning utensils etc. are adequately complied with. The importance of using freshly prepared dilutions of disinfectants in clean containers was emphasized.

5. *Stability and long-term effectiveness test*

Maurer (1969) devised this test to be used as a supplement to the capacity test and his results clearly show the need for this additional test. For example, some disinfectants were less effective when dilutions were prepared seven days before use than when freshly prepared. Other disinfectant dilutions may be effective on the first day of use but cease to be effective on subsequent use several days later. Small numbers of organisms which survive in a disinfectant may multiply rapidly and reach 10^6/ml in five or six days. Maurer chose *P. aeruginosa* for her test organism because of its resistance to most disinfectants and its greater ability to grow rapidly in low concentrations of disinfectants than other Gram-negative organisms. Basically the test consists of evaluating the activity of freshly prepared and seven-day-old use-dilutions of disinfectant in standard hard water (300 p.p.m. hardness) under 'clean' and 'dirty' conditions (1% dry weight yeast) against a final concentration of approximately 10^7 *P. aeruginosa*/ml. The disinfectant–*P. aeruginosa* reaction mixtures are sampled after seven days at room temperature using a '50-dropper' pipette and adding one drop to each of five tubes containing 10 ml nutrient broth for phenolic disinfectants and 10 ml inactivator-broth for non-phenolics. All subculture tubes are incubated for 48 hr at either 32 °C or 37 °C. No growth in at least two out of five subculture tubes is taken as a negative result. The test is carried out in triplicate and the disinfectant can be passed for use in both 'clean' and 'dirty' conditions or just for use in 'clean' conditions.

6. Conclusions

It appears that, as a result of the development of these recent test procedures, the Department of Public Health and Social Security believe they have the basis for differentiating between disinfectants suitable and unsuitable for hospital use (Kelsey, 1969). The same author stated that manufacturers will be asked to submit the following details: (i) formulation; (ii) minimum inhibitory concentrations; (iii) Kelsey–Sykes capacity test results for both 'clean' and 'dirty' conditions; (iv) stability and long-term effectiveness results for both 'clean' and 'dirty' conditions, unless the label specifically states that the disinfectant must be diluted immediately before use and the dilution discarded 24 hr after preparation; (v) recommendations for storage; (vi) results of toxicity tests; (vii) suitable inactivators; (viii) contraindications and effect on materials and (ix) incompatibilities.

Gardner, (1972) suggested the adoption in Australia of the disinfectant testing programme evolved by Kelsey and colleagues. That is, using the capacity test (Kelsey & Sykes, 1969) as the primary test for evaluation and estimation of the probable use-dilutions for clean and dirty conditions, plus a laboratory test for stability and long-term effectiveness (Maurer, 1969) and an in-use test (Kelsey & Maurer, 1966), carried out in the hospital.

Therefore it would appear that, with the use of approved disinfectants in accordance with the careful hospital disinfection policies, the contamination of the environment within our hospitals by *P. aeruginosa* and other undesirable bacterial contaminants should be severely restricted.

Preservation of Ophthalmic Solutions

It was widely recognized by the early 1950s that *P. aeruginosa* was sometimes brought to the eye in the preparations used for the treatment of various eye conditions (Bignell, 1951; Theodore, 1951; Theodore & Minsky, 1951; Allwn, 1952; Theodore & Feinstein, 1952; Soet, 1952; Theodore & Feinstein, 1953).

Starting with Garretson & Cosgrove (1927) a number of papers connected corneal ulcer caused by *P. aeruginosa* with the use of contaminated ophthalmic solutions. Lepard (1942) reported three cases of corneal ulcer and stated that one case resulted from using fluorescein eye drops contaminated with *P. aeruginosa*. McCulloch (1943) traced five cases of *Pseudomonas* infection to the use of contaminated eye drops.

Since this organism can be totally destructive to the eye and invariably causes rapid, severe and permanent damage it is obvious that the situation described above was very serious and many research workers in a number of countries have been challenged to attempt to solve the problem of preserving multi-dose ophthalmic solutions against contamination with *P. aeruginosa*. The preparation of the initial sterile product is not the problem. Sterilization in the final container by heat treatment is the method of choice for thermostable ingredients and there are satisfactory alternative methods for thermolabile substances (BPC 1968). Effective preservation throughout the period of use, however, has proved to be the difficulty. Sterile, single-dose units containing no preservative provide the answer for ophthalmic solutions needed to be used during eye surgery. However, this is not the answer to other aspects of eye medication such as long-term treatments and general eye medication for the vast populations represented by the world's poorer countries. In these situations multi-dose preparations will almost certainly be used and, because of this, adequately preserved multi-dose ophthalmic solutions must be formulated. Therefore, with ophthalmic solutions we have the situation that demands the *in vitro* elimination of *P. aeruginosa*. It is also the field of pharmaceutical and cosmetic preservation in which by far the most research has been published. For these reasons it will be reviewed in detail here. Lawrence (1955b), Brown & Norton (1965), Brown (1967, 1971) and Richards (1967a,b; 1972) have written reviews on this general subject of the preservation of ophthalmic solutions.

1. *Inadequate Methods of Evaluation*

(a) Inactivators. Inadequate inactivation of the antibacterial activity seems to be the reason for the very rapid sterilization times obtained with benzalkonium chloride by some of the early workers in this field (McPherson & Wood, 1949; Hind & Szekely, 1953; Scigliano & Skolaut, 1954; Heller, Foss, Shay & Ichniowski, 1955). Three of these four groups of workers appreciated the need to inactivate the carry-over effect of the organic mercurials but none seemed to appreciate the need of a similar procedure for benzalkonium chloride, despite the publications showing that quaternaries must also be inactivated (Quisno, Gibby & Foter, 1946; McCulloch, 1947; Armbruster & Ridenour, 1947; Weber & Black, 1948). Later work by Anderson, Lillie & Crompton (1964a) also seems open to question with regard to the inactivation procedures used. They did not use conventional inactivators in the recovery medium, but used a washing procedure, the efficiency of which was not demonstrated, and which is now known to be unsuitable for use with *P. aeruginosa* (Brown, 1968, 1971).

(b) Test organism. There is now widespread agreement about including *P. aeruginosa* as one of the test organisms when investigating the antibacterial activity of preservatives suitable for use in ophthalmic preparations. Hughson & Styron (1949) and Theodore & Feinstein (1953) did not take sufficient account of this and relied on chance contaminants as their inocula.

(c) Experimental details. Klein, Millwood & Walther (1954) gave only brief experimental details. It is therefore difficult to assess whether thioglycollate was used as an inactivator for their work with final preparations. It is also not obvious whether only one strain of *P. aeruginosa* was used for the work with the final preparations, or three strains, as in another aspect of their work. The temperature and pH of the reaction mixtures were not given and the extent to which inactivation of antibacterial carry-over effect was made is not clear.

Ridley (1958) and Jeffs (1959), both working in hospital pharmacies, reported on their experiences of successfully preserving ophthalmic solutions against bacterial contamination. Ridley used methyl hydroxybenzoate 0·1% and phenylmercuric nitrate 0·004% while Jeffs used chlorhexidine 0·005%. Both workers claimed that, in the concentrations used by them, these preservatives were effective against *P. aeruginosa* but, unfortunately, neither worker gave sufficient details of the bacteriological test procedures used for an accurate assessment of their results to be made.

Crompton (1962) in a general article on ophthalmic prescribing, stressed the necessity of having sterile ophthalmic solutions. The author stated that chlorhexidine was effective against *P. aeruginosa* and quoted two personal communications but no experimental details in support of the statement.

(d) Test procedure. Iannarone & Eisen (1961) investigated the activity of three chemicals alone, or in combination, dissolved in phosphate buffer pH 6·8. The method of evaluating the inhibitory properties was that of the 1·5 cm FDA agar cup plate as prescribed in Circular 198. The test organism used was *P. aeruginosa*, and three strains were used. This type of test, however, does not lend itself for use in this field as so much depends upon the diffusion characteristics of the agents tested and their activity in the presence of agar. It is also more valuable to know the concentrations that sterilize rather than inhibit the test inoculum since Riegelman *et al.* (1956) showed that organisms that were merely being inhibited could produce an infection when injected intracorneally. Since the results of workers using inadequate methods of evaluation are of reduced significance they have not been quoted in detail.

2. *Improved Methods of Evaluation*

(a) *In vitro* testing. Certain chemicals rapidly lose antibacterial activity on dilution and these agents do not necessitate the specific inactivators required by such antibacterials as the organic mercurials and the quaternary ammonium compounds. The fact that Murphy, Allen & Mangiaracine (1955) did not use an inactivator for chlorbutol and phenylethyl alcohol does not therefore invalidate their results. Table 1 gives a brief summary of the experimental procedure and findings of Murphy *et al.* (1955) and Lawrence (1955b). Both investigations used large numbers of strains of *P. aeruginosa* as the test organism and made a substantial contribution to this field of work. The contact time of 24 hr used by Murphy *et al.* (1955), however, is too long for a precise assessment of the time taken for a given chemical to effect sterilization. This sterilization time for a given chemical is very useful when comparing the results obtained by several different chemicals.

It is apparent from the results of Murphy *et al.* (1955) that chlorbutol 0·5%, when formulated in ophthalmic preparations of pH 5·0, is a useful antimicrobial agent. It was used in the Massachusetts Eye and Ear Infirmary from 1926 to 1955. No bacterial contamination was detected throughout this period and no ill effects upon the tissues of the eye were observed.

Table 1. Summary of the Work of Lawrence (1955a) and Murphy, Allen & Mangiaracine (1955)
(Reproduced with permission from R. M. E. Richards, Aust. J. Pharm., Science Supplement, **55**, (1967)

Workers	Chemicals and concentration	Organisms & approximate inoculum	Test solutions	Temperature	pH	Contact time	Inactivator	Pertinent results and comments
Lawrence (1955a)	Benzalkonium 0·02% and 0·01%	P. aeruginosa 26 strains Proteus 4 sp.	Phosphate buffer	24–26°	7·2	½; 1; 3; 6; 24 and 48 hr and sometimes 6 days	Thioglycollate Polysorbate-lecithin broth Combinations of first 2	Benzalkonium 0·02% sterilized within ½ hr Phenylethyl alcohol 0·5% had least activity of chemicals tested often more than 48 hr to sterilize
	Chlorbutol, Phenol, Phenylethyl alcohol all 0·5%							
	Phenylmercuric nitrate 0·01% and 0·005%	P. aeruginosa 4 strains 10⁸ cells/ml	7 F.P. in buffer	24–26°	7·2			
	Thiomersal 0·01% and 0·005%							
	Methyl and propyl hydroxybenzoates 0·16% and 0·02%		7 F.P. in distilled water	24–26°	?			

								Results
Murphy et al. (1955) (Tests in broth omitted)	Chlorbutol 0·5% Phenylethyl alcohol 0·5% Phenylmercuric nitrate 0·004%	P. aeruginosa 15 strains 10^6 cells/ml	Phosphate buffer	?	5·0	24 hr	Thio-glycollate	Chlorbutol 0·5% sterilized 15/15 strains Phenylmercuric nitrate 0·004% 13/15 and phenylethyl alcohol 12/15 (Preliminary tests with benzalkonium inconsistent)
	Chlorbutol 0·5%	P. aeruginosa 4–9 strains 10^6 cells/ml	8 F.P.	?	3·4 5·5 3·4 4·1 3·8 3·9 7·2 4·4	24 hr	None	Chlorbutol 0·5% sterilized all except 4/4 with fluorescein and 1/9 homatropine which took more than 48 hr

F.P. = Final ophthalmic preparation.

Lawrence (1955b) used inactivators for the benzalkonium chloride and for the mercurials tested, both in simple solution and in final ophthalmic preparations. Inactivators were not used for the other chemicals tested. This weighted the experimental procedure against the chemicals being inactivated. Nevertheless, of all the chemicals tested, benzalkonium chloride 0·02% was shown to have the shortest sterilization time against heavy inocula of *P. aeruginosa*. The pH of the unbuffered alkaloidal preparations used by Lawrence would be of the order of pH 4·0–5·0. Benzalkonium chloride was, however, shown to be as consistently active in these test solutions as in the buffered test solutions pH 7·2.

The work of Lawrence (1955b) shows the importance of testing the antimicrobial agents in final ophthalmic preparations in addition to simple solutions. Phenylethyl alcohol 0·5% v/v was apparently more active in final preparations than in simple solution. The mercurials, phenylmercuric nitrate and thiomersal, both at 0·01 and 0·005% exhibited the opposite effect by being less effective in final preparations. The results obtained by Lawrence with chlorbutol 0·5% and phenylethyl alcohol 0·5% v/v were in general agreement with the results obtained with these two chemicals by Murphy *et al.* (1955). It must be noted, however, that preliminary investigations by Murphy *et al.* of the antibacterial activity of benzalkonium chloride at concentrations of 0·02–0·002% gave 'decidedly variable' results. This is in contradiction to the findings of Lawrence.

Anderson & Stock (1958) made some preliminary investigations of the antibacterial activity of chlorhexidine acetate 0·01%. These workers compared its activity against *Micrococcus pyogenes* and *P. aeruginosa*. One strain of each was used at an approximate inoculum of 10^5 cells/ml. The chemicals tested were benzalkonium chloride 0·005%, phenylethyl alcohol 0·6% v/v, chlorbutol 0·5%, phenylmercuric nitrate 0·01%, cetrimide 0·005% and dequalinium chloride 0·02%. The results obtained, although containing admitted inconsistencies, indicated that chlorhexidine 0·01% had a sterilization time of 15–30 min and thus showed promise of being a useful preservative. Inactivators were used for the chlorhexidine, the quaternary ammonium compounds and for the phenylmercuric nitrate. The concentration of benzalkonium tested was less than that usually recommended for preserving ophthalmic solutions.

Kleinman & Huyck (1961) gave full experimental details of their investigations using benzalkonium chloride 0·02% and chlorbutol 0·5% made up in buffered ophthalmic solutions. The solutions were sterilized by filtration and subsequently contaminated with 10^8 cells/ml of one strain of *P. aeruginosa*. A suitable inactivating medium was used. Benzalkonium chloride 0·02% had a sterilization time of 30 min in both preparations. Chlorbutol 0·5% had a sterilization time of 30 min in one preparation and 180 min in the other.

During a prolonged correspondence in the *Lancet* on the sterility of eye medicaments, Crompton (1963b) implied that chlorhexidine was suitable for use as a preservative for ophthalmic solutions. Richards (1964) reported that chlorhexidine in final ophthalmic preparations was less effective against inocula of 10^8 *P. aeruginosa*/ml than it was in simple solution. Conversely, chlorocresol was more active in final preparations of acid pH than it was in simple solution. These results again stressed the need to evaluate the final preparations.

Foster (1964) evaluated eight chemical agents by testing the activity of their aqueous solutions against the following organisms: *P. aeruginosa, S. aureus, Streptococcus pyogenes, Bacillus subtilis, P. vulgaris* and *E. coli.* Low inocula of 10 organisms/ml and 100 organisms/ml were used. Inactivators were used for those chemicals which were considered to need inactivating. The results indicated that when the contamination was small then a whole range of chemical antibacterial agents in aqueous solution and at a concentration recommended in the literature were capable of sterilizing within 60 min. It is doubtful if such low contamination could always be guaranteed in practice, however, and Riegelman (1964) reported that contact of an eye dropper with an infected eye could result in the transmission of 10,000 organisms. Allowing the dropper to touch the eye is acknowledged bad practice, but it cannot be guaranteed not to happen. Therefore, a test inoculum larger than 100 organisms/ml is indicated since the test procedure must cater for the worst, or greatest contamination possible under the conditions of practice. A larger inoculum is also indicated to ensure that a true representation of the resistance of the culture is contained in each inoculum. This is because a bacterial culture may contain a small percentage of cells which are more resistant than the rest of the population (Chaplin, 1951).

(b) Correlation of *in vitro* with *in vivo* testing. The work of Riegelman *et al.* (1956) marked a definite advance in the experimental procedure for evaluating chemical antibacterial agents suitable for use in ophthalmic solutions. These workers emphasized the need of using efficient inactivators and developed an *in vivo* testing procedure, based on intracorneal injections into rabbits' eyes, which made it possible to evaluate the efficiency of various inactivating agents against specific antimicrobials. Riegelman *et al.* showed that thioglycollate medium, which was generally accepted as an efficient medium for inactivating the antimicrobial action of phenylmercuric nitrate, was not able, by itself, to neutralize the action of phenylmercuric nitrate on the particular strains of *P. aeruginosa* tested.

For example, *in vitro* subcultures into thioglycollate broth of phenylmercuric nitrate up to 0·01%, which had been contaminated with heavy inocula of *P. aeruginosa*, indicated that sterility had been achieved at the end of 1 hr exposure. However, intracorneal injections into rabbits' eyes of small volumes of these same phenylmercuric nitrate–*P. aeruginosa* reaction mixtures produced corneal ulcers even after one week's contact.

Riegelman *et al.* were eventually able to develop inactivating media for phenylmercuric nitrate, benzalkonium chloride, chlorbutol and polymyxin B sulphate which enabled *in vitro* determinations of the sterilization time for a given chemical to be made which was consistently the same as the sterilization time for that chemical determined by the *in vivo* method.

The results of Riegelman *et al.* (1956) are summarized in Table 2. It is interesting to note that the results obtained by these workers with benzalkonium chloride 0·02% are different from those obtained by Lawrence (1955b). The difference in the resistance of the strains of *P. aeruginosa* used could be a possible cause of the widely divergent results. For example, the strains of *P. aeruginosa* which Riegelman *et al.* used may have contained at least one strain which was highly resistant to benzalkonium chloride possibly through previous contact with the chemical. It has been shown by MacGregor & Elliker (1958) that it is possible to train *P. aeruginosa* to grow in the presence of increasingly concentrated solutions of a quaternary ammonium compound. MacGregor & Elliker were able by this means to grown *P. aeruginosa* in the presence of 0·2% of this quaternary.

It must be noted that the results obtained by Riegelman *et al.* (1956) and Lawrence (1955b), using chlorbutol 0·5% and phenylethyl alcohol 0·5%, are in good general agreement.

The results obtained by Riegelman *et al.* (1956) with polymyxin B sulphate confirm the results of Wiggins (1952a,b) that this antibacterial agent is very active against *P. aeruginosa*. Polymyxin B sulphate was in 1956, and still is one of the agents of choice in the treatment of *P. aeruginosa* infections. For this reason the wisdom of using polymyxin B sulphate as a preservative for ophthalmic preparations, as recommended by Riegelman *et al.* (1956) and the USP XVII (1965) is to be questioned. Presumably there is a relationship between the freedom of use of a given antimicrobial agent and the rate at which resistant strains of bacteria develop to that agent. Therefore, it would seem to be unwise to risk developing strains of *P. aeruginosa* resistant to the action of polymyxin B sulphate by using this antibacterial agent as a preservative in ophthalmic solutions. It may also be questioned whether it is justifiable to risk sensitizing patients who must use ophthalmic solutions to an antibiotic of such effectiveness.

Kohn, Gershenfeld & Barr (1963a,b) developed and extended the work begun by Riegelman *et al.* (1956). These authors did a vast amount of work evaluating a wide range of chemicals, many of which had not previously been examined with reference to their use in ophthalmic solutions. Full details of the experimental procedure was given and their work is summarized in Table 3.

Benzalkonium 0·02% was shown to be the fastest acting of the bactericides commonly used in ophthalmic solutions, sterilizing a heavy inoculum of 13 strains of *P. aeruginosa* within 45 min. These findings are in contradiction with those obtained by Riegelman *et al.* (1956), but are in agreement with those of Lawrence (1955b).

Polymyxin was shown to be slow acting, 1000 units/ml sterilizing within 18 hr. Riegelman *et al.* (1956) found polymyxin to be the fastest acting of the chemicals which they tested, 1000 units/ml sterilizing within 30 min. These conflicting results between workers using good experimental procedure may

Table 2. Summary of the work of Riegelman, Vaughan and Okumoto (1956). Reproduced with permission from R. M. E. Richards, *Aust J. Pharm., Science Supplement*, 55 (1967) Table 2.

Chemicals and concentration	Organisms and approximate inoculum	Test solutions	Temperature	pH	Contact time	Inactivator	Sterilizing time
Phenylmercuric Nitrate up to 0·01%	*P. aeruginosa* several strains 10^8 cells/ml	Sterile solutions in saline	?	?	Ranging from 5 min to 1 week	Specific inactivators for each chemical tested except in the case of phenylethyl alcohol	Phenylmercuric nitrate up to 0·01% did not sterilize within 1 week
Benzalkonium up to 0·02%							Benzalkonium up to 0·02% did not sterilize within 3 days
Phenylethyl alcohol 0·5% to 2·0%							Phenylethyl alcohol 0·5% to 2·0% did not sterilize within 8 hr. These were the longest contact times used in each case
Chlorbutol 0·5% to 0·8%							Chlorbutol 0·5% sterilized within 8 to 24 hr
Polymyxin B sulphate up to 1000 units/ml							Polymyxin B sulphate 1000 units/ml sterilized within 30 min

Table 3. Summary of work of Kohn, Gershenfeld and Barr (1963).

Reproduced with permission from R. M. E. Richards, *Aust. J. Pharm., Science Supplement,* **56**, (1967) Table 3.

Chemicals and concentration	Organisms and approximate inoculum	Test solutions	Temperature	pH	Contact time	Inactivator	Sterilizing time
Chlorbutol 0·5% and 0·7%	*P. aeruginosa* 13 strains 10^6 cells/ml	Sterile solutions in distilled water	24	?	Many ranging from 15 min to 24 hr	Specific inactivators for each chemical tested	Chlorbutol 0·5% 12 hr
Benzalkonium 0·02% and 0·01%							Benzalkonium 0·02% 45 min
Thiomersal 0·02% and 0·01%							Thiomersal 0·02% 6 hr
Methyl and propyl hydroxybenzoates 0·2% and 0·04% respectively and 0·18% and 0·02% respectively							Methyl hydroxybenzoate 0·2% in combination with Propyl hydroxybenzoate 0·04% sterilized in 3 hr
Phenylmercuric nitrate 0·01% and 0·005%							Phenylmercuric nitrate 0·01% and 0·005% 6 hr
Phenylethyl alcohol 0·5%							Phenylethyl alcohol 0·5% took longer than 24 hr
Polymyxin B sulphate 1000 and 2000 units/ml							Polymyxin B sulphate 2000 units/ml 12 hr 1000 units/ml 18 hr

37 quaternary ammonium compounds 8 amphoteric surface-active agents 3 iodophors Also a group of miscellaneous agents, including Chlorhexidine 0·002%, 0·004%, 0·01% and 0·02% Colistin 250, 500 and 1000 units/ml	*P. aeruginosa* 13 strains 10^6 cells/ml	Aqueous solutions and in some cases solutions in boric acid 1%	24	?	Many ranging from 15 min to 24 hr	Specific inactivators for each chemical tested	6 quaternary ammonium compounds at 0·02% 45 min 3 iodophors at 25 ppm iodine 15 min Chlorhexidine 0·004% 30 min: 0·005%, 0·01% and 0·02% 15 min Colistin 250 units/ml 45 min, 500 and 1000 units/ml 15 min

best be explained in terms of the varying resistance of the strains of *P. aeruginosa* used by the different workers. Strains of *P. aeruginosa* have been shown to have the capacity to be, or to become resistant to, the following antibacterial agents: (i) polymyxin (Newton, 1954); (ii) benzalkonium chloride and other quaternary ammonium compounds (Riegelman *et al.*, 1956; MacGregor & Elliker, 1958); (iii) phenylethyl alcohol (Murphy *et al.*, 1955); (iv) phenylmercuric nitrate (Riegelman *et al.*, 1956): (v) chlorhexidine (Brown, Watkins & Scott Foster, 1969) and even to decompose phenol (Davey & Turner, 1961) and *p*-hydroxybenzoates (Hugo & Foster, 1964). The case reports published by Cassady (1959), although showing that polymyxin B sulphate was used with success in ten cases of *Pseudomonas* corneal infection, also showed marked differences in the sensitivity to polymyxin of the *P. aeruginosa* cells recovered from the different cases.

The results obtained by Kohn *et al.* (1964a) with chlorbutol 0·5% and phenylethyl alcohol 0·5% are in general agreement with those obtained by Lawrence (1955b); Murphy *et al.* (1955) and Riegelman *et al.* (1956) and the results obtained with the mercurials are in general agreement with those obtained by Lawrence (1955b).

Chlorhexidine 0·005–0·02% in simple solution, as tested by Kohn *et al.* (1963b), was shown to be efficient with a sterilization time of 15 min. This supports the results of Anderson & Stock (1958).

Other chemicals not commonly used as preservatives in ophthalmic solutions were also shown to be highly active against *P. aeruginosa*. Kohn *et al.* (1963b) were careful to point out that the toxicity, ocular irritability, stability and compatibilities with common ophthalmic drugs and vehicles must also be determined for these agents. All the chemicals evaluated by Kohn *et al.* (1963a,b) also need to be evaluated in final ophthalmic solution because Lawrence (1955b) found that the antibacterial properties could be modified in the final preparation.

Anderson (1965), working with dodecyldi (aminoethyl) glycine, one of the chemicals tested by Kohn *et al.* (1963b), concluded that this agent justified further investigations to determine its effectiveness in slightly alkaline ophthalmic solutions.

It is interesting to note that the results obtained by Kohn *et al.* (1963a) in testing the efficiency of inactivators supported those of Riegelman *et al.* (1956). Both sets of workers found that thioglycollate medium alone was not as effective in inactivating the action of the mercurials as was the thioglycollate–lecithin–polysorbate 80 combination.

(c) Misunderstandings concerning benzalkonium chloride.

(i) Other than bacteriological. Klein *et al.* (1954) and Anderson *et al.* (1964a) have misquoted the literature concerning benzalkonium chloride (Brown *et al.*, 1965). Both groups of workers apparently misunderstood the work of Ginsburg & Robson (1949). Later Runti (1960) and Dale, Nook & Barbiers (1959) use Klein *et al.* (1954) as their authority that benzalkonium is irritant to the eye. Ginsburg & Robson (1949) did not use a quaternary ammonium compound, but worked with anionic and non-ionic wetting agents. They found that the anionic detergent dodecyl sodium sulphate 1% damaged the cornea. They also found that although 1% anionic Lissapol N caused slight oedema, which disappeared in 24 hr, 0·5% applied at 2-hr intervals caused no observable effect. These results are supported by those of Buschke (1949), who studied the effects of a wide variety of agents upon intercellular cohesion in sheets of corneal epithelium. Buschke found that six out of seven detergents '. . . produced marked effects in concentration of 1% or sometimes even in lower concentrations'. Not one of a large selection of non-ionic or cationic detergents caused loss of intercellular cohesion. Benzalkonium chloride was used at concentrations up to 10%.

Anderson *et al.* (1964b) stated '. . . Swan has shown that wetting agents such as benzalkonium chloride are injurious to the corneal epithelium and especially to the endothelium. . . .' Swan (1944) found that intraocular concentrations of benzalkonium chloride in excess of 0·01% caused serious damage. Instillation of 0·1% benzalkonium chloride produced a severe reaction, but 0·03–0·04% used over periods up to eight weeks produced a less severe reaction. In most cases the conjunctiva and cornea were normal within 12 hr. Concentrations as high as 0·025% were tolerated in the conjunctival sac.

Hughson & Styron (1949) replaced the aqueous humour of rabbits' eyes with benzalkonium chloride in saline and found that concentrations of 0·033% and 0·017% produced endothelial oedema which disappeared in six to eight weeks. The use of a concentration of 0·015% showed no visible evidence of damage when observed with a hand slit lamp.

Post (1949) routinely used benzalkonium chloride 0·033% to sterilize his instruments for eye surgery. For a period of one month a dilution of 0·33% was used by mistake, but at no time did any untoward ocular reactions occur.

Shafer (1950) used benzalkonium 0·1% to sterilize the surrounding skin before doing corneal grafts in rabbits. No mention is made of any untoward effects attributable to the benzalkonium chloride.

Bell (1951) for three years used a quaternary ammonium compound at a concentration of 0·01% as an irrigant before eye surgery. He did not observe any hypersensitivity or allergic reaction, nor was there any evidence of irritation that could be attributed to the solution.

It may therefore be concluded that, provided benzalkonium chloride is not introduced into the anterior chamber of the eye, then the concentration of 0·02% recommended by many workers is not likely to cause irritation, except in especially sensitive patients, or perhaps after prolonged usage.

(ii) Bacteriological. Theodore & Feinstein (1953) made the following statement: 'The cationic wetting agents (benzalkonium, cetyl benzalkonium and Phemerol) appear to be of questionable value for use as preservatives. Their bacteriostatic effect is too variable and at times unreliable, especially against *P. aeruginosa*.' No evidence was given to support this statement.

King (1953) stated: 'They (quaternaries) are not advised by authors for use against *Pseudomonas* and are not recommended in the New and Non-official

Remedies published by the Council of Pharmacy of the American Medical Association.' Lawrence (1955b) quoted from this official publication of the American Medical Association: 'Strains of *Pseudomonas aeruginosa* and *Mycobacterium tubercolosis* are particularly resistant to these agents. Bacterial spores remain viable even after prolonged contact with the solutions of the quaternaries.' Lawrence goes on to add: 'The absence of similar statements in the description and uses of the other chemical preservatives for ophthalmic solutions in official publications does not mean that such compounds are superior in their action against the organisms mentioned.' Thus, in the absence of relevant scientific evidence, the generalizations of Theodore & Feinstein (1953) and King (1953) can be given little significance.

Anderson *et al.* (1964b) stated: 'Our reservations regarding benzalkonium and cetrimide relate mainly to their well-known feeble activity against *Pseudomonas* species, one of the most virulent organisms in ocular infection, . . .' These authors went on to quote Allen (1959), Riegelman *et al.* (1956) and Lowbury (1951) in support of their statement. Lowbury was actually quoted via Williams, Blowers, Garrod & Shooter (1960). The investigations of Lowbury (1951) demonstrated the dangers of bad practices. Williams *et al.* stated '*Pseudomonas pyocyanea* has an especial ability to survive in solutions of the commonly used disinfectant cetrimide ('Cetavlon', cetyl trimethyl ammonium bromide) and wound infection has been clearly attributed to persistence of the organisms in bottles containing cleansing solutions of cetrimide, when bark corks were used to stopper them. This hazard was eliminated by the use of sterilizable bottle caps (Lowbury, 1951).' Therefore the conclusion made as the result of this work was to avoid stoppering cetrimide solutions with bark corks, not to abandon the use of cetrimide as a disinfectant.

Riegelman *et al.* (1956) did demonstrate the existence of strains of *P. aeruginosa* which were resistant to benzalkonium chloride, but it is interesting to note, however, that later Riegelman & Vaughan (1958) concluded that 'with all its limitations, benzalkonium chloride is among the most effective and rapidly acting preservatives when the conditions of its use are properly controlled'.

The report of Allen (1959) that bottles containing different concentrations of benzalkonium chloride were shown to be contaminated with *P. aeruginosa* indicates that the *P. aeruginosa* could have been inadvertently 'trained' to exist in solutions of benzalkonium chloride of increasing concentration.

It would seem therefore that the conclusions of Riegelman & Vaughan (1958) represent a more accurate assessment of the effectiveness of benzalkonium chloride than do the comments of Theodore & Feinstein (1953), King (1953) and Anderson *et al* (1964b).

The possibility, however, of producing strains of *P. aeruginosa* which are highly resistant to the action of benzalkonium chloride is very disturbing and therefore the finding of MacGregor & Elliker (1958) that the acquired resistance to a quaternary ammonium compound was eliminated in the presence of ethylenediaminetetraacetate (EDTA) is very important. The USNF XI (1960) subsequently suggested the use of EDTA for this purpose. Brown & Richards (1965) showed that log-phase cultures of *P. aeruginosa* and *E. coli* in nutrient broth were made less resistant to the action of benzalkonium chloride, chlorhexidine diacetate and polymyxin B sulphate by the action of EDTA. The action of the EDTA was correlated with its ability to chelate divalent cations.

(d) Summary of the usefulness of the chemicals tested.

(i) Benzalkonium chloride. Many investigations have been concerned with the use of benzalkonium chloride as a preservative in ophthalmic preparations (Lawrence, 1955b; Riegelman *et al.*, 1956; Kohn *et al.*, 1963a). Other investigations have included many other aspects of its use in such preparations (Buschke, 1949; Hughson & Styron, 1949; Swan, 1944). The only scientifically supported evidence challenging its bacteriological efficiency was produced by Riegelman *et al.* (1956) and it is interesting to note that two of these authors, Riegelman & Vaughan (1958), subsequently stated: 'with all its limitations, benzalkonium chloride is among the most effective and rapidly acting preservatives when the conditions of its use are properly controlled.' Since that time the finding of several workers, including Kohn *et al.* (1963a), have supported the use of benzalkonium chloride 0·02% and further supported the findings of Lawrence (1955b). The incorporation of 0·1–0·01% EDTA, as recommended by the USNF XI, should remove the possibility of having preparations contaminated with strains of *P. aeruginosa* which have acquired a resistance to benzalkonium chloride. Suitable care should be exercised to ensure that benzalkonium chloride is not introduced into the anterior chamber of the eye.

(ii) Chlorbutol. Chlorbutol 0·5% has been shown consistently to be an effective but relatively slow sterilizing agent (Murphy *et al.*, 1955; Riegelman *et al.*, 1956; Kohn *et al.*, 1963a). Other aspects of its use in ophthalmic solutions, such as its heat stability, compatibility and its effect on the tissues of the eye have been investigated (Murphy *et al.*, 1955).

(iii) Chlorhexidine. This chemical has been shown to be active in aqueous solution (Anderson & Stock, 1958; Kohn *et al.*, 1963b). Chlorhexidine was included in some formulations of the Australian Pharmaceutical Formulary 1964 in 0·01% concentration. There are problems of compatibility with chlorhexidine, however, and it is not uniformly satisfactory with all ophthalmic solutions (Anderson, 1964). Chlorhexidine has shown diminished activity when tested in final ophthalmic preparations (Richards, 1964).

(iv) Chlorocresol. This will be considered under the section dealing with antibacterial combinations. Earlier published work that evaluated this chemical as a preservative in ophthalmic solutions is very limited.

(v) Mercurials. Phenylmercuric nitrate and thiomersal 0·01% were both shown to be slow acting by Kohn *et al.* (1964a) and were even slower acting in final preparation (Lawrence, 1955b). Phenylmercuric nitrate 0·01% was also shown to be slow acting by Murphy *et al.* (1955) and Riegelman *et al.* (1956).

The mercurials on prolonged administration may give rise to deposition of mercury in ocular tissues known as mercurialentis (Editorial, 1963). As far as is known, however, the condition is not associated with impairment of vision and Abrams (1963) concluded: 'Whether any noxious effect can really be attributed to mercurials appears to be doubtful. . . .'

(vi) Phenylethyl alcohol. The available evidence does not support the use of this compound used alone as a preservative for ophthalmic solutions (Murphy *et al.*, 1955; Lawrence, 1955b; Riegelman *et al.*, 1956; Kohn *et al.*, 1963a). Evidence will be given later showing its usefulness when used in combination with other antibacterials.

(vii) Hydroxybenzoate Esters. The available evidence would suggest that these chemicals are efficient only at concentrations near the limit of their solubility and these concentrations are too irritant to the eye (Lawrence, 1955b; Kohn *et al.*, 1963a). Hugo & Foster (1964) showed that *P. aeruginosa* was able to utilize these chemicals as a source of carbon and this also would seem to preclude their recommendation for widespread use.

(viii) Polymyxin B sulphate. This antibiotic is one of the agents of choice in treating *P. aeruginosa* infections (Wiggins, 1952b; Cassady, 1959; Leopold & Apt, 1960) and therefore it is considered that it should not be used for preserving ophthalmic preparations. Polymyxin B sulphate is also limited by its relatively low activity against Gram-positive organisms and some species of Proteus (Wiggins, 1952a).

(e) Conclusions on the preservation of ophthalmic solutions. It is evident that no single substance is entirely satisfactory for use as a preservative for ophthalmic solutions.

Benzalkonium chloride 0·02% and chlorbutol 0·5% have been well-substantiated as being suitable for use in ophthalmic solutions when the conditions of their use are suitably controlled. Phenylmercuric nitrate has also been widely used and has been shown to have a slow antibacterial action in simple solution which is further reduced in certain final ophthalmic preparations. Benzalkonium chloride has the most rapid antibacterial action of these three chemicals.

EDTA has been shown to potentiate the antibacterial action of benzalkonium chloride, chlorhexidine acetate and polymyxin B sulphate. EDTA therefore shows promise of being used in combination with other chemical agents in the preservation of ophthalmic solutions.

3. *Antibacterial Combinations*

(a) The rationale for antibacterial combinations. In the field of chemotherapy the elucidation of the interaction between chemical agents has stimulated interest right from the early days (Ehrlich, 1913) until the present (Jawetz, 1968; Kabins, 1972; Stockley, 1973). The hoped-for advantages resulting from the use of two antibiotics include: (i) a larger spectrum of activity; (ii) prevention of the development of organisms resistant to one substance alone, (iii) a reduction of physiologically harmful effects without a reduction in therapeutic activity and (iv) a reduction of the total dose of antibiotics administered (Garrett, 1958; Maccacaro, 1961). The use of two antibacterials together in the preservation of pharmaceuticals and cosmetics offers the possibility of similar advantages.

(b) The use of antibacterial combinations.

(i) EDTA plus antibacterial. MacGregor & Elliker (1958) showed that EDTA reversed the acquired resistance of *P. aeruginosa* to a quaternary ammonium compound. They postulated that EDTA increased the permeability of the resistant cells to the quaternary. Subsequently the United States National Formulary (USNF XI, 1960; USNF XII, 1965) recommended the use of EDTA with benzalkonium chloride as a possible preservative for ophthalmic solutions. Later, EDTA was shown to potentiate the activity of polymyxin B sulphate, chlorhexidine diacetate and benzalkonium chloride against logarithmic-phase *P. aeruginosa* (Brown & Richards, 1965). The effect was considered to be the result of EDTA chelating divalent cations from the bacterial cell envelopes and thus altering the cells permeability properties to the test chemicals (see Chapter 5). Monkhouse & Groves (1967) found that the incorporation of EDTA 0·1% with benzalkonium chloride 0·015% reduced the mean single survivor time of *P. aeruginosa* from 45·5 min for benzalkonium alone to 7·0 min for the combination. Nevertheless, there appears to be no advantage in using EDTA in combination with phenylmercuric nitrate or thiomersal (Brown, 1968; Richards, Suwanprakorn, Neawbanij & Surasdikul, 1969; Richards & McBride, 1972a; Richards & Reary, 1972). Richards (1971) found that EDTA 0·05% in combination with either benzalkonium 0·01% or chlorocresol 0·05% reversed the resistance of *P. aeruginosa* to these two antibacterials. EDTA 0·05% chlorbutol combinations, however, appear to have no advantage over chlorbutol alone (Richards, 1971; Richards & McBride, 1972a). The comment was made that the mode of action of the antibacterial and the state of resistance of the *P. aeruginosa* seem to be important factors in determining whether or not EDTA enhances antibacterial activity. Brown (1971 and see Chapter 3) discussed the mode of action of EDTA in detail. In the preservation of sulphacetamide eye-drops, EDTA with phenylethyl alcohol (phenylethanol) plus a third antibacterial (phenylmercuric nitrate, chlorocresol, or chlorhexidine) gave better sterilization times against heavy inocula of *P. aeruginosa* than either one agent alone or two component combinations (Richards & McBride, 1973a).

(ii) Non-ionic plus antibacterial. Polyoxyethylene sorbitan mono-oleate (polysorbate 80), depending on the concentration used, possesses the rather confusing property of either potentiating or antagonizing the activity of benzalkonium chloride and chlorhexidine diacetate against *P. aeruginosa* (Richards & Brown, 1964; Brown & Richards, 1964b). The activity of polymyxin B sulphate against *P. aeruginosa* and *E. coli* is potentiated by all concentrations of polysorbate in the range 0·02–0·5% (Brown & Richards, 1964; Richards, 1965). Polysorbate 80 alone had no inhibitory effect on the test cells. Potentiation of the activity of chlorhexidine and benzalkonium against *E. coli* was not observed. This was probably due to the ratio of non-ionic to antibacterial agent being more critical in the *E. coli* test system and the correct ratio not being found.

Gershenfeld & Stedman (1949) were not able to show any potentiation of the action of cationics against *P. aeruginosa* and *E. coli* at any concentration of non-ionic used. Moore & Hardwick (1956), however, using combinations of a quaternary ammonium compound and a non-ionic, found that an increased antibacterial activity against Gram-negative organisms occurred at ratios of non-ionic to quaternary of about 2:1. Higher ratios of non-ionic to quaternary than about 4:1 caused inactivation of the antibacterial activity. Moore & Hardwick (1956) interpreted their results in terms of critical micelle concentration (CMC) but no evidence of the CMC of the system was given.

The effect of polysorbate 80, at different concentrations, on the antibacterial action of benzalkonium, chlorhexidine and polymyxin against *P. aeruginosa* was not considered by Richards (1965) to be directly related to the CMC because of the following observations. Firstly, the CMC for polysorbate 80 is reported to be 0·001% (Vidal-Paruta & King, 1964), but the potentiation of antibacterial activity against *P. aeruginosa* occurred at 0·02% polysorbate, which was considered to be many times the CMC for the polysorbate 80, bacterial culture, antibacterial agent mixture(s). Secondly, 0·02% polysorbate 80 did not potentiate the antibacterial activity of benzalkonium and chlorhexidine against *E. coli*. Thirdly, all concentrations of polysorbate 80 tested potentiated the action of polymyxin against cultures of *P. aeruginosa* and *E. coli*. Therefore, in these test systems, the permeability properties of the bacterial cell were thought to be largely responsible for the resistance of *P. aeruginosa* (and *E. coli*) to inactivation by the antibacterials under test. Polysorbate 80 at selected concentrations was thought to assist the penetration of the test antibacterials into *P. aeruginosa*.

The results of Brown & Winsley (1969) supported the hypothesis that polysorbate has an immediate effect on the permeability barrier of *P. aeruginosa*. These workers studied the effect of polysorbate 80 on cell leakage and viability of *P. aeruginosa* exposed to rapid changes of pH, temperature and tonicity.

Brown (1966) found that selected concentrations of polysorbate 80 could enhance the activity of *p*-hydroxybenzoates against *P. aeruginosa* and Brown and Winsley (1968, 1971) showed that polysorbate 80 potentiated the effect of polymyxin against this organism. As Brown (1971) concludes, it would seem that polysorbate renders *P. aeruginosa* and *E. coli* more sensitive to antibacterial agents by altering an otherwise relatively impermeable barrier. Polysorbate 80 is one of the most commonly used wetting agents in contact lens wetting solutions (Krezanoski, 1970; Richards, 1972) but, because of its potential to inactivate chemical antibacterials also contained in the wetting solution, care must be exercised in the choice of polysorbate concentration used. An adequate knowledge of the properties of polysorbate 80, however, should make it possible to select a polysorbate concentration which has suitable wetting action without diminishing the antibacterial activity of the preservative.

(iii) 2-Phenylethanol plus antibacterial. Phenylethanol was first recommended for use as a preservative for ophthalmic solutions by Brewer, Goldstein & McLaughlin (1953) following a report that it was active against Gram-negative organisms (Lilly & Brewer, 1953). Grote & Woods (1955) found that 2-phenylethanol was not irritating to the rabbit eye and that a 0·3% solution does not destroy the activity of the lysozyme normally present in the lachrymal fluid. Kohn *et al.* (1963a) found phenylethanol to have too slow an action against *P. aeruginosa* for phenylethanol to be recommend for use in ophthalmic solutions. Nevertheless, phenylethanol is one of the four antibacterials recommended for preserving ophthalmic solutions in the USNF XIII (1970). Deeb & Boenigk (1958) were the first workers to evaluate the use of phenylethanol in combination with other antibacterials (chlorbutol and benzylalcohol) and their results showed that the combinations had greater antibacterial activity than the single substances. Foster (1965) investigated combinations of phenylethanol with several other antibacterials used as preservatives in ophthalmic solutions. Filter paper strips were saturated with either phenylethanol or one of the antibacterials, and the strips laid at right-angles to each other on the surface of nutrient agar seeded with *P. aeruginosa*. The zones of growth inhibition so obtained indicated enhanced activity between phenylethanol and phenylmercuric nitrate but not between phenylethanol and any of the other antibacterials. Richards *et al.* (1969) investigated the effect of phenylethanol on the activity of phenylmercuric nitrate against *P. aeruginosa* by three different methods. Firstly, 2% fluorescein solutions preserved with either phenylethanol 0·6% or 0·4% v/v plus phenylmercuric nitrate 0·002% were shown to have faster sterilization times against $3 \cdot 10^5$ cells/ml *P. aeruginosa* than either phenylmercuric nitrate 0·002% alone, or phenylethanol 0·6% alone. Secondly, *P. aeruginosa* cells grown on nutrient agar containing 0·25% v/v phenylethanol were shown to be much more sensitive to the action of fluorescein solutions preserved with phenylmercuric nitrate or phenylethanol plus phenylmercuric nitrate, than were *P. aeruginosa* cells which had been grown on plain nutrient agar. Thirdly, when 0·26% v/v phenylethanol was added to log.-phase *P. aeruginosa* growing in nutrient broth, and to log.-phase cells in nutrient broth plus phenylmercuric nitrate 0·001%, a 45% kill of *P. aeruginosa* resulted in the nutrient broth but an 80% kill was obtained in the nutrient broth plus phenylmercuric nitrate 0·001%. It was concluded from these three sets of results that phenylethanol had an effect on the permeability of the *P. aeruginosa* cells, thus enabling concentrations of phenylmercuric nitrate which could not, on their own, effect penetration into the cell to pass into the cell and exert an antibacterial effect. These findings are in general agreement with those of Silver & Wendt (1967) who found that the uptake of acriflavine and efflux of potassium ions by *E. coli* cells was increased in the presence of phenylethanol. Silver & Wendt concluded that the main action of phenylethanol was on the permeability properties of the *E. coli*.

Richards *et al.* (1969) suggested that phenylethanol might be used with advantage in combination with phenylmercuric nitrate and possibly in combination with other antibacterials in the preservation of pharmaceuticals against contamination with *P. aeruginosa*. Richards & McBride (1971a,b; 1972a,b; 1973a,b) and Richards & Hardie (1972) confirmed this hypothesis and showed that, in addition to enhancing the activity of phenylmercuric nitrate phenylethanol was also able to enhance the activity of benzalkonium, chlorhexidine, chlorocresol, chlorbutol, fentichlor and a hydroxybenzoate mixture against *P. aeruginosa* in a variety of test systems. In addition, Richards (1971) showed that phenylethanol–antibacterial combinations were able to inactivate *P. aeruginosa* resistant, or trained to be resistant, to the 'antibacterial' component of the combination. Later Richards & McBride (1972b) found that phenylethanol-antibacterial combinations were also effective against *P. aeruginosa* trained to be resistant to the phenylethanol component of the combination.

(c) Desirable properties of antibacterial combinations. Richards & McBride (1972b) suggested that the following properties seemed to be desirable for a preservative combination in order that it could be considered suitable for using in pharmaceutical solutions.

(1) The antibacterial combination should have a faster sterilization time against the test organism than the same concentration of either of the antibacterials used individually. For ophthalmic solutions this sterilization time should be 1 hr or less for an inoculum of *P. aeruginosa* having a final concentration in the test system of not less than 10^6 cells/ml (Kohn *et al.*, 1963b; Richards & McBride, 1971a; 1972a).

(2) The antibacterial combination should still be effective when the test organism has acquired a resistance to either one of the antibacterials.

(3) The spectrum of activity of the combination should include pathogenic Gram-positive and Gram-negative bacteria and fungi.

In addition, the following properties were suggested as being desirable for the individual members of the combination.

(1) One member of the combination should be chosen for its rapid action against a wide spectrum of microorganisms.

(2) The other member of the combination should have properties that enable it to potentiate the action of the first antibacterial, particularly against organisms that have developed a resistance to the first antibacterial.

(d) The place for antibacterial combinations. There is world-wide acceptance that two or more chemicals should be used in combination in the initial treatment of tuberculosis (Ross & Horne, 1969), and combinations of two bactericidal antibiotics are of great value in bacterial endocarditis (Editorial, 1966b) but there is no such widespread agreement in the treatment of other infections with antibacterial combinations. The logical policy in general infections is first to carry out the appropriate *in vitro* tests. Kabins (1972) states 'there is no substitute for adequate *in vitro* studies to determine the precise effect obtained by antibiotic combinations against specific bacterial isolates'. In the preservation of ophthalmic solutions I would suggest that the problem is more akin to the treatment of tuberculosis than it is to the treatment of general infections in the examples from clinical chemotherapy quoted above. That is, in both tuberculosis and the preservation of ophthalmic solutions the main target organism is known and is difficult to inactivate with a single antibacterial. This being so, it would seem as appropriate to use selected antibacterial combinations for the preservation of ophthalmic solutions as it is to use two or more antibacterials in the treatment of tuberculosis. The combinations for ophthalmic solutions should have been shown to have a rapid bactericidal activity against *P. aeruginosa*, including strains which are known to be especially resistant to commonly used ophthalmic preservatives. In addition to increasing the antipseudomonal activity of ophthalmic solutions, antibacterial combinations can also be a means of overcoming irritancy problems by reducing the concentration of the main antibacterial agent. For example, in contact lens wetting solutions the concentration of benzalkonium chloride usually used is 0·004%. This is because higher concentrations are too irritant (Richards, 1972) and may also adversely affect the wetting properties of the lens surface, transforming it from hydrophilic to hydrophobic (Szekely, Riegelman & Petricciani, 1959). Benzalkonium 0·004%, however, does not provide sufficient antibacterial cover for the solution. Antibacterial combinations offer the best possibility of solving this problem by reducing irritancy without impairing antibacterial activity.

(e) Evaluation of antibacterial combinations. Methods of evaluating the interaction between two antibacterials are quite numerous. Twelve different methods which had been reported in the literature at the time were very well described and evaluated by Maccacaro (1961). A similar treatment will not be attempted here but methods using growth-rate determinations and sterilization time determinations will be described.

(i) Growth-rate determinations. Garrett (1958) reviewed the chaotic position existing in the literature at that time on the classification of combined action. Most authors had their own definition for synergistic, antagonistic, additive or indifferent interactions between two antibiotics. Garrett proposed a scheme for the classification of the responses to antibiotic combinations based on 'additivity' and 'equivalence'. Additivity was for situations where the combined response was additive with respect to the separate responses of the antibiotics. Equivalence was for the system where the two substances acted in the same manner with the same response curve whether they were used separately or in combination. The only difference in the response with equivalent drugs is the difference in the weight of an arbitrarily defined therapeutic 'unit dose'.

The second area of confusion dealt with by Garrett (1958) was the choice of a suitable response to characterize combined antibiotic action. Garrett stated that the logarithmic viable-time curve slopes that are functions of rate constants are a good criteria for drug action but that a better criteria would be the rate constants themselves, determined for rates of kill and inhibition of growth of microorganisms. It was suggested that this latter method could be used to classify and evaluate combined antibiotic activity. Garrett & Brown (1963) and Brown & Garrett (1964) subsequently investigated the action of tetracycline and chloramphenicol, both alone and in combination, on the growth of *E. coli*. These authors added the antibacterial agent during the exponential phase of growth and measured the growth rates with a Klett–Summerson colorimeter and by plate counts. Brown & Richards (1964a,b, 1965) and Richards (1965) adapted this method for use with *P. aeruginosa* and investigated the effect of antibacterials, both alone and in combination with either polysorbate 80 or EDTA. The growth rate was measured by determining the extinction measurements in 1 cm cells at 420 nm with a Unicam SP600 spectrophotometer. Therefore, care was taken to make comparisons between suspensions of the same organism grown under exactly similar growth conditions and taken from the same stage of the growth cycle. Extinction readings were compared with total counts to confirm that Beer's law was being obeyed by the particular bacterial suspensions under test. The blanks used in making the spectrophotometric measurements consisted of samples of the particular batch of growth medium being used and tests were made to check that the absorption of the growth medium was not affected by the growth of the organisms.

Basically, the technique was as follows. A broth culture from an isolated colony of *P. aeruginosa* was used to inoculate replicate agar stabs which were stored in a refrigerator. A fresh stab culture was used to prepare an overnight culture for each experiment. A sample of the overnight broth culture was inoculated into pre-warmed broth at 37 °C and the extinction was then measured at intervals. At a suitable value, such that the cells were known to be dividing exponentially, 1 ml samples were added to replicate 250 ml conical flasks containing 99 ml pre-warmed nutrient broth. Samples were again removed at timed intervals for extinction determinations to be made. When the growth rate had been established, 0·5 ml of suitable concentrations of the prewarmed antibacterial(s) were added to all except the control culture, which received 0·5 ml pre-warmed water. Subsequent extinction measurements were made and the growth rates determined. Brown (1966) used the same method to investigate the effect of polysorbate 80 on the activity of several antibacterials against *P. aeruginosa*. Richards & McBride (1971b; 1972b; 1973b) used adaptations of the method of Brown & Richards (1964a) for the evaluation of phenylethanol both alone and in combination with a variety of antibacterial agents against growing cultures of *P. aeruginosa*.

The advantages of using extinction measurements to determine the effects of antibacterials used alone and in combination against growing cultures of bacteria include the rapidity and sensitivity of the method. Results are obtained on the day of the investigation and relatively subtle changes in growth rate detected which would be difficult to determine by other means. Therefore, provided that the cultures obey Beer's Law, the interactions between antibacterials can be screened by this method and specific effects can be confirmed using another method such as counting procedures or sterilization-time determinations.

(ii) Sterilization-time determinations. Sterilization times are particularly valuable for investigating final preparations of ophthalmic solutions. Basically, a known high inoculum of the test organism is added to a fixed volume of the antibacterial test system at known pH. The test organism–antibacterial system, known as the reaction mixture, is maintained at a constant temperature and at pre-determined times samples are removed to inactivator-recovery broth and incubated at 37 °C for at least three days. The test is carried out in duplicate and the sterilization time is the time of the first replicate samples to show no growth, followed by no growth in subsequent samples. Controls are included to demonstrate the efficiency of the inactivating medium. Lawrence (1955b), Riegelman *et al.* (1956) and Kohn *et al.* (1963a,b) all used this type of experiment for evaluating single antibacterials and Brown (1968), Richards *et al.* (1969), Richards & McBride (1971a; 1972a; 1973a), Richards & Reary (1972) and Richards & Hardie (1972) used this type of experiment for evaluating combinations. Richards & McBride (1972a; 1973a) used two separate inocula of *P. aeruginosa* to test the preservative capacity of the formulations under investigation. Table 4 gives a summary of the work using antibacterial combinations for the preservation of ophthalmic solutions. It can also be seen from Table 4 that suitable concentrations of either benzalkonium, chlorbutol or chlorocresol alone are capable of sterilizing certain ophthalmic solutions within 1 hr. Phenylmercuric nitrate is again shown to be slow-acting and in these final preparations chlorhexidine is also quite slow-acting. Phenylethanol in combination with each of the antibacterial agents is consistently effective but EDTA–antibacterial combinations are not always more effective than the antibacterial used alone.

Sodium metabisulphite contained in the physostigmine and sulphacetamide solutions seems to inactivate the chlorhexidine and the phenylmercuric nitrate respectively. The sodium metabisulphite, however, does not appear to inactivate the phenylmercuric nitrate in the physostigmine solutions at acid pH. Richards & Reary (1972) and Richards, Fell & Butchart (1972) showed that sodium metabisulphite and phenylmercuric nitrate form a complex on autoclaving together. This complex had reduced antibacterial activity at alkaline pH (8·4) when compared with the activity of phenylmercuric nitrate alone at the same pH. The activity of the complex at acid pH (3·9) was greater than the activity of phenylmercuric nitrate alone at the same pH.

(f) Conclusions. It can be concluded that antibacterial combinations have a place in the preservation of ophthalmic solutions against contamination with *P. aeruginosa*. Phenylethanol seems to offer the greatest possibilities for use in combination with a suitable broad spectrum antibacterial such as benzalkonium chloride or chlorocresol and to a lesser extent with chlorhexidine and phenylmercuric nitrate. EDTA-benzalkonium and EDTA-chlorocresol combinations are also very effective combinations for the preservation of ophthalmic solutions.

Table 4. Summary of the work using antibacterial combinations for the preservation of ophthalmic solutions against contamination with *P. aeruginosa*

| | Sterilization times (min) | | | | | | | | | | | | | | | |
Ophthalmic solutions	Bzk[a]	Bzk + EDTA[b]	Bzk + PEA[c]	Chb[d]	Chb + EDTA	Chb + PEA	Chc[e]	Chc + EDTA	Chc + PEA	Chh[f]	Chh + EDTA	Chh + PEA	PMN[g]	PMN + EDTA	PMN + PEA	Workers
Fluorescein	—	—	—	—	—	—	—	—	—	—	—	—	180	300	60	Brown (1968); Richards *et al.* (1969)
Sodium bicarbonate	—	—	—	—	—	—	30	45	15	—	—	—	240	180	60	Richards & McBride (1971a)
Pilocarpine hydrochloride	15	15	15	15	15	15	45	45	15	60	30	15	240	120	60	
Atropine sulphate	60	15	15	—	—	15	30	15	15	60	—	—	24 hr	300	90	Richards & McBride (1972a)
Physostigmine sulphate	15	15	15	45	60	30	30	45	15	—	90	30	90	90	45	
Physostigmine salicylate	—	—	—	30	60	15	45	30	15	180	90	30	90	60	45	
Sulphacetamide 10%	—	—	—	—	—	—	—	45	30	—	30	15	—	120	45	
Sulphacetamide 10% + sodium metabisulphite 0·1%	—	—	—	—	—	—	90	45	30	120	60	60	300	>300	120	Richards & McBride (1973a)
Sulphacetamide 30%	—	—	—	—	—	—	—	15	15	—	45	15	—	45	30	
Sulphacetamide 30% + sodium metabisulphite 0·1%	—	—	—	—	—	—	—	30	15	—	60	60	—	90	60	

[a] Benzalkonium chloride 0·01%. [b] Sodium edetate 0·05%. [c] Phenylethanol 0·4% v/v. [d] Chlorbutol 0·5%. [e] Chlorocresol 0·05%. [f] Chlorhexidine 0·01%. [g] Phenylmercuric nitrate 0·002%.

Preservation of Multiphase Systems

This section includes certain sterile ophthalmic suspensions but consists mainly of the preservation of non-sterile oral and topical preparations, such as mixtures and emulsions for internal use and lotions, applications, ointments and creams for external use. Two distinct areas are in need of evaluation. Firstly, there is the problem of whether these latter products should be required to be sterile or whether a certain predetermined level of contamination should be accepted. This could be referred to as the philosophical area of evaluation. Secondly, there is the practical area of evaluation, involving the determination of the interactions occurring between the preservatives and the components of the various formulations, so that the formulations can be designed to ensure the effective functioning of the preservatives.

1. *Philosophical*

Kallings *et al.* (1966) felt it was possible to recommend a general bacterial hygienic level for constituents of non-sterile medical preparations of not more than 100 bacteria/gram. Henry (1969) reviewed the microflora of man and his environment and made a plea for a reasoned approach to the subject of what is an acceptable bacterial content in consumer goods. Henry is concerned not to eliminate organisms which are not harmful to man from non-sterile products and not to unnecessarily eliminate man's indigenous micro-organisms by using 'preservative-supercharged' products. Parker (1970) states: '. . . a cosmetic preparation should not present any greater hazard to health than the rest of man's normal environment'.

Wedderburn (1970), however, states: 'Ideally, cosmetics should be self-sterilizing; any organisms present either in the ingredients, the water, or the empty containers at the time of packaging should die out within a short time'. Bean (1972) thought it desirable to have a preservative performance test to measure the ability of the product to destroy invading organisms. The Monograph (1970) contains the recommendation that cosmetic products should preferably be self-sterilizing.

The foregoing situation is reflected in the USP XVIII (1970), which shows an awareness of the need for greater microbiological control in the area of these non-sterile preparations but also indicates that the position has not yet been reached where total numerical limits for microbial counts can be made for all products. The USP XVIII contains the following statement on the attributes of non-sterile pharmaceuticals: 'Among the desirable attributes of a suitable product is freedom from viable harmful microorganisms examples of which are *Salmonella* species *Escherichia coli*, certain species of *Pseudomonas* including *P. aeruginosa*, and *Staphylococcus aureus*.' In this context 'harmful' refers to human infections or disease caused by these organisms or their toxins (Bruch, 1972).

'Objectionable' micro-organisms is another term that is used in connection with microbial contamination. This term includes damage to the medicaments as well as direct damage to the user.

Bruch (1971) gave the following ranking for objectionable organisms in topical products:

A Eye products. 1. *P. aeruginosa*. 2. All other *pseudomonads*. 3. *S. aureus*.

B Genito-urinary tract products. 1. *E. coli*. 2. *P. mirabilis*. 3. *S. marcescens*. 4. *Klebsiella*. 5. *P. aeruginosa* and *P. multivorans*.

C. Topical products used over extensive parts of the body other than the eye or genito-urinary tract. 1. *P. aeruginosa*. 2. *S. marcescens*. 3. *Klebsiella*. 4. *P. multivorans* and *P. putida*. 5. *S. aureus*.

2. *Practical*

In general, multi-phase systems are more difficult to preserve than simple aqueous solutions. This is usually because the preservative present in the aqueous phase of the multi-phase system is reduced below an effective level by such physical interactions as adsorption by solids, partitioning by oils and association with surfactants and emulsifying agents. The fact that a multi-phase system is often highly nutritious adds to the problem of preservation.

(a) Emulsions. The preservation of emulsions against microbiol attack was extensively reviewed by Wedderburn (1964). Partition of the preservative into the oil phase and association of the preservative with the emulsifying agent are two of the main interactions resulting in loss of preservative activity in emulsions.

Most of the investigations in this field have been of an empirical nature but Kostenbauder and associates and Bean and associates have made more fundamental studies. For example, Patel & Kostenbauder (1958) used equilibrium dialysis to determine free and bound methylparabenzoate and propylparabenzoate in the presence of polysorbate 80. They demonstrated that the interaction of the antimicrobial agent with the micellar surfactant can be treated as a Langmuir-type adsorption, and in effective preservative concentration ranges could be described by a fairly simple equation. Microbiological studies by Pisano & Kostenbauder (1959) confirmed that the antimicrobial activity is a function of the activity of the unbound preservative. With a knowledge of the required parabenzoate concentration in the absence of surfactant and the ratio of total to free parabenzoate concentration at a given surfactant concentration, a prediction can be made, with the aid of an equation, of the increased concentration of preservative needed. Agreement was obtained between predicted and experimentally determined inhibitory concentrations of preservatives in these particular test systems. Deluca & Kostenbauder (1960) investigated the binding of quaternary ammonium compounds by non-ionic agents.

Bean and associates studied the influence of emulsion components on preservative activity using simplified models involving a minimum of components (Bean, Richards & Thomas, 1962; Bean & Heman-Ackah, 1964; Bean, Konning & Malcolm, 1969). It can be concluded from their work that, with the aid of mathematical models and a knowledge of the appropriate parameters, it is possible to predict the antibacterial activity of a fluid containing surface-active agents or an emulsified preparation with acceptable accuracy (Bean, 1972).

(b) Suspensions. Bean & Dempsey (1971) studied the effect of suspensions of light kaolin and procaine penicillin on the bactericidal activity of *m*-cresol and benzalkonium chloride. *m*-Cresol was shown to have the same activity, both in aqueous solution and in kaolin suspension, but benzalkonium chloride was less active in the kaolin suspension than in aqueous solution. This indicated that benzalkonium was adsorbed on to kaolin whereas *m*-cresol was not. The supernatant taken from a suspension of kaolin containing benzalkonium, however, had less bactericidal activity than the suspension. This indicated that some benzalkonium chloride adsorbed on to the kaolin was, or became, available to the bacteria. Procaine penicillin gave results with benzalkonium similar to those obtained for light kaolin.

Clarke & Armstrong (1972) found that benzoic acid was adsorbed to a significant extent by kaolin and suggested ways of overcoming this by making suitable pH adjustments to the kaolin–benzoic acid system.

Dale *et al.* (1959) tested the sterilization times of 10 commercially prepared ophthalmic suspensions of adrenal cortical hormones. *P. aeruginosa* 10^3 cells/ml was one of the test organisms, but specific inactivators were not used. Under the conditions of the test benzalkonium chloride 0·02% was thought to be a suitable preservative for these suspensions.

Lee (1972) studied the formulation of hydrocortisone eye-drops and found that it was possible to inactivate 10^6 *P. aeruginosa*/ml in less than 1 hr using formulations preserved with benzalkonium chloride 0·01%, either alone on in combination with phenylethanol 0·4% v/v. Suitable inactivators were used in the test procedure.

3-Phenylpropan-1-ol has been suggested as having potential usefulness in the preservation of oral medicaments (Richards, McBride & Gunn, 1972). The investigations, which were of a preliminary nature, determined the preservative capacity of 3-phenylpropanol alone and in combination with either chloroform water, or a mixture of hydroxybenzoates, in the preservation of kaolin suspensions against contamination with *P. aeruginosa*, or *E. coli.* or *S. aureus.*

Manufacturing Technique

This subject is mentioned briefly because it is well-known that products contamined with *P. aeruginosa* have reached the user through inadequacies at the production level (Baker, 1959; Kallings *et al.*, 1966). This also applies to the hospital pharmacy situation (Report, 1971). Brennan, Baker & Gasdia (1968) outlined a number of steps to reduce the possibility of contamination of pharmaceuticals produced in the hospital pharmacy.

The 'Guide to good pharmaceutical manufacturing practice', (Guide, 1971) describe measures for the control of quality during manufacture and assembly of pharmaceuticals and a very substantial guide has been produced for the cosmetic industry entitled 'The hygienic manufacture and preservation of toiletries and cosmetics' (Monograph, 1970). In addition Davis (1972) has written an excellent article on the fundamentals of microbiology in relation to cleansing in the cosmetic industry.

General Conclusions

Failures in the *in vitro* elimination of *P. aeruginosa* from pharmaceuticals and cosmetics have been humbling for all concerned and no doubt this organism has further stern lessons to teach us. Nevertheless, the cumulative knowledge acquired in the areas of sources of contamination, mechanisms of resistance, activity and mode of action of antibacterials, properties and formulation requirements of different dosage forms, and improved manufacturing techniques and packaging should ensure that contamination by this organism is severely restricted.

REFERENCES

Abrams, J. D. (1963). Iatrogenic mercurialentis. *Transactions of the Ophthalmological Societies of the United Kingdom*, **83**, 263–269.

Allen, H. F. (1952). Contributing to a discussion. *American Journal of Ophthalmology*, **35**, 99–100.

Allen, H. F. (1959). Aseptic technique in ophthalmology. *Transactions of the American Ophthalmological Society*, **57**, 383–472.

Anderson, K., Lillie, S. & Crompton, D. (1964a). Efficiency of bacteriostats in ophthalmic solutions. *The Pharmaceutical Journal*, **192**, 593–594.

Anderson, K., Lillie, S. & Crompton, D. (1964b). Preservation of ophthalmic solutions. *The Pharmaceutical Journal*, **193**, 165.

Anderson, R. A. (1964). Bacteriostats in ophthalmic solutions. *The Pharmaceutical Journal*, **193**, 148.

Anderson, R. A. (1965). The bactericidal effect of some ophthalmic vehicles: III Cation-active preservatives against *Pseudomonas aeruginosa*. *The Australasian Journal of Pharmacy, Science Supplement Number 27*, S25–S27.

Anderson, R. A. & Stock, B. H. (1958). The bactericidal effect of some ophthalmic vehicles. *The Australasian Journal of Pharmacy*, **39**, 1110–1112.

Armbruster, E. H. & Ridenour, G. M. (1947). A new medium for study of quaternary bactericides. *Soap and Sanitary Chemicals*, **23**, 119–143.

Australian Pharmaceutical Formulary, (1964). Wilke and Co., Clayton, Victoria.

Ayliffe, G. A. J., Lowbury, E. J. L., Hamilton, J. G., Small, J. M., Asheshov, E. A. & Parker, M. T. (1965). Hospital infection with *Pseudomonas aeruginosa* in neurosurgery. *The Lancet*, **ii**, 365–368.

Ayliffe, G. A. J., Barry, D. R., Lowbury, E. J. L., Roper-Hall, M. J. & Walker, W. M. (1966). Postoperative infection with *Pseudomonas aeruginosa* in an eye hospital. *The Lancet*, **i**, 1113–1117.

Ayliffe, G. A. J., Brightwell, K. M., Collins, B. J. & Lowbury, E. J. L. (1969). Varieties of aseptic practice in hospital wards. *The Lancet*, **ii**, 1117–1120.

Baker, J. H. (1959). That unwanted cosmetic ingredient-bacteria. *Journal of the Society of Cosmetic Chemists*, **10**, 133–143.

Bassett, D. C. J., Stokes, K. J. & Thomas, W. R. G. (1970). Wound infection with *Pseudomonas multivorans*; a water-borne contaminant of disinfectant solutions. *The Lancet*, **i**, 1188–1191.

Bean, H. S. (1972). Preservatives for pharmaceuticals. *Journal of the Society of Cosmetic Chemists*, **23**, 703–720.

Bean, H. S. & Dempsey, G. (1971). The effect of suspensions on the bactericidal activity of *m*-cresol and benzalkonium chloride. *Journal of Pharmacy and Pharmacology*, **23**, 699–704.

Bean, H. S. & Farrell, R. C. (1967). The persistence of *Pseudomonas aeruginosa* in aqueous solutions of phenols. *Journal of Pharmacy and Pharmacology*, **19**, *Supplement* 183S–188S.

Bean, H. S. & Heman-Ackah, S. M. (1964). Influence of oil:water ratio on the activity of some bactericides against *Escherichia coli* in liquid paraffin and water dispersions. *Journal of Pharmacy and Pharmacology*, **16**, *Supplement*, 58T–67T.

Bean, H. S., Konning, G. H. & Malcolm, S. A. (1969). A model for the influence of emulsion formulation on the activity of phenolic preservatives. *Journal of Pharmacy and Pharmacology*, **21**, *Supplement*, 173S–181S.

Bean, H. S., Richards, J. P. & Thomas, J. (1962). The bactericidal activity against *Escherichia coli* of phenol in water dispersions. *Bolletino Chimico Farmaceutico*, **101**, 339–346.

Beatson, S. H. (1972). Pharaoh's ants as pathogen vectors in hospitals. *The Lancet*, **i**, 425–427.

Bell, R. P. (1951). A new ophthalmic irrigating solution. *American Journal of Ophthalmology*, **34**, 1321–1322.

Bergan, T. & Lystad, A. (1971). Disinfectant evaluation by capacity use-dilution test. *Journal of Applied Bacteriology*, **34**, 741–750.

Berry, H. (1951). A review of disinfectants and disinfection. *Journal of Pharmacy and Pharmacology*, **3**, 689–699.

Bignell, J. L. (1951). Infection of the cornea with *B. pyocyaneus*. Clinical study and summary of ten cases personally observed. *British Journal of Ophthalmology*, **35**, 419–423.

BPC (1968). *British Pharmaceutical Codex*, London, The Pharmaceutical Press, p. 1076.

Brennan, C. E., Baker, D. E. & Gasdia, S. D. (1968). Bacteriological purity; a consideration in the manufacture and packaging of pharmaceuticals. *American Journal of Hospital Pharmacy*, **25**, 302–304.

Brewer, J. H., Goldstein, S. W. & McLaughlin, C. B. (1953). Phenylethyl alcohol as a bacteriostatic agent in ophthalmic solutions. *Journal of the American Pharmaceutical Association, Scientific Edition*, **42**, 584–586.

Brown, M. R. W. (1966). Turbidimetric method for the rapid evaluation of antimicrobial agents. Inactivation of preservatives by nonionic agents. *Journal of the Society of Cosmetic Chemists*, **17**, 185–195.

Brown, M. R. W. (1967). Control of contamination in ophthalmic solutions. *Proceedings of the Royal Society of Medicine*, **60**, 354–357.

Brown, M. R. W. (1968). Survival of *Pseudomonas aeruginosa* in fluorescein solution. Preservative action of PMN and EDTA. *Journal of Pharmaceutical Sciences*, **57**, 389–392.

Brown, M. R. W. (1971). Inhibition and destruction of *Pseudomonas aeruginosa*. In *Inhibition and Destruction of the Microbial Cell*, (Ed. W. B. Hugo), Academic Press, London and New York, p. 307.

Brown, M. R. W., Foster, J. H. S., Norton, D. A. & Richards, R. M. E. (1965). *The Lancet*, **i**, 604.

Brown, M. R. W. & Garrett, E. R. (1964). Kinetics and mechanisms of action of antibiotics on microorganisms I. Reproducibility of *Escherichia coli* growth curves and dependence on tetracycline concentration. *Journal of Pharmaceutical Sciences*, **53**, 179–183.

Brown, M. R. W. & Norton, D. A. (1965). The preservation of ophthalmic preparations. *Journal of the Society of Cosmetic Chemists*, **16**, 369–393.

Brown, M. R. W. & Richards, R. M. E. (1964a). The effect of Polysorbate (Tween) 80 on the growth rate of *Pseudomonas aeruginosa*. *Journal of Pharmacy and Pharmacology*, **16**, *Supplement* 41T–45T.

Brown, M. R. W. & Richards, R. M. E. (1964b). Effect of Polysorbate (Tween) 80 on the resistance of *Pseudomonas aeruginosa* to chemical inactivation. *Journal of Pharmacy and Pharmacology*, **16**, *Supplement*, 51T–55T.

Brown, M. R. W. & Richards, R. M. E. (1965). Effect of Ethylenediamine Tetraacetate on the resistance of *Pseudomonas aeruginosa* to antibacterial agents. *Nature, London*, **207**, 1391–1393.

Brown, M. R. W., Watkins, W. M. & Scott Foster, J. H. (1969). Stepwise resistance to polymyxin and other agents by *Pseudomonas aeruginosa*. *Journal of General Microbiology*, **55**, xvii.

Brown, M. R. W. & Winsley, B. E. (1968). Synergistic action of polysorbate 80 and polymyxin B sulphate on *Pseudomonas aeruginosa*. *Journal of General Microbiology*, **50**, ix.

Brown, M. R. W. & Winsley, B. E. (1969). Effect of polysorbate 80 on cell leakage and viability of *Pseudomonas aeruginosa* exposed to rapid changes of pH, temperature and tonicity. *Journal of General Microbiology*, **56**, 99–107.

Brown, M. R. W. & Winsley, B. E. (1971). Synergism between polymyxin and polysorbate 80 against *Pseudomonas aeruginosa*. *Journal of General Microbiology*, **68**, 367–373.

Brown, W. R. L. (1971). The preparation of pharmaceutical products with a low level of microbial contamination in hospital pharmacy. *Joint Symposium on Microbial Control*, organized by the Pharmaceutical Society and the Society of Cosmetic Chemists, Great Britain.

Bruch, C. W. (1971). Microbiological products of topical quality. Types *vs* numbers of microorganisms. *Drug and Cosmetic Industry*, **109**, 26–30, 105–110.

Bruch, C. W. (1972). Possible modifications of USP microbial limits and tests, *Drug and Cosmetic Industry*, **110**, 32–37, 116–121.

Buck, A. C. & Cooke, E. M. (1969). The fate of ingested *Pseudomonas aeruginosa* in normal persons. *Journal of Medical Microbiology*, **2**, 521–525.

Burdon, D. W. & Whitby, J. L. (1967). Contamination of hospital disinfectants with *Pseudomonas* species. *British Medical Journal*, **2**, 153–155.

Buschke, W. (1949). Studies of intercellular cohesion in corneal epithelium. *Journal of Cellular and Comparative Physiology*, **33**, 145–176.

Cantor, A. & Shelanski, H. A. (1951). A 'capacity' test for germicidal action. *Soap and Sanitary Chemicals*, **27**, 133, 135, 137.

Cassady, J. V. (1959). *Pseudomonas* corneal ulceration. *American Journal of Ophthalmology*, **48**, 741–747.

Chambers, C. W. & Clarke, U. A. (1966). In *Advances in Applied Microbiology*, Vol. 8, Academic Press, London & New York.

Chaplin, C. E. (1951). Observations on quaternary ammonium disinfectants. *Canadian Journal of Botany*, **29**, 373–382.

Clarke, C. D. & Armstrong, N. A. (1972). Influence of pH on adsorption of benzoic acid by kaolin. *The Pharmaceutical Journal*, **209**, 44–45.

Cook, A. M. (1960). Phenolic disinfectants. *Journal of Pharmacy and Pharmacology*, **12**, 19T–28T.

Cooke, E. M., Shooter, R. A., O'Farrell, S. M. & Martin, D. R. (1970). Faecal carriage of *Pseudomonas aeruginosa* by newborn babies. *The Lancet*, **ii**, 1045.

Cooper, L. (1942). Contributing to a discussion on: Bacillus pyocyaneus ulcer; report of three cases; results of sulpha- pyridine therapy in one case. *Archives of Ophthalmology*, **28**, 183–184.

Crompton, D. O. (1961). Some factors in the prevention of sepsis in ophthalmic surgery. *The Medical Journal of Australia*, **i**, 356–362.

Crompton, D. O. (1962). Ophthalmic prescribing. *The Australasian Journal of Pharmacy*, **43**, 1020–1026.

Crompton, D. O. (1963a). Scientifically prepared eye-drops. *The Medical Journal of Australia*, **ii**, 29.

Crompton, D. O. (1963b). Sterility of eye medicaments. *Lancet*, **ii**, 1013.

Crompton, D. O., Anderson, K. F. & Kennare, M. A. (1962). Experimental infection of the rabbit anterior chamber. *Transactions of the Ophthalmological Society of Australia*, **22**, 81–98.

Curtin, J. A., Petersdorf, R. G. & Bennet, I. L. (1961). *Pseudomonas bacteremia*: Review of ninety-one cases. *Annals of Internal Medicine*, **54**, 1077–1107.

Dale, J. K., Nook, M. A. & Barbiers, M. A. (1959). Effectiveness of preservatives in commercial ophthalmic preparations. *Journal of the American Pharmaceutical Association, Practical Pharmacy Edition*, **20**, 32–33.

Dallas, J. & Hughes, W. H. (1972). Sterilization of hydrophilic contact lenses. *British Journal of Ophthalmology*, **56**, 114–119.

Darmady, E. M., Hughes, K. E. A., Burt, M. M., Freeman, B. M. & Powell, D. B. (1961). Radiation Sterilization. *Journal of Clinical Pathology*, **14**, 55–58.

Darrell, J. H. & Wahba, A. H. (1964). Pyocine-typing of hospital strains of *Pseudomonas pyocyanea*. *Journal of Clinical Pathology*, **17**, 236–242.

Davey, B. B. & Turner, M. (1961). Some phenol decomposing strains of *Pseudomonas*. *Journal of Applied Bacteriology*, **24**, 78–82.

Davis, J. G. (1960). Chemical sterilization. *Journal of Pharmacy and Pharmacology*, **12**, Supplement, 29T–39T.

Davis, J. G. (1972). Fundamentals of microbiology in relation to cleansing in the cosmetics industry. *Journal of the Society of Cosmetic Chemists*, **23**, 45–71.

Deeb, E. N. & Boenigk, J. W. (1958). Preservative action of combined bacteriostatic agents I. Preservative action of chlorbutanol in combinations with certain other bacteriostatic agents. *Journal of the American Pharmaceutical Association, Scientific Edition*, **47**, 807–809.

Deeley, S. (1962). In *Developments in Industrial Microbiology*, Vol. 3, Plenum Press, New York.

Deluca, P. P. & Kostenbauder, H. B. (1960). Interaction of preservatives with macromolecules IV. Binding of quaternary ammonium compounds by nonionic agents. *Journal of the American Pharmaceutical Association, Scientific Edition*, **49**, 430–437.

Drewett, S. E., Payne, D. J. H., Tuke, W. & Verdon, P. E. (1972). Eradication of *Pseudomonas aeruginosa* infection from a special-care nursery. *The Lancet*, **i**, 946–948.

Dunnigan, A. P. (1968). Microbiological control of cosmetics. *Drug and Cosmetic Industry*, **102**, 43–45, 152–158.

Editorial (1963). Codex amendments. *The Pharmaceutical Journal*, **191**, 575–576.

Editorial (1966a). Pseudomonas aeruginosa. *The Lancet*, **i**, 1139–1140.

Editorial (1966b). Antibiotic combinations. *The Lancet*, **i**, 863.

Ehrlich, P. (1913). Chemotherapeutics: scientific principles, methods, and results. *The Lancet*, **ii**, 445–451.

Falcão, D. P., Mendonça, C., Scrassolo, A., De Almeida, B. B., Hart, L., Farmer, L. H. & Farmer, J. J. (1972). Nursery outbreak of severe diarrhoea due to multiple strains of *Pseudomonas aeruginosa*. *The Lancet*, **ii**, 38–40.

Farrand, R. J. & Williams, A. (1973). Evaluation of single-use packs of hospital disinfectants. *The Lancet*, **i**, 591–593.

Favero, M. S., Band, W. W., Paterson, N. J. & Carsen, L. A. (1970). *Bacteriological Proceedings*, Abstract No. 75, p. 11.

Fisher, E. & Allen, J. H. (1958). Corneal ulcers produced by cell-free extracts of *Pseudomonas aeruginosa*. *American Journal of Ophthalmology*, **46**, 21–24.

Foster, J. H. S. (1964). Studies in the preservation of ophthalmic solutions. *Master of Pharmacy Thesis*, University of Nottingham.

Gardner, J. F. (1972). Which disinfectant for Australian hospitals? *The Medical Journal of Australia*, **ii**, 1229–1236.

Garretson, W. T. & Cosgrove, K. W. (1927). Ulceration of the cornea due to *Bacillus pyocyaneus*. *Journal of the American Medical Association*, **88**, 700–702.

Garrett, E. R. (1958). Classification and evaluation of combined antibiotic activity. *Antibiotics and Chemotherapy*, **8**, 8–20.

Garrett, E. R. & Brown, M. R. W. (1963). The action of tetracycline and chloramphenicol alone and in admixture on the growth of *Escherichia coli*. *Journal of Pharmacy and Pharmacology*, **18**, Supplement, 185T–191T.

Gerke, J. R. & Magliocco, M. V. (1971). Experimental *Pseudomonas aeruginosa* infection of the mouse cornea. *Infection and Immunity*, **3**, 209–216.

Gershenfeld, L. & Stedman, R. L. (1949). The potentiating effects of various compounds on the antibacterial activities of surface active agents. *American Journal of Pharmacy*, **121**, 249–267.

Gibson, G. L. (1971). In *Infection in Hospital: a Code of Practice*, E. and S. Livingstone, Edinburgh and London.

Ginsburg, M. & Robson, J. M. (1949). Further investigations on the action of detergents on the eye. *British Journal of Ophthalmology*, **33**, 574–579.

Gould, J. C. (1963). *Pseudomonas pyocyanea* infections in hospital. In *Infection in Hospitals: Epidemology and Control*, Blackwell Scientific Publications, Oxford.

Grote, I. W. & Woods, M. (1955). Beta-phenylethyl alcohol as a preservative for ophthalmic solutions. *Journal American Pharmaceutical Association, Scientific Edition*, **44**, 9–11.

Guide (1971). *Guide to good pharmaceutical manufacturing practice*, Her Majesty's Stationery Office, London.

Hardy, P. C., Ederer, G. M. & Matsen, J. M. (1970). Contamination of commercially packaged urinary catheter kits with the pseudomonad E0-1. *New England Journal of Medicine*, **282**, 33–35.

Hare, R., Raik, E. & Gash, S. (1963). Efficiency of antiseptics when acting on dried organisms. *British Medical Journal*, **1**, 496–500.

Heller, W. M., Foss, D. N. E., Shay, D. E. & Ichniowski, C. T. (1955). Preservatives in solutions. *Journal of the American Pharmaceutical Association, Practical Pharmacy Edition*, **16**, 29, 30, 36.

Henry, S. M. (1969). The microflora of man and his environment. *TGA Cosmetic Journal*, **1**, 6–11.

Herbold, M. (1943). *American Perfumer*, **45**, 36. Cited by Wedderburn, D. L. (1964).

Hess, H. & Speiser, P. (1959a). Comparative efficacy of bactericidal compounds in buffer solutions. Part I. *Journal of Pharmacy and Pharmacology*, **11**, 650–658.

Hess, H. & Speiser, P. (1959b). Comparative efficacy of bactericidal compounds in buffer solutions. Part II. *Journal of Pharmacy and Pharmacology*, **11**, 694–702.

Hind, H. W. & Szekely, I. J. (1953). Self sterilizing ophthalmic solutions. *Journal of the American Pharmaceutical Association, Practical Pharmacy Edition*, **14**, 644–645.

Hooper, W. L. (1971). The nature and extent of microbial contamination of pharmaceutical preparations in hospitals. Joint symposium on microbial control, organised by the Pharmaceutical Society and the Society of Cosmetic Chemists, Great Britain.

Hughson, D. T. & Styron, N. C. (1949). The use of alkyl-dimethyl-benzyl ammonium chloride for maintenance of sterility of solutions. *American Journal of Ophthalmology*, **32**, (June Pt. 2), 102–109.

Hugo, W. B. & Foster, J. H. S. (1964). Growth of *Pseudomonas aeruginosa* in solutions of esters of *p*-hydroxybenzoic acid. *Journal of Pharmacy and Pharmacology*, **16**, 209.

Iannarone, M. & Eisen, J. (1961). Ophthalmic solutions. *Journal of the American Pharmaceutical Association*, **NS1**, 696–697.

International Dairy Federation (1963). Standard capacity test for the evaluation of the disinfectant activity of dairy disinfectants. *Dairy Industries*, **28**, 610–613.

Jawetz, E. (1952). Infections with *Pseudomonas aeruginosa* treated with Polymyxin B. *Archives of Internal Medicine*, **89**, 90–98.

Jawetz, E. (1968). The use of combinations of antimicrobial drugs. *Annual Review of Pharmacology*, **8**, 150–170.

Jeffs, P. L. (1959). Modified A. P. F. ophthalmic vehicles for hospital use. *The Australasian Journal of Pharmacy*, **40**, 218–219.

Jellard, C. H. & Churcher, G. M. (1967). An outbreak of *Pseudomonas aeruginosa* (pyocyanea) infection in a premature baby unit with observations on the intestinal carriage of *Pseudomonas aeruginosa* in the newborn. *Journal of Hygiene Cambridge*, **65**, 219–228.

Kabins, S. A. (1972). Interactions among antibiotics and other drugs. *Journal of the American Medical Association*, **219**, 206–212.

Kallings, L. O., Ringertz, O., Silverstolpe, L. & Ernerfeldt, F. (1966). Microbiological contamination of medical preparations. *Acta Pharmaceutica Suecica*, **3**, 219–228.

Kelsey, J. C. (1969). Disinfectants in hospital practice. *British Hospital Journal and Social Service Review*, **79**, 2180–2182.

Kelsey, J. C., Beeby, M. M. & Whitehouse, C. W. (1965). A capacity use-dilution test for disinfectants. *Monthly Bulletin of the Ministry of Health and the Public Health Laboratory Service*, **24**, 152–160.

Kelsey, J. C. & Maurer, I. M. (1966). An in-use test for hospital disinfectants. *Monthly Bulletin of the Ministry of Health and the Public Health Laboratory Service*, **25**, 180–184.

Kelsey, J. C. & Maurer, I. M., (1967). The choice of disinfectants for hospital use. *Monthly Bulletin of the Ministry of Health and the Public Health Laboratory Service*, **26**, 110–114.

Kelsey, J. C. & Maurer, I. M. (1972). *The Use of Chemical Disinfectants in Hospitals*, Her Majesty's Stationery Office, London.

Kelsey, J. C. & Sykes, G. (1969). A new test for the assessment of disinfectants with particular reference to their use in hospitals. *The Pharmaceutical Journal*, **202**, 607–609.

Kelsey, J. C. & Wagg, R. E. (1969). The disinfection of textiles in laundering in hospitals. *British Launderers' Research Association Bulletin*, **9**, 225, 337.

King, J. H. (1953). Contamination of eye medications. Practical methods of prevention. *American Journal of Ophthalmology*, **36**, 1389–1397.

Klein, M., Millwood, E. G. & Walther, W. W. (1954). On the maintenance of sterility in eye-drops. *Journal of Pharmacy and Pharmacology*, **6**, 725–732.

Kleinman, K. & Huyck, C. L. (1961). Preparation on a small scale . . . ophthalmic solutions. *Journal of the American Pharmaceutical Association*, **NS1**, 162–166.

Kohn, S. R., Gershenfeld, L. & Barr, M. (1963a). Effectiveness of antibacterial agents presently employed in ophthalmic preparations as preservatives against *Pseudomonas aeruginosa*. *Journal of Pharmaceutical Sciences*, **52**, 967–974.

Kohn, S. R., Gershenfeld, L. & Barr, M. (1963b). Antibacterial agents not presently employed as preservatives in ophthalmic solutions found effective against *Pseudomonas aeruginosa*. *Journal of Pharmaceutical Sciences*, **52**, 1126–1129.

Kominos, S. D., Copeland, C. E., Grosiak, B. & Postic, B. (1972). Introduction of *Pseudomonas aeruginosa* into a hospital via vegetables. *Applied Microbiology*, **24**, 567–570.

Krezanoski, J. Z. (1970). Contact lens products. *Journal of the American Pharmaceutical Association*, **NS10**, 13–18.

Kronig, B. & Paul, T. (1897). Die chemischen grundlagen der lehre von der gift wirkung und disinfektion. *Z. f. hyg. und infektionskransh*, **25**, 1–112. Cited by Bass, G. K. & Stuart, L. S. (1968). In Disinfection, Sterilisation and Preservation. (Ed. C. A. Lawrence & S. S. Block) Lea and Febinger, Philadelphia, p. 135.

Lawrence, C. A. (1955a). Chemical preservatives for ophthalmic solutions. *American Journal of Ophthalmology*, **39**, 385–394.

Lawrence, C. A. (1955b). An evaluation of chemical preservatives for ophthalmic solutions. *Journal of the American Pharmaceutical Association, Scientific Edition*, **44**, 457–464.

Lee, A. S. (1972) Formulation studies on hydrocortisone eye-drops. Master of Science Thesis, Heriot-Watt University, Edinburgh.

Leopold, I. H. & Apt, L. (1960). Post-operative intraocular infections. *American Journal of Ophthalmology*, **50**, 1225–1247.

Lepard, C. W. (1942). *Bacillus pyocyaneus* ulcer: report of three cases; results of sulfapyridine therapy in one case. *Archives of Ophthalmology*, **28**, 180–184.

Lilley, A. B. & Bearup, A. J. (1928). Generalised infections due to *Pseudomonas aeruginosa (Bacillus pyocyaneus)*, with a study of the characteristics of the local strains of the organism. *Medical Journal of Australia*, **1**, 362.

Lilley, B. D. & Brewer, J. H. (1953). The selective antibacterial action of phenylethyl alcohol. *Journal of the American Pharmaceutical Association, Scientific Edition*, **42**, 6–8.

Lowbury, E. J. L. (1951). Contamination of cetrimide and other fluids with *Pseudomonas pyocyanea*. *British Journal of Industrial Medicine*, **8**, 22–25.

Lowbury, E. J. L. & Fox, J. (1954). The epidemiology of infection with *Pseudomonas pyocyanea* in a burns unit. *Journal of Hygiene Cambridge*, **52**, 403–416.

Lowbury, E. J. L. & Lilly, H. A. (1960). Disinfection of the hands of surgeons and nurses. *British Medical Journal*, **1**, 1445–1450.

Lowbury, E. J. L., Lilly, H. A. & Bull, J. P. (1960). Disinfection of the skin of operation sites. *British Medical Journal*, **2**, 1039–1044.

Lowbury, E. J. L., Lilly, H. A. & Bull, J. P. (1963). Disinfection of hands: removal of resident bacteria. *British Medical Journal*, **1**, 1251–1256.

Lowbury, E. J. L., Lilly, H. A. & Bull, J. P. (1964a). Disinfection of hands: removal of transient organisms. *British Medical Journal*, **2**, 230–233.

Lowbury, E. J. L., Lilly, H. A. & Bull, J. P. (1964b). Methods for disinfection of hands and operation sites. *British Medical Journal*, **2**, 531–536.

Maccacaro, G. A. (1961). The assessment of the interaction between antibacterial drugs. In *Progress in Industrial Microbiology*, Vol. 3, Heywood & Company Limited, London, pp. 175–210.

MacGregor, D. R. & Elliker, P. R. (1958). A comparison of some properties of strains of *Pseudomonas aeruginosa* sensitive and resistant to quaternary ammonium compounds. *Canadian Journal of Microbiology*, **4**, 499–503.

Marzulli, F. N., Evans., J. R. & Yoder, P. D. (1972). Induced Pseudomonas keratitis as related to cosmetics. *Journal of the Society of Cosmetic Chemists*. **23**, 89–97.

Maurer, I. M. (1969). A test for stability and long-term effectiveness in disinfectants. *The Pharmaceutical Journal*, **203**, 529–534.

McCulloch, J. C. (1943). Origin and pathogenicity of *Pseudomonas pyocyanea* in conjunctival sac. *Archives of Ophthalmology*, **29**, 924–935.

McCulloch, E. C. (1947). False disinfection velocity curves produced by quaternary ammonium compounds. *Science*, **105**, 480–481.

McLeod, J. W. (1958). The hospital urine bottle and bedpan as reservoirs of infection by *Pseudomonas pyocyanea*. *The Lancet*, **i**, 394–397.

McPherson, S. D. & Wood, R. M. (1949). Self-sterilizing ophthalmic solutions. *American Journal of Ophthalmology*, **32**, 675–678.

Meyers, J. A. (1972). Hospital infections caused by contaminated fluids. *The Lancet*, **ii**, 282.

Mitchell, R. G. & Hayward, A. C. (1966). Postoperative urinary-tract infections caused by contaminated irrigating fluid. *The Lancet*, **i**, 793–795.

Monkhouse, D. C. & Groves, G. A. (1967). The effect of EDTA on the resistance of *Pseudomonas aeruginosa* to benzalkonium chloride. *The Australasian Journey of Pharmacy Science, Supplement Number*, **53**, S70–S75.

Monograph (1970). The hygienic manufacture and preservation of toiletries and cosmetics. *Journal of the Society of Cosmetic Chemists*, **21**, 719–800.

Moore, C. D. & Hardwick, R. B. (1956). Germicides based on surface–active agents: their nature and mechanism of action. *Manufacturing Chemist*, **27**, 305–309.

Murphy, J. T., Allen, H. F. & Mangiaracine, A. B. (1955). Preparation, sterilisation and preservation of ophthalmic solutions. *Archives ophthalmology*, **53**, 63–78.

Newton, B. A. (1954). Site of action of polymyxin on *Pseudomonas aeruginosa*: Antagonism by cations. *Journal of General Microbiology*, **10**, 491–499.

Niven, C. F. Jr. (1958). Microbiological aspects of radiation preservation of food. *Annual Review of Microbiology*, **12**, 507–524.

Noble, W. C. & Savin, J. A. (1966). Steroid cream contaminated with *Pseudomonas aeruginosa. The Lancet*, **i**, 347–349.

Noble, W. C. & White, P. M. (1969). Pseudomonads and man. *Transactions and Reports of St. John's Hospital Dermatological Society*, **55**, 202–208.

Olson, S. W. (1967). The application of microbiology to cosmetic testing. *Journal of the Society of Cosmetic Chemists*, **18**, 191–198.

Ortenzio, L. F. & Stuart, L. S. (1961). Adaptation of the use-dilution method to primary evaluations of disinfectants. *Journal of the Association of Official Agricultural Chemists*, **44**, 416–421.

Parker, M. S. (1970). Some factors in the hygienic manufacture of cosmetics and their preservation. *Soap, Perfumery & Cosmetics*, **43**, 483–485.

Parker, M. T. (1972). The clinical significance of the presence of microorganisms in pharmaceutical and cosmetic preparations. *Journal of the Society of Cosmetic Chemists*, **23**, 415–426.

Patel, N. K. & Kostenbauder, H. B. (1958). Interaction of preservatives with macromolecules. I. Binding of parahydroxybenzoic acid esters by polyoxyethylene–20 sorbitan monooleate (Tween 80). *Journal of the American Pharmaceutical Association, Scientific Edition*, **47**, 289–293.

Perry, E. T. & Nichols, A. C. (1956). *J. invest. Derm.*, **27**, 165. Cited by Noble, W. C. & White, P. M. (1969).

Phillips, I., Eykyn, S., Curtis, M. A. & Snell, J. J. S. (1971). *Pseudomonas cepacia (Multivorans)* septicaemia in an intensive-care unit. *The Lancet*, **i**, 375–377.

Phillips, I., Eykyn, S. & Laker, M. (1972). Outbreak of hospital infection caused by contaminated autoclaved fluids. *The Lancet*, **i**, 1258–1260.

Phillips, I. & Spencer, G. (1965). *Pseudomonas aeruginosa* cross-infection due to contaminated respiratory apparatus. *The Lancet*, **ii**, 1325–1327.

Pisano, F. D. & Kostenbauder, H. B. (1959). Interaction of preservatives with macromolecules. II. Correlation of binding data with required preservative concentrations of *p*-hydroxybenzoates in the presence of Tween-80. *Journal of the American Pharmaceutical Association, Scientific Edition*, **48**, 310–314.

Post, M. H. (1949). Prevention of infection in eye surgery. *American Journal of Ophthalmology*, **31**, 862–863.

Quisno, R., Gibby, I. W. & Foter, M. J. (1946). A neutralizing medium for evaluating the germicidal potency of the quaternary ammonium salts. *American Journal of Pharmacy*, **118**, 320–323.

Report (1909). The standardisation of disinfectants. With special reference to the disinfectant preparations commonly sold to the public. A chemical and bacteriological inquiry. *The Lancet*, **ii**, 1454–1458; 1516–1531; 1612–1616.

Report (1965). Use of disinfectants in hospitals. *British Medical Journal*, **1**, 408–413.

Report (1970). *The Bacteriological Examination of Water Supplies,* Her Majesty's Stationery Office, London.

Report (1971). Microbial contamination of medicines administered to hospital patients. *The Pharmaceutical Journal,* **207**, 96–99.

Richards, R. M. E. (1964). The sterility of eye medicaments. *The Lancet,* **i,** 42.

Richards, R. M. E. (1965). Investigations of the resistance of *Pseudomonas aeruginosa* to chemical antibacterial agents. Doctor of Philosophy Thesis, University of London.

Richards, R. M. E. (1967a). An evaluation of the literature on the effectiveness of antibacterial agents used as preservatives in ophthalmic solutions Part I. *The Australasian Journal of Pharmacy, Science Supplement Number,* **55,** S86–S89.

Richards, R. M. E. (1967b). An evaluation of the literature on the effectiveness of antibacterial agents used as preservatives in ophthalmic solutions Part II. *The Australasian Journal of Pharmacy, Science Supplement Number,* **56,** S96–S101.

Richards, R. M. E. (1971). Inactivation of resistant *Pseudomonas aeruginosa* by antibacterial combinations. *Journal of Pharmacy and Pharmacology,* **23,** *Supplement,* 136S–140S.

Richards, R. M. E. (1972). Contact lenses and their solutions. *The Pharmaceutical Journal,* **208,** 314–316.

Richards, R. M. E. & Brown, M. R. W. (1964). Resistance of *Pseudomonas aeruginosa* to chemical inactivation, *Journal of Pharmacy and Pharmacology,* **16,** 360–361.

Richards, R. M. E., Fell, A. F. & Butchart, J. M. E. (1972). Interaction between sodium metabisulphite and PMN. *Journal of Pharmacy and Pharmacology,* **24,** 999–1000.

Richards, R. M. E. & Hardie, M. P. (1972). Effect of polysorbate 80 and phenylethanol on the antibacterial activity of fentichlor. *Journal of Pharmacy and Pharmacology,* **24,** *Supplement,* 90P–93P.

Richards, R. M. E. & McBride, R. J. (1971a). Preservation of sodium bicarbonate eye lotion BPC against contamination with *Pseudomonas aeruginosa. British Journal of Ophthalmology,* **55,** 734–737.

Richards, R. M. E. & McBride, R. J. (1971b). Phenylethanol enhancement of preservatives used in ophthalmic preparations. *Journal of Pharmacy and Pharmacology,* **23,** *Supplement,* 141S–146S.

Richards, R. M. E. & McBride, R. J. (1972a). The preservation of ophthalmic solutions with antibacterial combinations. *Journal of Pharmacy and Pharmacology,* **24,** 145–148.

Richards, R. M. E. & McBride, R. J. (1972b). Cross-Resistance in *Pseudomonas aeruginosa* resistant to phenylethanol. *Journal of Pharmaceutical Sciences,* **61,** 1075–1077.

Richards, R. M. E. & McBride, R. J. (1973a). Preservation of sulphacetamide eye-drops B.P.C. *The Pharmaceutical Journal,* **210,** 118–120.

Richards, R. M. E. & McBride, R. J. (1973b). Effect of 3-phenylpropan-1-ol, 2-phenylethanol and benzylalcohol on *Pseudomonas aeruginosa. Journal of Pharmaceutical Sciences,* **62,** 585–587.

Richards, R. M. E., McBride, R. J. & Gunn, M. A. (1972). Preliminary investigation of the preservative properties of 3-phenylpropanol. *Journal of Pharmacy and Pharmacology,* **24,** *Supplement,* 158P–159P.

Richards, R. M. E. & Reary, J. M. E. (1972). Changes in antibacterial activity of thiomersal and PMN on autoclaving with certain adjuvants. *Journal of Pharmacy and Pharmacology,* **24,** *Supplement,* 84P–89P.

Richards, R. M. E., Suwanprakorn, P., Neawbanij, S. & Surasdikul, N. (1969). Preservation of fluorescein solutions against contamination with *Pseudomonas aeruginosa. Journal of Pharmacy and Pharmacology,* **21,** 681–686.

Rideal, S. & Walker, J. T. A. (1903). The standardization of disinfectants. *Journal of the Royal Sanitary Institute,* **24,** 424–441.

Ridley, F. (1958). Sterile drops and lotions in ophthalmic practice. *British Journal of Ophthalmology*, **42**, 641–654.

Riegelman, S. (1964). Contributing to a discussion. *The Pharmaceutical Journal*, **193**, 297.

Riegelman, S. Vaughan, D. G. & Okumoto, M. (1956). Antibacterial agents in *Pseudomonas aeruginosa* contaminated ophthalmic solutions. *Journal of the American Pharmaceutical Association, Scientific Edition*, **45**, 93–98.

Riegelman, S. & Vaughan, D. G. (1958). A rational basis for the preparation of ophthalmic solutions. *Journal of the American Pharmaceutical Association, Practical Pharmacy Edition*, **19**, 474–477; 537–540; 665–666.

Ringen, L. M. & Drake, C. H. (1952). A study of the incidence of *Pseudomonas aeruginosa* from various natural sources. *Journal of Bacteriology*, **64**, 841–845.

Robinson, E. P. (1971). *Pseudomonas aeruginosa* contamination of liquid antacids: a survey. *Journal of Pharmaceutical Sciences*, **60**, 604–605.

Rogers, K. B. (1960). *Pseudomonas* infections in a children's hospital. *Journal of Applied Bacteriology*, **23**, 533–537.

Ross, J. D. & Horne, M. W. (1969). In *Modern Drug Treatment in Tuberculosis*, Health Horizon Limited, London, pp. 38–48.

Runti, C. (1960). Preparazione E conservazione dei colliri. *Bollettino Chimico Farmaceutico*, **99**, 286–376.

Rupp, C. A. & Forni, P. (1972). Formic I. V. therapy. *New England Journal of Medicine*, **286**, 894–895.

Samish, Z. & Etinger-Tulczynska, R. (1963). Distribution of bacteria within the tissue of healthy tomatoes, *Applied Microbiology*, **11**, 7–10.

Schiller, I., Kuntscher, H., Wolff, A. & Mekola, M. (1968). Microbial content of nonsterile therapeutic agents containing natural or seminatural active ingredients. *Applied Microbiology*, **16**, 1924–1928.

Scigliano, J. A. & Skolaut, W. (1954). Preparation of ophthalmic medication. *Bulletin of the American Society of Hospital Pharmacy*, **11**, 37–41.

Shafer, D. M. (1950). Experimental corneal grafts of the lamellar particle type. *American Journal of Ophthalmology*, **33**, 26–31.

Shooter, R. A., Cooke, E. M., Gaya, H., Kumar, P., Patel, N., Parker, M. T., Thom, B. T. & France, D. R. (1969). Food and medicaments as possible sources of hospital strains of *Pseudomonas aeruginosa*. *The Lancet*. **i**, 1227–1229.

Shooter, R. A., Walker, K. A., Williams, V. R., Horgan, G. M., Parker, M. T., Asheshov, E. H. & Bullimore, J. F. (1966). Faecal carriage of *Pseudomonas aeruginosa* in hospital patients; possible spread from patient to patient. *The Lancet*, **ii**, 1331–1334.

Shrewsbury, J. F. D. (1934). *B. pyocyaneus* meningitis with recovery. *British Medical Journal*, **i**, 280–281.

Silver, S. & Wendt, L. (1967). Mechanism of action of phenylethyl alcohol: breakdown of the cellular permeability barrier. *Journal of Bacteriology*, **93**, 560–566.

Soet, J. C. (1952). Crisis in a Michigan plant. *Sight saving Review*, **22**, 202–204. Cited by King, J. H. (1953).

Speller, D. C. E., Stephens, M. E. & Viant, A. C. (1971). Hospital infection with *Pseudomonas cepacia*. *The Lancet*, **i**, 798–799.

Stockley, I. H. (1973). Drug Interactions 8. Interactions with anti-infective agents. Part 1. Antibiotics. *The Pharmaceutical Journal*, **210**, 36–43.

Stuart, L. S., Ortenzio, L. F. & Friedl, J. L. (1955). Use-dilution confirmation tests for results obtained by phenol coefficient methods. *Journal of the Association of Official Agricultural Chemists*, **36**, 466–480.

Sutter, V. L., Hurst, V. & Landucci, A. O. J. (1966). *Pseudomonads* in human saliva. *Journal of Dental Research*, **45**, 1800–1803.

Swan, K. C. (1944). Reactivity of the ocular tissue to wetting agents. *American Journal of Ophthalmology*, **27**, 1118–1122.

Sykes, G. (1962). The philosophy of the evaluation of disinfectants and antiseptics. *Journal of Applied Bacteriology*, **25**, 1–11.

Szekely, I. J., Riegelman, S. & Petricciani, M. A. (1959). World contact lens standard committee report, part III. Ophthalmic microbial hazards, antimicrobial agents and use of contact lens solutions. *Contacto*, **3**, 258–267.

Tenenbaum, S. (1971). Significance of pseudomonads in cosmetic products. *American Perfumer and Cosmetics*, **86**, 33–37.

Theodore, F. H. (1951). Contamination of eye solutions. *American Journal of Ophthalmology*, **34**, 1764.

Theodore, F. H. & Feinstein, R. R. (1952). Practical suggestions for the preparation and maintenance of sterile ophthalmic solutions. *American Journal of Ophthalmology*, **35**, 656–659.

Theodore, F. H. & Feinstein, R. R. (1953). Preparation and maintenance of sterile ophthalmic solutions. *Journal of the American Medical Association*, **152**, 1631–1633.

Theodore, F. H. & Minsky, H. (1951). Lack of sterility of eye medicaments. *Journal of the American Medical Association*, **147**, 1381.

Thornley, M. J. (1963). Radiation resistance among bacteria. *Journal of Applied Bacteriology*, **26**, 334–345.

Tinne, J. E., Gordon, A. M., Bain, W. H. & Mackay, W. A. (1967). Cross-infection by *Pseudomonas aeruginosa* as a hazard of intensive surgery, *British Medical Journal*, **4**, 313–315.

USNF XI (1960). United States National Formulary, Mack Publishing Company, Easton Pennsylvania, p. 502.

USNF XII (1965). United States National Formulary, Mack Publishing Company, Easton Pennsylvania, p. 481.

USNF XIII (1970). United States National Formulary, Mack Publishing Company, Easton Pennsylvania, p. 835.

USP XVII (1965). United States Pharmacopoeia, Mack Publishing Company, Easton Pennsylvania, p. 792.

USP XVIII (1970). United States Pharmacopoeia, Mack Publishing Company, Easton Pennsylvania, p. 800.

Vaughan, D. G. (1955). The contamination of fluorescein solutions. With special reference to *Pseudomonas aeruginosa (Bacillus pyocyaneus)*. *American Journal of Ophthalmology*, **39**, 55–61.

Victorin, L. (1967). An epidemic of otitis in newborns due to infection with *Pseudomonas aeruginosa*. *Acta Paediatrica Scandinavica*, **56**, 344–347.

Vidal-Paruta, M. R. & King, L. D. (1964). Critical micelle concentration of nonionic surfactants in water and carbon tetrachloride. *Journal of Pharmaceutical Sciences*, **53**, 1217–1220.

Weber, G. R. & Black, L. A. (1948). Laboratory procedure for evaluating practical performance of quaternary ammonium and other germicides proposed for sanitizing food utensils. *American Journal of Public Health*, **38**, 1405–1417.

Wedderburn, D. L. (1964). Preservation of emulsions against microbial attack. In *Advances in Pharmaceutical Sciences I*, Academic Press, London and New York, pp. 195–268.

Wedderburn, D. L. (1965). Hygiene in manufacturing plant and its effect on the preservation of emulsions. *Journal of the Society of Cosmetic Chemists*, **16**, 395–403.

Wedderburn, D. L. (1970). Interactions in cosmetic preservation. *American Perfumer and Cosmetics*, **85**, 49–53.

Wedderburn, D. L., Flawn, P. C., Malcolm, S. A. & Woodroffe, R. C. S. (1971). Assessment of the preservative capacity of pharmaceutical and cosmetic preparation.

Joint symposium on microbial control, organised by the Pharmaceutical Society and the Society of Cosmetic Chemists, Great Britain.

Whitby, J. L. & Rampling, A. (1972). *Pseudomonas aeruginosa* contamination in domestic and hospital environments. *The Lancet*, **i**, 15–17.

White, P. M. (1971). *Pseudomonas aeruginosa* in a skin hospital. *British Journal of Dermatology*, **85**, 412–417.

Wiggins, R. L. (1952a). Experimental studies on the eye with polymyxin B. *American Journal of Ophthalmology*, **35**, 83–89.

Wiggins, R. L. (1952b). Treatment of *Pseudomonas* corneal ulcer with polymyxin B. *Archives of Ophthalmology*, **48**, 522.

Williams, R. E. O., Blowers, R., Garrod, L. R. & Shooter, R. A. (1960). In *Hospital Infection: Causes and Prevention*, Lloyd-Duke, Medical Books Limited, London, p. 98.

Wilson, L. A., Kuehone, J. W., Hall, S. W. & Ahearn, D. G. (1971). Microbial contamination in ocular cosmetics. *American Journal of Ophthalmology*, **71**, 1298–1302.

Wilson, W. J. (1929). In *A System of Bacteriology in Relation to Medicine*, Vol. 4, His Majesty's Stationery Office, London.

Wilson, G. S. & Miles, A. A. (1964). In *Principles of Bacteriology and Immunity*, Vol. 1, Arnold, London, p. 636.

Yasufuku, M., Hashimoto, K., Hamai, J. & Uesugi, J. A. (1968). 5th Cong. Int. Fed. Soc. Cosmet, Chem. Tokyo. Cited by Wedderburn, D. L., Flawn, P. C., Malcolm, S. A. & Woodroffe, R. C. S. (1971).

Subject Index

Acetic acid, resistance to, 41
Achromobacter sp, resistance of, 93
Actinomycin D, 44, 76, 78
  cytoplasmic membrane effects, 96
Aerobacter aerogenes, see Klebsiella aerogenes
Aminoglycoside antibiotics, 14
  chemical basis, 14
  modifying enzymes, 14–19, 51
  physiological expression, 18
  reactions catalysed, 14
  R-factor mediated resistance, 17–18
  species-specific antagonism by cations, 82, 90
Ampicillin, 7, 8
  outer membrane activity, 86
  sensitization by EDTA, 151
1-Anilinonaphylamine-8-sulphonic acid (ANS)
  penetration of, 75
Anionic detergents, corneal damage, 297
Antibiotic degrading enzymes, *see* Enzymes *and also* named enzymes
Antibiotic testing, disc method, 50
Antibiotics, *see also* named compounds
  crypticity studies, 20, 77
  enzymatic destruction of, 51
  exclusion of, 75
  lack of uptake, 85
  pH effects, 49
  prevention of resistance to, 252
  problems in use of, 251–252
Antibodies
  assessment of, 260
  importance of, 260
  in serum, 260
  protective, 136–137
Antigens, *see also* O-antigens
  vaccines from, 257
Autolysin
  peptidoglycan degradation by, 170
Azotobacter agile, 55
A. vinelandii
  action of EDTA on, 148, 156

Bacillus cereus
  β-lactamases in, 3, 8
B. licheniformis
  β-lactamases in, 3, 8
B. megaterium
  polymyxin sensitivity, 87
B. polymyxa, 239
B. subtilis, 291
  cell wall composition, 50
  cold shock, 57
Bacitracin, 76
Bacteriophages
  action, 190
  attachment, 190
  LPS specific, 87
  receptors, 85, 197
  typing, 190–196
    composition of sets, 194
    historical development, 191
    interpretation, 191–193
    method, 194–196
    new typing set, 193–194
    reproducibility, 212–214
Bacteroides fragilis, 50
Benzalkonium chloride
  elimination of resistance by EDTA, 299
  irritation of eyes by, 296–297
  ophthalmic solutions, 296–299
  rabbits' eyes, 297
  resistance to, 94, 298
  usefulness of, 299
Benzyl penicillin, 7, 8, 96
  and sensitization by EDTA, 151
Binding affinity, 46
Blood
  protective effect of, 57
Buffers, effect on resistance, 56

Calcium
  effect on resistance, 38
Carbenicillin, 7, 8, 35, 94, 246–252
  clinical use, 246–247
  in vitro, 248
  resistance to, 247–252

325

Epidemiology, *continued*
relationship between methods, 215
serological typing, 205–212
Erythromycin, 44, 76, 77
Escherichia coli 20, 41, 246, 249, 291,
309, 310, 311
cationics, action of, 302
cell wall, structure of, 54, 79, 92, 162,
171
chloramphenicol, action of, 306
DNA-dependent, RNA polymerase, 76
EDTA action, 149, 150, 155, 158,
160, 167
enzymes in, 37, 53
erythromycin sensitivity, 76
gentian violet, penetration of, 76
β-lactamases in, 3, 77
LPS in, 163–164
lipoprotein in, 169
lysozyme, sensitivity to, 165
outer membrane, 134, 172
penicillin, resistance to, 94, 95
peptidoglycan, role of, 96
phenyl ethanol, action of, 303
phospholipid, degrading enzymes in,
169
polymyxin, sensitivity to, 87, 88
polysorbate 80 action, 301, 302
R-factors in, 25, 28
spheroplasts, 77
survival of, 55, 59
tetracycline action, 306
E. coli J5
LPS in, 164
E. coli K12
outer membrane of, 166
Ethylenediaminetetraacetic acid, 38–43,
145–177
antibiotic combination with, 177
antibiotic potentiation by, 177
autolysin stimulation by, 170
autolytic enzyme activated by, 169
bactericidal activity of, 146–148
benzyl penicillin, permeability of, 154
cation target for, 38–43, 159
cell:EDTA ratio, 156
cell envelope, effect on, 79, 87,
159–176
cell swelling, 154
characteristic sensitivity to, 82, 89
chelating ability of, 153–168
clinical significance, 177
composition of complex extracted by,
162

Ethylenediaminetetraacetic acid, *cont.*
culture age effect, 154
detergent-like action of, 168
disinfectant potentiation by, 177
dissociation, effects of, 164
dissociation of cell envelopes by,
164–167
E. coli spheroplasts effects on, 165
E. coli spheroplasts formed by, 165
endotoxic protein release by, 162
factors affecting action, 152–159
growth media, effects, 38–43, 154
intracellular products released by, 148
ionic complex, properties of, 168
ionic strength of media, effect on activity, 156
kinetics of lysis by, 40
location of complex extracted by, 173
LPS release by, 114, 160, 164
lysis by, 117, 148–150
lysozyme, in combination with, 133
medium pH of, 156
Mg affinity for, 153, 160
Mg concentration and sensitivity of,
154–155
mode of action, 167–176
nucleotide pool, loss of, 149
O-antigens, effect on, 167
ophthalmic solutions, 299, 300, 301
osmoplasts, preparation of, 157
osmotic shock, 149
outer membrane proteins affected by,
162
peptidoglycan, lack of action on, 160
periplasmic enzymes released by, 149
permeability changes caused by, 150,
164
polymyxin, relationship to, 168
protein-LPS released by, 121, 160–161
pseudomonads resistant to, 164
resistance to, 74, 147
RNA breakdown by, 149
salt effects, 157
sensitizing effects of, 73, 150–152
slime, effect on sensitivity to, 81
species resistant to, 176
species sensitive to, 147
specificity of action, 173
spheroplast production by, 149
temperature, modification of action,
158–159
tissue damage, 42
treatment prior to exposure to, 155
tris buffer, 157–158